Developmental Exercise Physiology

Thomas W. Rowland, MD
Baystate Medical Center

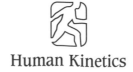

Human Kinetics

Library of Congress Cataloging-in-Publication Data

Rowland, Thomas W.
    Developmental exercise physiology / Thomas W. Rowland.
       p.   cm.
    Includes bibliographical references and index.
    ISBN 0-87322-640-2
    1. Motor ability in children--Physiological aspects.   2. Exercise-
-Physiological aspects.   I. Title.
    RJ133.R679   1996
    612'.044'083--dc20   96-10886
                                           CIP

ISBN: 0-87322-640-2

Permission notices for material reprinted in this book from other sources can be found on pages 257-260.

Developmental Editor: Holly Gilly; **Assistant Editors:** Chad Johnson, Jacqueline Blakley, and Lynn Hooper; **Editorial Assistant:** Amy Carnes; **Copyeditor:** Joyce Sexton; **Proofreader:** Erin Cler; **Indexer:** Margie Towery; **Typesetters and Layout Artists:** Impressions and Kathy Boudreau-Fuoss; **Text Designer:** Judy Henderson; **Cover Designer:** Jack Davis; **Photographer (cover):** Dave Black; **Illustrator:** Jennifer Delmotte; **Printer:** Braun-Brumfield

Human Kinetics books are available at special discounts for bulk purchase. Special editions or book excerpts can also be created to specification. For details, contact the Special Sales Manager at Human Kinetics.

Printed in the United States of America   10 9 8 7 6 5 4 3 2 1

Human Kinetics
Web site: http://www.humankinetics.com

United States:
Human Kinetics, P.O. Box 5076, Champaign, IL 61825-5076
1-800-747-4457
e-mail: humank@hkusa.com

Canada:
Human Kinetics, Box 24040, Windsor, ON N8Y 4Y9
1-800-465-7301 (in Canada only)
e-mail: humank@hkcanada.com

Europe:
Human Kinetics, P.O. Box IW14, Leeds LS16 6TR, United Kingdom
(44) 1132 781708
e-mail: humank@hkeurope.com

Australia:
Human Kinetics, 57A Price Avenue, Lower Mitcham, South Australia 5062
(08) 277 1555
e-mail: humank@hkaustralia.com

New Zealand:
Human Kinetics, P.O. Box 105-231, Auckland 1
(09) 523 3462
e-mail: humank@hknewz.com

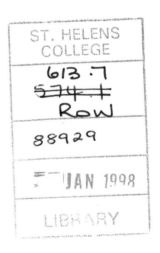

CONTENTS

PREFACE

Nothing marks the child's remarkable journey to adulthood more than the process of *change*. Consider: During the time an infant grows to become a mature adult, body mass increases over 25-fold, paralleling the development of skeletal size, muscle bulk, and the generation of metabolic energy. A neuromuscular system capable of nothing more than gross movements of the arms and legs develops the ability to play Paganini, or throw a basketball through an 18 in. hoop from 20 ft out. A mind that can discern only vague shapes learns to do ninth-grade algebra and then to meditate, imagine, and create. An isolated, totally dependent organism becomes a self-reliant member of society, capable of interacting lovingly or destructively with his or her fellow humans.

This is a book about a part of this extraordinary metamorphosis. It deals with the changes in the physiology of locomotion as the child grows—the field of *developmental exercise physiology*. In doing so, its concern is with the process of maturation— the progression toward attaining the adult state. Its central themes are the natural evolution of the physiologic responses to exercise as the child grows and the individual variability that characterizes the normal progression of biological maturation.

Developmental exercise physiology addresses responses to exercise that—at any age—serve one of two functions. These processes either (1) support the performance of the muscle "motor" (i.e., provide an energy substrate and the mechanics of muscular contraction), or (2) assure homeostasis during the stresses of physical exercise (temperature regulation, elimination of metabolic by-products). Uniquely, though, the developmental exercise physiologist studies the means by which these processes operate in a subject of increasing size and functional sophistication.

Physiologic changes during exercise as a child ages can reflect increase in dimension (cardiac output rises with age mainly from enlargement of ventricular dimensions), or development of function (improvements

in anaerobic capacity may be effected by quantitative changes in glycolytic enzymes), or integration of systems (improvements in neuromuscular coordination may increase submaximal running economy). It follows that an examination of these types of responses to exercise in children provides an insight into biologic maturation different in kind from that offered by traditional static measures of growth and development as obtained in the physician's office. Developmental exercise physiology concerns the changes during childhood of physiologic function under stress; it is the study of the maturation of the body's functional capacities.

WHY DEVELOPMENTAL EXERCISE PHYSIOLOGY?

The roots of research involving exercise physiology in children can be traced back to studies conducted by Robinson in the Harvard Fatigue Laboratory in the 1930s. His landmark report on variations in cardiopulmonary responses to maximal treadmill exercise relative to age continues to be corroborated by studies today (2). These concepts were expanded by Åstrand in his 1952 monograph, *Experimental Studies of Physical Working Capacity in Relation to Sex and Age*, which again identified children as a unique exercising population (1).

It was not until contemporary times, however, that a series of concerns regarding children and exercise prompted a dramatic interest in the study of developmental exercise physiology. These issues all possess a certain immediacy; they are practical concerns that have led parents, children, and coaches to seek guidance from the scientific community. Each calls for certain insights into the physiologic responses of children to exercise and/or sport training—insights that at the current time are largely nonexistent. Clearly a major gap exists between our understanding of exercise physiology in children and the information that is necessary to address these issues. Several examples can be cited:

1. **Are there risks to intensive sport training and competition in the prepubertal athlete?** Some of these concerns are anatomic (will repetitive microtrauma to the epiphyses of long bones from endurance training impair bone growth?). Others relate to the effects of vigorous training regimens on physiologic function. Such training is specifically designed to place high stress on skeletal muscle, heart, and lungs. Will this stress be injurious to processes of growth and functional change that are unique features of the child athlete? Despite the increasing number of young athletes involved in highly intense training regimens, the research literature offers little insight into these concerns.

Similarly, physical training in females can clearly interrupt normal reproductive hormonal patterns, leading to oligomenorrhea and risk of decreased bone mineralization. Are there long-term implications regarding fertility and osteoporosis for the intensely training young athlete? These questions are only just beginning to be addressed.

2. **What is the relationship between physical fitness and health, and how can this be addressed through field fitness testing of children in the school setting?** Creation of field fitness tests of children in the schools followed concerns generated in the 1950s that American youngsters were "unfit" compared to children in other countries. Considerable controversy surrounds the rationale, composition, and interpretation of such testing. For example, 1-mile run time is considered indicative of cardiorespiratory fitness since results reflect reasonably well a child's maximal oxygen uptake (relative to body weight) measured in the laboratory. What is unclear, however, is the extent to which $\dot{V}O_2$max per kg and mile run time are (a) indicative of present or future health and (b) simply a reflection of factors such as amount of body fat and subject motivation.

Mile run time improves significantly with age during childhood, while $\dot{V}O_2$max per kg remains unchanged (boys) or declines (girls). Deciphering the meaning of run test scores in a group of children of different stages of biological development (even if the same chronological age) is problematic. Compounding the problem, there is no study in children (or adults) identifying a threshold value of maximal aerobic power that lowers risk for adult cardiovascular disease. That risk (at least in adults) seems more closely linked to level of habitual physical activity than to fitness. Lack of an accurate yet feasible means of measuring physical activity hampers those investigating children's activity habits, particularly their re-

lationship to physical fitness, adult activity levels, and health outcomes.

Are field fitness tests in children useful in promoting health? Is activity more important than fitness? There is little information available from the research laboratory. Yet the concern over the perceived "fitness crisis" in children continues to support the testing yearly of many thousands of youngsters.

3. **Is exercise a valuable therapeutic modality for children with chronic cardiopulmonary and musculoskeletal disease?** A number of investigations have indicated that physical rehabilitation programs may prove beneficial to children with chronic conditions such as congenital heart disease, cystic fibrosis, and muscular dystrophy. But there is little information to provide guidance regarding the forms of exercise and structure of programs that can be expected to produce salutary results.

Moreover, it is not altogether clear what the benefits are expected to be. Does a rehabilitation program for a child with a cardiomyopathy improve cardiac function or work only to increase peripheral muscle aerobic capacity? Will physical training of this child affect the natural course of his/her illness? Are benefits to be expected in functional ability? Or does the program offer benefit predominantly from an emotional and social perspective? The many rehabilitative programs currently being conducted for such children could be more appropriately structured (and justified) if the answers to these questions were available.

4. **Can the study of developmental exercise physiology provide insights into adaptive responses to physical training at all ages?** It has been noted that many of the expected changes in physiologic responses to exercise in children as they grow closely mirror the adaptations that occur in response to exercise training (3). Likewise, the developmental changes in children occur in parallel with improvements in endurance performance. It is conceivable, then, that investigations into developmental exercise physiology might serve as a model for understanding physiologic and performance adaptations that would be equally applicable to adults. What is the physiologic explanation for the observation that boys improve their 1-mile run time by almost 100% between the ages of 6 and 15 years? What is the physiologic basis for improvement of distance running performance with training in adults? What type of training do I need to do to improve my 10K race time? Could all these answers be the same?

This potpourri of questions-without-answers is presented to underscore the deficiencies in our current understanding of exercise physiology in children. It illustrates, too, the weaknesses of the scientific foundations upon which significant clinical decisions and major public health policies have been formulated. Clearly there is a critical need for greater knowledge of the physiologic responses of children to exercise and their relationship to health and well-being.

GOALS, SCOPE, AND CAVEATS

The goal of this book is to provide the reader with a comprehensive state-of-the-art review of our current knowledge of the physiologic responses to exercise in children. The dramatic growth of information in this field, however, precludes a truly encyclopedic approach. The author has thus endeavored to provide pertinent references that will allow the reader to pursue particular areas of interest in more depth. This book has also been written with the open intention of highlighting deficiencies in our understanding of exercise physiology in children. This has been motivated by a desire to indicate those areas where future research efforts might be appropriately directed.

Physical activity takes many forms, yet the pediatric exercise literature is reasonably well demarcated into categories by the duration of the activity and metabolic pathways involved: (a) endurance activity, which utilizes aerobic metabolism; (b) short-burst activity, which uses energy derived from anaerobic sources; and (c) more static activity, which involves muscle strength. The approach of this book will be similarly divided.

An understanding of the nature of biologic maturation is critical for conducting exercise research in children. Appropriately, this issue is addressed in the opening chapter. Particularly important is the concept that at any given chronological age, biological developmental status among a group of children can be expected to vary widely. For many research questions, a mismatch of biologic maturation between or among groups of subjects will strongly influence physiologic comparisons. Ignoring such differences is likely to produce misleading results and lead to erroneous conclusions.

As developmental exercise physiology denotes change, the discussions in this book will address the period of time encompassing childhood through the age of puberty to the fully mature state. Many physiologic changes in children advance in a progressive continuum through the growing years (e.g., maximal oxygen uptake); other physiologic functions, such as muscle strength, are related to endocrinologic influences that become accelerated at puberty. Attention is therefore focused in this book not only on changes in exercise physiology in the growing child but also on the importance of patterns and rates of change in these functions.

While this book strives to provide an encompassing view of developmental exercise physiology, it is important to recognize what it is not. First, its content presupposes that the reader possesses an understanding of the basic principles of exercise physiology. No attempt is made to review these concepts. In addition, the discussions will be restricted primarily to physiologic characteristics of the healthy childhood population.

Considerable interest has focused on understanding exercise responses in children with chronic illness; likewise, the physiologic profiling of childhood athletes has received increasing research attention. However, this book will not endeavor to review these important areas. Similarly, the epidemiologic and public health aspects of physical activity and fitness in children, the influence of nutrition on exercise performance, field fitness testing, and the psychological and biomechanical features of activity in children will be largely ignored.

Several important caveats are in order as the reader considers the features of exercise responses in children reviewed in this book. It is necessary to recognize that studies of children's responses to exercise have been necessarily limited to subjects old enough (and motivated enough) to test effectively in the laboratory. Likewise, children who will volunteer for treadmill or cycle testing can be expected to represent a sample of the population skewed toward those who are athletically oriented. As a consequence, our current view of the characteristic physiologic responses to exercise in "normal" children is clearly a limited one, confined for the most part to youngsters age 10 and older, predominantly males, who are relatively fit and motivated toward physical activity.

Forming generalizations from the current body of pediatric research literature is hampered by other considerations. Insights are limited by ethical constraints in utilizing children as exercise subjects. The use of invasive methodologies, radiation, and nontherapeutic medications is improper in children. The difficulties surrounding "normalizing" physiologic data for body size in the growing child are particularly perplexing. Selecting one of several alternative choices for the "denominator" to factor out size may dramatically alter the conclusions of the study. These issues of ethical research in children and factoring for body size are sufficiently critical in developmental exercise physiology to warrant discussion in two chapters of this book.

The problem of establishing causality adds further complexity to understanding developmental exercise physiology. A great number of factors influencing exercise can be expected to progressively increase as a child grows; not surprisingly, then, one can often demonstrate a statistically significant association between any two of these variables. But other means must be employed to establish a causal relationship, since covariance with other factors, particularly body size, is common. The correlation between shoe size and maximal cardiac output during childhood is presumably high, but there is little to suspect a causal relationship between the two.

The reader will undoubtedly be impressed with the limited scientific dogma surrounding our concepts of the physiologic responses to exercise in children. Variations in subject population, the ethical restriction of methodologies, and differences in testing techniques have produced a body of often inconclusive, conflicting information. The challenge for the future is to surmount these problems: to develop new noninvasive techniques, standardize testing methods, and involve a broader scope of children by fitness, age, and gender.

REFERENCES

1. Åstrand, P.O. Experimental studies of physical working capacity in relationship to sex and age. Copenhagen: Munksgaard; 1952.
2. Robinson, S. Experimental studies of physical fitness in relation to age. Arbeitsphysiologie 10:251-323; 1938.
3. Rowland, T.W. Exercise and children's health. Champaign, IL: Human Kinetics; 1990.

ACKNOWLEDGMENTS

While this is a single-author text, the contributors are, in fact, as numerous as those listed in the references at the end of each chapter. To these exercise scientists who have extended our knowledge of children and exercise, this book is dedicated. I would like to extend a special thanks to those who have given me their generous assistance with particular chapters: Geraldine Naughton, William Thorland, Neil Armstrong, Ed Winter, Emmanuel Van Praagh, and Frank Cerny. This also provides me the opportunity to extend my appreciation to colleagues and mentors who have provided me with encouragement and support through the years in my professional career. Without these special people, I would not have had the opportunity to write this book: Rainer Martens, Oded Bar-Or, Lee Cunningham, Patty Freedson, Bill Byrnes, Steve Siconolfi, and Vicky Foster. I am also grateful to a cadre of students, including Vish Unnithan, Jill Auchinachie, Nisha Charkoudian, Michelle Borkuis, Leslie Martel, and Tiki Rimany, who were deluded into thinking they were simply receiving education and supervision. In fact, in their enthusiasm they have given me inspiration and energy for both my professional and personal growth. Holly Gilly, my developmental editor at Human Kinetics, was a constant source of encouragement, guidance, and support during the creation of this book. My secretary, Jackie Fournier, has my gratitude for her tireless efforts in preparing the manuscript. And my wife, Margot, for the many sacrifices for the time her husband spent secluded at the word processor, deserves my deepest appreciation.

PART I

EXPERIMENTAL APPROACH TO THE EXERCISING CHILD

If we are to understand the physiological responses of children to exercise, we must have accurate tools for measuring and interpreting these variables. Indeed, for the developmental exercise physiologist measurement becomes a particularly critical issue. That's because the assessment of body composition, creation of exercise testing protocols, and accounting for body size must always be conducted in the context of subjects who are invariably growing and undergoing biological maturation. They are also subjects who are emotionally immature and who must be protected from both physical and psychological injury during research studies.

A knowledge of how children grow and develop, how ethical constraints during research become important, and how exercise studies must be adapted for small body size are critical issues for all investigators dealing with children. Pediatric research subjects are not simply small adults; they require special consideration in order for meaningful physiologic data to be obtained.

The first part of this book reviews these issues. These chapters on biological maturation, size, exercise testing, body composition, and ethical issues are "required reading" before the second part of the book surveys the physiologic data accumulated with these considerations in mind.

CHAPTER 1

THE PROCESS OF BIOLOGICAL MATURATION

Biological maturation is a critical determinant of physiological responses to exercise. In this chapter, we will address (1) the characteristics of normal biological maturation during childhood; (2) the morphologic, sexual, and skeletal manifestations of this maturation; and (3) the factors that influence normal biological development.

Put simply, developmental exercise physiology is the study of curves—curves that describe the normal changes in physiologic responses to exercise as the child grows to adulthood. Changes in both size and function contribute to this process of biological maturation (15), which culminates in the mature adult state (although it is apparent that changes occur in exercise physiology throughout one's life span). There is an expectation that the evolution of physiologic changes during childhood will be reflected in similar patterns in motor performance. Just how physiologic and performance maturation are linked, however, remains problematic.

Mechanisms for the development of physiologic function in children are multiple: increase in cell number, enlargement of cell size, and differentiation of cell function may all contribute to alterations in particular physiologic responses to exercise. For example, multiplication of cartilage cells in the epiphyseal centers of long bones is responsible for growth in stature and leg length. Consequent changes in stride frequency and stride length may influence the metabolic cost of submaximal running.

Muscle strength, on the other hand, is a direct consequence of muscle fiber cross-sectional area; improvements in strength as a child grows are largely related to the increasing size of individual muscle fibers. Secondary sexual characteristics at puberty appear as the hypothalamus-pituitary-gonadal machinery is activated. The resulting hormonal alterations affect compositional changes (increased body fat in the female, greater skeletal muscle bulk in the male) that prominently influence exercise capacity.

CHARACTERISTICS OF BIOLOGICAL MATURATION

It is important that the student of developmental exercise physiology be aware of the complexity posed by certain characteristics of biological maturation:

1. **Physiologic and anatomic values at maturity exhibit a high degree of interindividual variability.** Consistent with the definition of biological maturation, all children achieve the same end point (reaching full maturity) (4). That is, each child will demonstrate a curve for the development of a particular physiologic function, which eventuates in the 100% mature state. But in the world of real numbers, this is obviously not true. Body height is an easy example to cite, for in accordance with everyone's personal experience, stature in a crowd of mature adults varies greatly.

Take three children, A, B, and C, all of whom have the same height of 130 cm. Is their level of biological maturity for stature identical? By no means can this be assumed. If the future adult height of A will be 190 cm, that of B 175 cm, and that of C 160 cm, C will currently be at 81% maturity (an early developer), B at 74%, and A at 68% (a delayed maturer).

2. **The rate of development of a particular physiologic variable differs significantly from one child to the next.** While progressive change is the hallmark of biological maturation, the characteristics of the developmental curves for different anatomic and

physiologic variables can be very distinct. Figure 1.1, a depiction of system growth suggested by Scammon (23), illustrates this well. The curve of general growth reflects the pattern of change typical of body dimensions such as height and weight. Most body systems involved in exercise physiology (muscle mass, strength, heart, and lung size) follow this type of curve. Growth of the brain and nervous system follows the neural curve, characterized by rapid early development in the preschool years and then little change throughout childhood. Reproductive function and mechanisms for secondary sexual characteristics (genital curve) are dormant during childhood until the time of puberty. Function of lymphoid tissue (tonsils, thymus gland, lymph nodes) actually declines during late childhood.

Significant interindividual variability in the rate and shape of developmental curves is also observed within exercise physiology variables. Figure 1.2 depicts the changes observed in vertical jump height (a measure of explosive strength of the legs) in five children studied longitudinally for 5 years (Rowland and

Cunningham, unpublished data). Clearly the shapes of the developmental curves for vertical jump for these children are dissimilar. The mechanisms for this variability in the healthy childhood population are obscure, but presumably the changes are influenced by both genetic and environmental factors.

The lesson from this observation is that chronological age is not typically a reliable indicator of biological age for any given physiologic marker. Within any given school grade, a wide diversity of levels of biological maturation can be expected, and these differences may significantly influence physiologic responses to exercise. As Malina and Bouchard have emphasized, "Biological processes have their own timetables and do not celebrate birthdays" (15, p. 6).

Two common examples of the importance of this lesson can be cited, and the author will avert criticism by using one of his own articles as an illustration (22). The ratio of tidal volume to respiratory rate at a given level of minute ventilation during exercise normally increases as the child grows. This same ventilatory finding is characteristic of trained adult athletes compared to nonathletes, suggesting that the ratio increases as part of a "training effect." We reported that ratios in child distance runners were higher than those for nonrunners who had the same average age but were 6.5 cm shorter in stature. The conclusion that child runners demonstrate the same ventilatory training effect as adults could be contested, since the same results would have been observed if the runners were simply more biologically mature.

A similar dilemma arises in the interpretation of field fitness tests in children. Consider the boy who finishes the 1-mile run at the 10th percentile for his age (or below any criterion standard felt to be consistent with good cardiovascular health). Is this a laggard youth whose developmental curve for aerobic fitness has been shifted to the right because of a sedentary lifestyle (and who needs encouragement for more exercise)? Or a normal child who is simply following a delayed biologic curve (no action necessary)? Or a child whose genetic potential is sufficiently limited that his finish time actually represents a relatively high degree of physical fitness (deserving of a pat on the back)? The testing results provide little insight in differentiating the three possibilities.

3. **It is not clear how much the developmental curves of different physiologic functions may vary within the same child.** One cannot assume a priori that maturation of a particular physiologic variable in a given subject will progress along the same curve that other variables do. There is reason to expect, however, that maturation patterns for various exercise physiologic functions might be similar; that is, the early-maturing child typically is stronger and faster

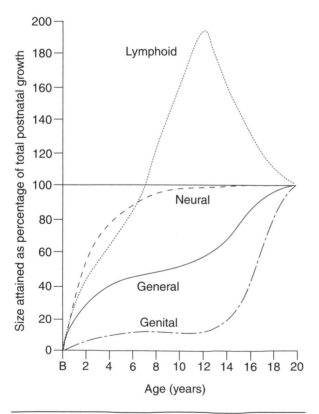

Figure 1.1 Different patterns of system growth during childhood. Growth of each system is expressed on the vertical scale as a percentage of the total gain between birth and age 20 years. Adapted from Scammon 1930.

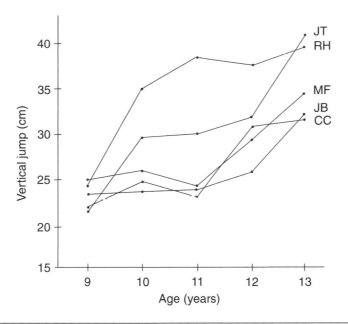

Figure 1.2   Developmental curves for performance on vertical jump in five children over 5 years (Rowland and Cunningham, unpublished data).

and has a higher aerobic capacity than the child whose maturation is delayed. Those who score well on tests of aerobic function tend to do better on anaerobic tests as well (2). If true, these observations suggest that similar intrinsic and extrinsic mechanisms are responsible for maturational rates of widely disparate physiologic functions.

Temporal clustering of developmental curves for different physiologic variables would at least partially explain the observation of Bar-Or that children—as opposed to adults—tend to be exercise "non-specialists" (2, p. 16). The youngster who is the high school's star football player and swimmer will probably do well in cross-country running as well, perhaps in relation to early development of varying physiologic capacities. Once maturity is reached, these links may be lost (the typical adult marathon runner would not survive long as a defensive end).

4. **Extrinsic factors may alter the timing and shape of developmental curves.** Extrinsic factors will be discussed in a later section of this chapter. Most obvious are such influences as athletic participation, level of physical activity, body composition, and nutritional status on factors like aerobic fitness or muscle strength. Other potential determinants of the growth of exercise performance, including socioeconomic level, cultural background, parental influence, self-esteem, testing conditions, and gender, have been less extensively studied.

5. **The family of physiological developmental curves for each form of physical activity is extra-**ordinarily complex. A given physiologic variable may include myriad components, each with its own maturational curve. To consider maximal O_2 uptake as an example: the contributions of factors such as cardiac and pulmonary function, blood volume and hemoglobin content, distribution of blood vessels, muscle aerobic capacity, muscle contractile function, temperature control, neuromuscular coordination, and cognitive abilities together form a composite $\dot{V}O_2$max curve. But the pattern of change with growth might be different for each. Alterations in the rate or shape of the developmental curve of any of these determinants may prominently alter one's level of aerobic fitness.

It is not difficult to comprehend how these features of biological maturation impede our progress in understanding developmental exercise physiology. At any given chronological age each child is unique—is characterized physiologically by a large multitude of biologic ages (11). The challenge for the developmental exercise physiologist lies in deciphering normal adaptations to exercise while accepting the dilemmas posed by these intra- and interindividual variations in human development.

Compounding this difficulty is our inability to directly determine a child's maturational level for any given physiologic factor. As an alternative means of estimating biological age, the investigator relies on those forms of maturation that can be more easily recognized. The following sections describe the features of these markers—morphological, sexual, and skeletal maturation—and how they can be assessed. The relationship of different forms of physiological function to these markers of biological maturation will be addressed subsequently throughout this book; the discussion here of these extensive areas of interest can be only an abbreviated one. For those wishing more comprehensive reviews, there are excellent sources (13, 15).

MORPHOLOGICAL MATURATION

Increase in body size, manifested by a progressive rise in body weight and height, is visually the most obvious expression of biological maturation of the child. The course of these changes clearly has significant bearing on exercise performance and is of great interest to the exercise physiologist.

In contrast to indicators for other forms of biological maturation, markers of morphological change are easily and accurately measured. Still, certain considerations in determining weight and height are important. The physiologist usually ascertains the subject's weight before testing and with the child wearing exercise clothing but no shoes. Height is obtained with the child standing, again without shoes. In some investigations—particularly longitudinal studies—it may be important to measure children at the same time each day, since there may be significant diurnal variation in stature. According to Malina and Bouchard, height can diminish by as much as 1 cm during the course of a day because of compression of intervertebral fibrous disks (15).

The shape of the growth curve from infancy through adolescence is not greatly different from one child to the next, but considerable interindividual variation exists in the timing of these changes as well as in values for height and weight among different children at the same chronological age. The most rapid rate of growth occurs in early infancy, as the birth weight is usually doubled by 3-4 months and tripled by age 1 year; thereafter there is a steady deceleration of growth rate until the school years, when the yearly gains in height and weight remain stable (see fig. 1.3).

In early adolescence, both height and weight accelerate in response to the hormonal changes of puberty. This pubertal growth spurt typically occurs earlier in girls—at about 10 to 12 years of age—with peak acceleration in boys appearing about 2 years later. The duration of the growth spurt is short, typically 1.0-1.5 years, but during this time the rate of height growth almost doubles. Virtually all muscle and skeletal dimensions contribute to the growth spurt, but there are some asymmetries. For instance, trunk length accelerates faster than length of the legs. The timing of peak growth rates during adolescence varies widely, with normal but late maturers showing acceleration of height and weight as many as 3 years later than early-maturing children. There is a tendency for children who exhibit an early growth spurt to have a higher maximal height velocity, but there is no association between the age of the growth spurt and ultimate adult height. However, early-maturing youngsters can be expected, on average, to weigh more as adults and to exhibit differences in body proportions (broader hips, narrow shoulders, and

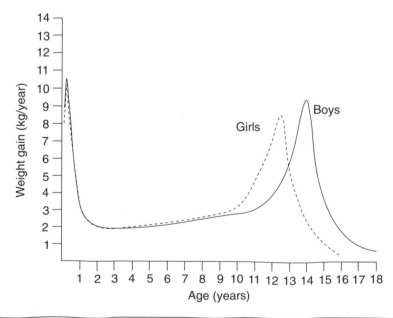

Figure 1.3   Velocity curves for weight during childhood and adolescence for boys and girls. Adapted from Tanner, Whitehouse, and Takaishi 1966.

shorter legs relative to height) compared to late maturers (15). After the pubertal growth spurt, the rate of linear growth decelerates abruptly, and little change in height is observed after the age of 16 years for most girls and after 18 years for boys.

Average values for height and weight are similar between sexes during childhood, but boys tend to be slightly heavier and taller than girls. With their earlier growth spurt, girls become temporarily taller than boys during late childhood. The boys rapidly catch up, however, achieving greater stature at maturity because (1) they have a longer growing period prior to the pubertal growth spurt and (2) their growth rate at the point of maximal velocity during puberty is greater (9.2 vs. 8.3 cm in the maximal year) (13).

Determining where the values for a given child's height and weight stand relative to his or her peers can be accomplished through percentile ranking in relation to normative data. A child whose stature is at the 20th percentile for her age is taller than 20 out of every 100 children that age and shorter than 80 of the 100. A youngster at the 50th percentile for weight is at the median value for his age; half the child's peers will be heavier and half will be lighter.

This information indicates the child's relative ranking in comparison to other children of the same age, but it tells little about the child's rate of linear growth. To determine this, one measures the child serially on charts that connect percentiles for height or weight at different ages. Figures 1.4 and 1.5 are examples of such charts commonly used in the United States, based on measurements of large numbers of normal healthy children. In using growth charts one must be certain, of course, that the subjects being assessed are similar in cultural, racial, and socioeconomic characteristics to the children on whom the normative data were based. The charts in figures 1.4 and 1.5, derived from measurements compiled by the United States Public Health Service, include both black and white children. Racial differences were felt to be insignificant for general clinical usage of these charts (13).

From age 2 to the beginning of adolescence, the normal child can be expected to track progressively along a particular percentile curve. That is, a 4-year-old whose height is at the 65th percentile for age will be expected to remain at the 65th percentile throughout the course of childhood. Deviations are used by physicians to detect disease: a downward "crossing of percentiles" in weight, for instance, is typically observed in infants with congestive heart failure, while a falloff in percentiles for height might be a sign of inadequate pituitary gland function. The child with obesity will demonstrate a progressive rise across weight percentiles whereas the height usually tracks normally. The degree to which a child maintains growth at a particular percentile, then, is a more important marker of normal morphological maturation than percentile ranking at a given age.

In early infancy, height and weight values may cross percentiles as the child gets on his or her "genetic track." At the other end of childhood, adolescents do not always follow published normal percentile curves for height and weight because of individual variations in the timing of the pubertal growth spurt, which can differ as much as 3 years between normal youngsters.

Comparing percentiles for height and weight of a child at a given age can provide quantitative information regarding the child's body habitus. A 6-year-old girl whose weight is at the 10th percentile and whose height is at the 60th percentile can be expected to be strikingly slender. Conversely, the boy with weight at the 60th percentile and height at the 10th percentile is either very "stocky" or obese.

Besides increasing body mass, the growing child shows alterations in body proportions. Most obvious is a progressive increase in the relative length of the legs in relation to height. This change is reflected in a decreasing ratio of sitting height to stature as the child grows, with a value of approximately 68% at birth falling to 52% at age 13 years. Few differences in relative leg length are observed, however, in the age group usually involved in exercise testing (over age 8) (20).

Children have a relatively large body surface area in relation to their mass, and the ratio between the two diminishes with increasing age (see fig. 1.6). It is important to recognize that the magnitude of these differences is not minor; the ratio changes by almost 50% between age 5 years and maturity. The principles of dimensionality theory that describe this phenomenon will be discussed in chapter 2; the implications of changes in the relationship between the growing child's mass and surface area to energy metabolism and thermoregulation will be addressed in chapters 6 and 15.

While ease and accuracy of measurement make morphological markers attractive as indicators of biological maturity, the use of height and weight to indicate a child's biological age has major drawbacks. Most significantly, both of these measures demonstrate marked interindividual variability at maturity: it is thus impossible to determine with any accuracy where an 8-year-old girl "is" in terms of maturity level (i.e., percentage of her ultimate adult value) on the basis of her height and weight alone.

In a given child, do increases in height and weight bear a relationship to changes in exercise physiology variables? For many variables the answer is, in general, yes, and this is not unexpected. Physiologic determinants of exercise provide for locomotion—locomotion that often involves the movement of body mass against the force of gravity. But the relationships between

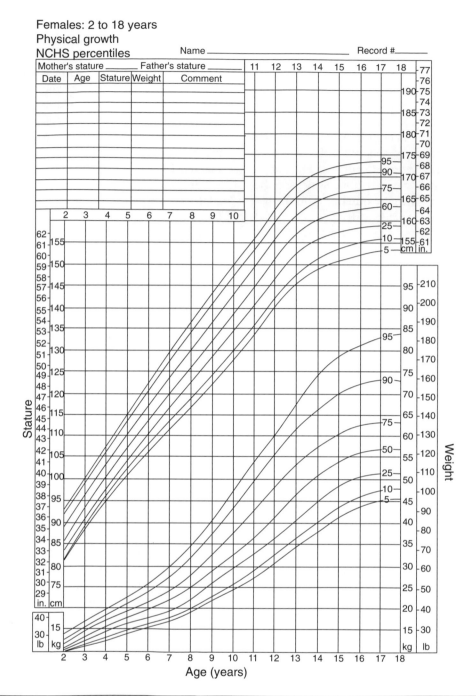

Figure 1.4 National Center for Health Statistics percentile curves for height and weight of girls 2-18 years of age. Adapted from Hamill et al. 1979.

physiologic markers and body height, weight, and/or surface area in the growing child are often not simple. This issue is discussed in detail in chapter 2; subsequent chapters will address the development of aerobic, anaerobic, and strength variables with respect to growing body size.

A common use of morphologic maturation by exercise physiologists is the determination of physiologic variables relative to the age of *peak height velocity*

(PHV, the age at the maximum growth rate during the adolescent spurt). This method allows physiologic comparisons between individuals, or groups of individuals, at similar levels of somatic maturation, and has been particularly useful in evaluating the influence of puberty on maximal aerobic power and muscle strength (see chapters 6 and 13). However, the determination of age at PHV requires longitudinal measurements, and this approach therefore has no utility as a maturity

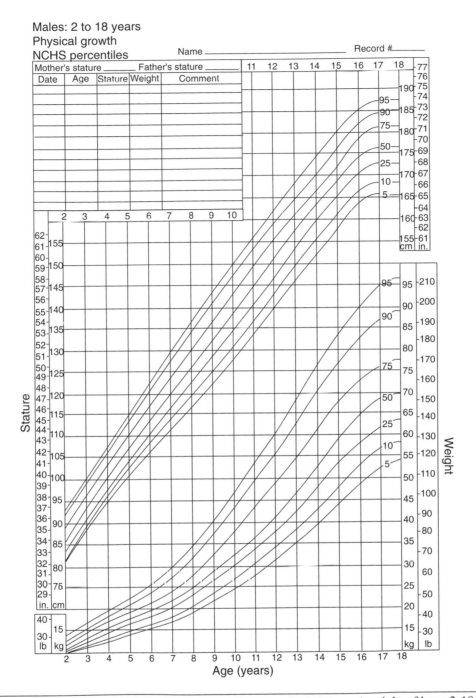

Figure 1.5 National Center for Health Statistics percentile curves for height and weight of boys 2-18 years of age. Adapted from Hamill et al. 1979.

marker in, for instance, a cross-sectional comparison of anaerobic capacity in 12-year-old basketball players and nonathletic controls.

SEXUAL MATURATION

Puberty can be defined as a succession of anatomic and physiologic changes in early adolescence that culminate in fertility. When puberty ends, the adolescent has achieved full sexual maturity, the adult reproductive state. The events of puberty, which are triggered by secretion of hormones from the hypothalamus, pituitary gland, and gonads, also produce a number of changes not directly related to sexual function. These include (1) the adolescent growth spurt, (2) a set of physical features collectively termed *secondary sexual characteristics* (including facial hair and deepening of the voice in

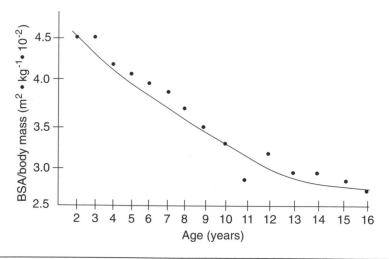

Figure 1.6   Ratio of body surface area to mass in children 2 through 16 years of age.

males, breast development in females), and (3) alterations in body composition (in particular, augmented muscle mass in males and increased deposition of body fat in females).

Because many of these features may influence exercise capacity, the parallels between sexual maturation and physiologic development are of particular interest. On the basis of this association, too, markers of sexual development have been utilized to match experimental subjects by biological age.

Stages of Sexual Maturation

Although pubertal changes progress in a continuum, the process has been divided for clinical purposes into a series of physical stages based on identifiable secondary sexual characteristics. The most commonly used rating system is that devised by Tanner (16, 17, 25), which describes features of breast development, pubic hair, and genitalia separately for boys and girls in five stages (see table 1.1). In the Tanner classification, stage 1 represents the immature, prepubertal state, while the adolescent with stage 5 findings is fully mature.

The average child progresses through these pubertal stages over a period of approximately 4 years. The process begins sooner in girls, usually with breast development (thelarche) starting at age 10 1/2 to 11 years. Puberty is initiated by boys with genital enlargement at age 11 to 12 1/2 years. Menarche, the most discrete observable point in pubertal development, typically occurs at age 12.6 years in the United States. The initiation of menses, then, is a relatively late event in the course of puberty, occurring usually at stage 4 breast and pubic

hair development and more than a year after PHV. Girls usually do not become fertile, however, until 1 to 2 years after menarche.

Table 1.1   Stages of sexual maturation

Breast development *(female)*

Stage
1 Preadolescent; breasts flat
2 Breast buds (small mound beneath areola)
3 Increased areolar and breast size with
     no separation of contours
4 Areola projects above breast plane
5 Mature stage; recession of areola to breast
     contour

Pubic hair *(male and female)*

Stage
1 Preadolescent; no pubic hair
2 Scant growth of long, straight or slightly
     curled hair at base of penis or along
     labia
3 Hair darker, more abundant, curled, and
     coarser
4 Adult pattern but does not extend to medial
     surface of thighs
5 Mature stage; extends to medial surface of
     thighs

Adapted from Marshall and Tanner 1969, 1970.

It is important to note that exceptions to these "rules" of normal pubertal development are common. In fact, Lowrey suggested that no more than 60% can be expected to follow the standard progression outlined by Tanner (13). The total duration of puberty may be as short as 18 months or as long as 8 years. One individual may pass a pubertal stage in less than 6 months, while another may stay fixed in that stage for 2 years. And developmental stages are not necessarily followed in the prescribed order. For instance, breast development reaches stage 2 or 3 in 75% of girls before the appearance of pubic hair, but in 10%, pubic hair is at stage 2 or 3 before breasts reach stage 2.

Maturity ratings for other secondary sexual characteristics such as axillary hair, voice change, and facial hair have been described (15). These are not often used in clinical practice both because they lack precision and because they are usually late events in pubertal progression.

Hormonal Regulation of Puberty

The hormonal alterations responsible for sexual maturation at puberty are complex and are not fully understood. A comprehensive description of these changes is not within the scope of this discussion. The following represents a brief summary; further detail can be obtained from standard references (7, 9).

In the adult, reproductive function is mediated by two hormones produced by the pituitary gland, follicle-stimulating hormone (FSH) and luteinizing hormone (LH), and by others secreted by the gonads (estrogen and progesterone in the female and testosterone in the male). Follicle-stimulating hormone and luteinizing hormone are released from the anterior pituitary after stimulation by releasing factors from the hypothalamus in the brain. These hormones are responsible for ovulation and stimulate secretion of estrogen by the ovary in the female; in the male they stimulate sperm production and secretion of testosterone by the testes. Testosterone and estrogen are important in spermatogenesis and ovulation, respectively, but are also responsible for the development of secondary sexual characteristics. The timing and quantity of secretion of these hormones are precisely regulated by a system of negative feedback upon the producing organ.

Before puberty, this system lies dormant. The factor that increases FSH and LH secretion at the onset of puberty appears to be a reduction in the sensitivity of the pituitary feedback receptors to circulating levels of reproductive hormones. The rise in FSH and LH triggers production of estrogen and testosterone by the gonads.

Serum testosterone levels in the prepubertal child are barely detectable. At the onset of puberty (ages 10-12 years), these rapidly rise in the male, reaching levels over 20-fold that of the prepubertal years; females show a much smaller increase (28). Similarly, serum estrogen levels are near zero before age 8-10 years. Puberty is associated with a rise to about 8 micrograms percent in the female and 2 micrograms percent in the male.

Testosterone is responsible for the virilizing changes of puberty in the male: enlargement of the testes, penis, and prostate; growth and coarseness of pubic, facial, and axillary hair; voice change; development of sebaceous and sweat glands; increase in linear growth; and skeletal muscle hypertrophy. In the normal female, estrogen causes breast development, uterine growth, body fat accumulation, and bone maturation.

Assessment of Sexual Maturation

Estimating level of sexual maturation has been approached through several methods:

1. **Direct observation of secondary sexual characteristics.** This involves grading breast, pubic hair, and genitalia characteristics in the nude subject by the Tanner staging method described earlier. Photographic guidelines are provided in standard texts (15, 25). Malina and Bouchard pointed out the imprecision of this five-stage system in noting that subjects just entering a stage and those leaving will be given the same score although they may be significantly different in level of sexual maturation (15).

While this approach is often satisfactory in the practice of medicine, considerations of invasion of privacy may cause the researcher to be hesitant to use Tanner staging in healthy volunteers for exercise testing. Likewise, the measurement of testicular volume in boys through comparisons with models of known volume (Prader orchidometer) is unlikely to be acceptable for most exercise physiology studies.

2. **Self-report.** It has been reported that children's assessment of their own sexual maturity through use of Tanner staging photographs can provide an adequate estimate of pubertal status (6, 18). Further studies will be important to determine the feasibility and validity of this approach.

3. **Age of menarche.** The timing of a girl's initial menstrual period is often used as a marker of sexual maturity (14). To obtain this information, one can determine how many girls in a group have achieved menarche (the status quo method), ask girls at what age they reached menarche (the retrospective method), or determine age of menarche prospectively (the most accurate). This approach, of course, provides no information about level of sexual maturity beyond a single marker (i.e., one can categorize the subjects only as pre- or postmenarcheal). There is no similar discreet reproductive marker in males.

4. **Serum hormone levels.** Levels of reproductive hormones have been utilized as indicators of pubertal status relative to exercise physiology variables (27). The large diurnal fluctuations and interindividual differences in serum hormone values limit their precision for estimations of pubertal development. However, with careful consideration of timing of phlebotomy, identification of children as pre- or postpubertal is reasonable.

It is clear that the use of expressions of sexual development as a means of matching individuals for level of biological maturity is problematic. Sexual indicators of biological maturity are limited, too, in that they are useful only during the period of pubertal development (approximately ages 10 to 16 years). Consequently, these markers are more commonly used to define groups of subjects as prepubertal, pubertal, or postpubertal in studies in which the hormonal influences of puberty might be expected to be influential.

To be defined as truly prepubertal, subjects should (1) be at Tanner stage 1 for pubic hair, genitalia, and breast development; (2) have not yet entered a growth spurt; (3) show low serum levels of testosterone or estrogen; and (4) have no menses. Most boys below the age of 12 years will fit these criteria. Females, on the other hand, begin puberty earlier, and a significant number will show beginning breast development by age 10. Studies designed to evaluate variables during exercise testing of prepubertal females may therefore be hampered by the young age and size of the subjects. For this reason, many investigators have defined their female population as "premenarcheal" rather than prepubertal. This resolves the issue of adequate patient age and size for treadmill or cycle testing but introduces the possibility of pubertal influences on exercise performance.

SKELETAL MATURATION

The bony skeleton grows progressively during childhood and serves as an easily identifiable indicator of biological maturation (1). Bones of the extremities develop progressively during the growing years by the process of ossification of cartilage, and growth of these long bones occurs through proliferation of cartilage cells in the epiphyseal plate. The mature adult state is reached when multiplication of these cells ceases and the bone becomes fully ossified.

Assessment of Skeletal Maturity

The x-ray appearance of the ossification status of bones provides an index of biological maturity, since these changes occur in a reasonably consistent pattern from birth to adult maturity. The bones of the wrist have been used most commonly because the wrist contains multiple bones for examination and radiation exposure is minimal.

The atlas method of Greulich and Pyle has been used most extensively in the United States (10). With this technique, one compares ossification features observed on radiographs of the wrists (such as bone size, shape, density) to published standards related to chronological age. On the basis of these findings one can assign a "bone age" to the child, with a typical standard deviation of 6 months at age 3 years and 16 months at 11 years. That is, a 5-year-old boy whose wrist and hand bones are characteristic of an 8-year-old has a bone age of 8 years. This approach allows the examiner to determine, then, whether a child is biologically advanced or delayed for his or her chronological age.

Other methods have been used for determining skeletal maturity. Tanner et al. devised a system for evaluating bone maturity at the hand and wrist that avoided reference to chronological age (26). This method involves comparison of bone features to a maturity scale, divided into seven to eight stages, with dissimilarities in the maturation rates of different bones taken into account. The method of Roche et al. involves findings on anteroposterior x-rays of the knee (21). This area has been considered more valuable for skeletal maturity assessment from birth to age 7 years (19).

Skeletal Maturity and Exercise Research

Many consider skeletal maturity the best indicator of biological maturity. Skeletal age has strong links with both sexual and morphological development (see discussion later in this chapter); one can easily determine bone development by x-ray with reasonable precision; and, most importantly, one can measure skeletal maturation throughout the pediatric years. Because of the expense and inconvenience as well as the radiation exposure (albeit minimal), however, determining skeletal maturation is not feasible for most research studies.

Correlational studies examining the influence of skeletal age on physiologic and motor performance findings in children are difficult to interpret. Simple correlations between skeletal age and fitness are typically high. For instance, Hollman and Bouchard reported a correlation of .89 between bone age and maximal O_2 uptake in children (12). But, as Malina and Bouchard have emphasized, correlations are of similar magnitude between $\dot{V}O_2max$ and height, weight, or chronological age. Therefore each of these markers by itself may not contribute highly to the variance of the test item (15).

Shephard et al. demonstrated this in their study of muscle strength and aerobic power in a large group of

French Canadian children (24). Multiple regression analysis with age, height, and weight as early independent variables indicated that chronological age accounted for 85% of the variance. Bone age added little to the predictability of fitness measures (4-7%). The correlation between wrist bone age and chronological age was $r = 0.88$.

When children of the same chronological age are placed into differing maturity categories by skeletal age, however, differences in fitness are observable. Early maturers are typically stronger and faster than late maturers and have a higher absolute maximal O_2 uptake. Such differences are less obvious in females (4, 15).

ASSOCIATION OF MARKERS OF BIOLOGICAL MATURITY

How closely in time do the curves of different forms of biological maturity track together in a given child? A close linkage would suggest that similar genetic and environmental factors are responsible for determining the rates of morphologic, skeletal, and sexual maturation. It is intuitively obvious that just such a close relationship is observed at least during the pubertal years: hormonal changes associated with sexual maturation also stimulate bone growth and muscle bulk, with subsequent acceleration in body height and weight. One would expect, then, that children who are early maturers in sexual development would also mature sooner than their peers in body size and skeletal dimensions.

Research data reviewed by Malina and Bouchard support this conclusion (15). Correlation coefficients between variables such as PHV, age of menarche, Tanner staging, and skeletal age are generally moderate to high (typically 0.60 to 0.80). Thus a youngster who is advanced in one indicator of biological maturity will be highly likely to show early development in the others. These correlations are not perfect, however, indicating some variability in timing of different forms of biological maturation during adolescence.

In the prepubertal years, skeletal maturity (bone age) is associated with somatic growth (expressed as percentage of adult stature) (3). But bone age at the onset of puberty does not strongly relate to markers of sexual and morphological maturation later in adolescence. This association becomes stronger as puberty progresses, however. These findings imply that mechanisms that control the tempo of maturation during the prepubertal years are different from those involved during puberty. This concept is consistent with the facts that (1) before puberty, growth hormone is responsible for bone and somatic growth and (2) during puberty, the influences of sex hormones become superimposed on the effects of growth hormone.

Cluster analysis of the Wroclaw Growth Study of Polish Children, tracked longitudinally from age 8 to 18, supports this idea (5). These data confirmed the clustering of maturity factors during adolescence. The study also identified clustering of skeletal age during late childhood and the age of attainment of 80% of adult height, both indicators of prepubertal maturation. It provided further evidence, then, that prepubertal growth is independent of rates of biological development during adolescence.

One of the tasks of the exercise physiologist is to ascertain the extent to which developmental curves for physiologic variables conform to these clusters of biological maturation. Again, a commonsense approach would say they should, since much of exercise capacity is linked to factors such as body dimensions and muscle size. The data available to confirm or deny this notion will be examined relative to specific physiologic variables throughout this book.

DETERMINANTS OF BIOLOGICAL MATURATION

The mechanisms that drive biological maturation are multiple, complex, and resistant to simplistic explanations. At the same time, this is a potentially fertile area of inquiry, since an examination of factors that influence the rates of skeletal, somatic, and sexual maturation might be expected to provide insight into the determinants of exercise physiology in the growing child. This subject has been extensively reviewed by Malina and Bouchard (15).

Genetics

It is assumed that children, who have inherited genetic information from their parents, will resemble their mothers or fathers both in size and in physical characteristics. Investigations regarding the degree of genetic influence on body dimensions indicate that while this is largely true, there are many exceptions. Comparative studies of identical twins (who share the same genetic information) and fraternal twins (who don't) suggest that the genetic contribution to a child's stature as well as his or her eventual adult height is approximately 60%.

The correlation coefficient between a child's height at age 3 years and that at maturity is 0.80. The effect of hereditary factors is lower with weight, about 40% (15). Genetic influences are greater in well-nourished and Caucasian children.

The power of the genetic influence on growth is suggested by the tenacity with which a child follows a given height or weight percentile with age. When illness causing a falloff of percentiles (congestive heart failure, malnutrition) is rectified, the child experiences "catch-up growth" and returns to the original percentile.

Hereditary influences are also significant with respect to other markers of biological maturity. The genetic contribution to length and diameter of long bones appears to be about 60% (following that of body stature). The correlation coefficient for age at menarche between identical (monozygotic) twins is reportedly .90, whereas that for nonidentical (dizygotic) twins is .60. And coefficients for age and extent of PHV in monozygotic twins are twice those for dizygotic (8).

Endocrine

The prominent role that reproductive hormones play in sexual, morphologic, and skeletal development during puberty was highlighted earlier in this chapter. Other endocrine functions also contribute in an important way to normal biological maturation. Growth hormone, secreted by the pituitary gland, is responsible for normal growth. As indicated previously, this hormone is the major factor contributing to skeletal and somatic maturation in the prepubertal years, and its function becomes supplemented by the effects of the reproductive hormones at puberty. The effects of growth hormone are mediated by the somatomedins, substances produced by the liver that respond to increased growth hormone levels by stimulating tissue cell division and protein synthesis.

Thyroid hormone is necessary for normal biological maturation. Depressed thyroid function (hypothyroidism) results in delay in growth and sexual function. Parathormone, secreted by the parathyroid glands in the neck, maintains normal blood calcium levels, a requisite for skeletal development. Anabolic steroids secreted by the adrenal gland are important in reproductive function. Clearly, the normal multiple functions of the endocrine glands are necessary for optimizing biological maturation.

Nutrition

An appropriate food intake is probably the most critical environmental factor influencing normal biological development. Caloric demands parallel increases in body size, as the child must consume sufficient food to provide for normal growth. At the same time, the diet must be composed of an appropriate balance of protein, fat, carbohydrates, vitamins, and minerals to support growth processes. An inadequate caloric intake (malnutrition) or deficiency in any specific dietary component can impair normal biological maturation.

Physical Activity

The amount of habitual physical activity has no effect on body height, but daily caloric expenditure can be a major determinant of weight. Increased physical activity or training can result in diminished levels of body fat and increased muscle mass. Bone mineralization responds directly to physical stressors, and some evidence indicates that adults who are more active are at less risk for osteoporosis (bone demineralization). Likewise, prolonged training may result in increased bone density. However, physical activity or sport participation does not appear to affect rate of skeletal maturation.

Other Factors

Social conditions, including socioeconomic status, family size, and social environment, can influence the progression of biological maturation. Likewise, differences in race, culture, climate, and geographical location can affect these changes. And, finally, it should be remembered that this discussion has focused on the healthy child. Childhood illness can be expected to profoundly affect normal rates of growth and maturation, and deviations from these expected curves can serve as an indication of disease.

BIOLOGICAL MATURATION AND RESEARCH IN CHILDREN

Most research on the normal evolution of physiologic function during exercise in children has involved cross-sectional data of youngsters at different ages. This study design obscures maturational changes, and the developmental patterns described might therefore not typify those expected for individual children. This effect is apparent in growth curves for adolescents that are based on cross-sectional values for height and weight; the growth spurt is "smoothed out," and the rise of mean percentile is considerably less than the accelerations in height and weight for a given youngster.

Comparing physiological findings in a group of prepubertal subjects with findings for mature, postpubertal individuals provides information about the effects of biological maturation. But such a comparison yields little insight into the rate and nature of changes during the course of childhood or the influence of puberty itself.

Cross-sectional comparisons in relation to a maturational marker provide a means of contrasting data in two groups relative to a biological rather than a chronological age. As noted previously, the most common use of this design is in examining data in children relative to their age at PHV. Children can then be lumped into groups of PHV age minus 1 year, minus 2 years, and so on. While this procedure allows matching for somatic maturity, it requires longitudinal data of several years on all groups for identification of PHV.

Longitudinal studies of the same children examined over time provide the best data, since this approach makes it possible to assess changes in mean values with respect to both chronological and biological age. In addition, the extent to which the patterns and timing of developmental curves differ between individual children can be more clearly assessed.

SUMMARY

The development of physiologic variables in the growing child that influence exercise is an example of biological maturation. The task for the developmental exercise physiologist is to identify and characterize these normal patterns of development. Since level of physiologic maturation is difficult to determine, the exercise scientist turns to more obvious markers to help define a child's biological age.

The ideal indicator of biological age would be (1) easy, safe, and accurate to measure, (2) closely associated with the development of physiological variables, and (3) equally appropriate and useful for all age groups. Unfortunately, no such marker has yet been identified.

Chronological age is not a reliable indicator of biological maturity. The stages in progression toward adult physiologic function can be expected to vary widely at any given age. Use of morphological markers such as height and weight has limited value because of the large interindividual variability at maturity. Age of the PHV, however, is useful for comparison of biological maturity levels between individuals.

Secondary sexual characteristics help define level of sexual maturity, but these are useful markers only in the adolescent age group. Skeletal age can be assessed at any age, but this requires x-rays of the wrist bones. Morphological, sexual, and skeletal maturity are linked during adolescence. In the prepubertal years, skeletal age is associated with body size, but there is little relationship with changes that occur later at puberty. Thus, there appear to be two separate periods of biological growth: the prepubertal years, when growth is controlled by growth hormone, and the pubertal years, or adolescence, when the influence of reproductive hormones becomes superimposed on the actions of growth hormone.

References

1. Acheson, R.M. Maturation of the skeleton. In: Falkner, F., ed. Human development. Philadelphia: Saunders; 1966:p. 465-502.
2. Bar-Or, O. Pediatric sports medicine for the practitioner. New York: Springer-Verlag; 1983:p. 16-18.
3. Bayley, N. The accurate prediction of growth and adult height. Mod. Prob. Paediatr. 7:234-255; 1962.
4. Beunen, G. Biological age in pediatric exercise research. In: Bar-Or, O., ed. Advances in pediatric sport sciences. Vol. 3. Champaign, IL: Human Kinetics; 1989:p. 1-40.
5. Bielicki, T.; Koniarek, J.; Malina, R.M. Interrelationships among certain measures of growth and maturation rate in boys during adolescence. Ann. Hum. Biol. 11:201-210; 1984.
6. Duke, P.M.; Litt, I.F.; Gross, R.T. Adolescent's self assessment of sexual maturation. Pediatrics 66:918-920; 1980.
7. Emans, S.J.H.; Goldstein, D.P. Pediatric & adolescent gynecology. 3rd ed. Boston: Little, Brown; 1990.
8. Fischbein, S. Onset of puberty in MZ and DZ twins. Acta Genet. Med. Gemel. 26:151-158; 1977.
9. Gardner, L.I. Endocrine and genetic diseases of childhood and adolescence. 2nd ed. Philadelphia: Saunders; 1975.
10. Greulich, W.W.; Pyle, I. Radiographic atlas of skeletal development of the hand and wrist. 2nd ed. Palo Alto, CA: Stanford University Press; 1959.
11. Hebbelinck, M. Methods of biological maturity assessment. In: Borms, J.; Hebbelinck, M., eds. Pediatric work physiology. Basel: Karger; 1978:p. 108-117.
12. Hollman, W.; Bouchard, C. Relations between chronological, skeletal age and ergometric characteristics, heart volume, anthropometric dimensions and muscle strength in 8 to 18 year old boys. Zeitschrift fur Kreislaufforschung 59:160-176; 1970.
13. Lowrey, G.H. Growth and development of children. 8th ed. Chicago: Year Book Medical; 1986.
14. Malina, R.M. Menarche in athletes: a synthesis and hypothesis. Ann. Hum. Biol. 10:1-24; 1983.
15. Malina, R.M.; Bouchard, C. Growth, maturation, and physical activity. Champaign, IL: Human Kinetics; 1991.
16. Marshall, W.A.; Tanner, J.M. Variations in pattern of pubertal changes in girls. Arch. Dis. Child. 44:291-303; 1969.
17. Marshall, W.A.; Tanner, J.M. Variations in the pattern of pubertal changes in boys. Arch. Dis. Child. 45:13-23; 1970.
18. Neinstein, L.S. Adolescent self-assessment of sexual maturation. Clin. Pediatr. 21:482-484; 1982.
19. Roche, A.F. The measurement of skeletal maturation. In: Johnston, F.E.; Roche, A.F.; Suzanne, C., eds. Human physical growth and maturation. Methodologies and factors. New York: Plenum Press; 1980:p. 61-82.
20. Roche, A.F.; Malina, R.M. Manual of physical status and performance in childhood. Vol. 1, Physical status. New York: Plenum Press; 1983.
21. Roche, A.F., Wainer, H.; Thissen, D. Skeletal maturity: knee joint as a biological indicator. New York: Plenum Press; 1975.
22. Rowland, T.W.; Green, G.M. The influence of biological maturation and aerobic fitness on ventilatory responses to treadmill exercise. In: Dotson, C.O.; Humphrey, J.H., eds. Exercise physiology. Current selected research. Vol. 4. New York: AMS Press; 1990:p. 52-61.

23. Scammon, R.E. The measurement of the body in childhood. In: Harris, J.A.; Jackson, C.M.; Paterson, D.G.; Scammon, R.E., eds. The measurement of man. Minneapolis: University of Minnesota Press; 1930:p. 193.
24. Shephard, R.J.; Lavallee, H.; Rajic, K.M.; Jequier, J.C.; Brisson, G.; Beaucage, C. Radiographic age in the interpretation of physiological and anthropological data. Med. Sport 11:124-133; 1978.
25. Tanner, J.M. Growth and endocrinology of the adolescent. In: Gardner, L.I. Endocrine and genetic disease of childhood and adolescence. 2nd ed. Philadelphia: Saunders; 1975:p. 14-63.
26. Tanner, J.M.; Whitehouse, R.H.; Marshall, W.A.; Healy, M.J.R.; Goldstein, H. Assessment of skeletal maturity and prediction of adult height (TW2 method). London: Academic Press; 1975.
27. Welsman, J.R.; Armstrong, N.; Kirby, B.J. Serum testosterone, peak $\dot{V}O_2$, and submaximal blood lactate responses in 12-16 year old males. Pediatr. Exerc. Sci.; in press.
28. Winter, J.S.D.; Falman, C. Pituitary-gonadal relations in male children and adolescents. Pediatr. Res. 6:126–135; 1972.

CHAPTER 2

ACCOUNTING FOR SIZE: THE PHYSIOLOGIST'S DILEMMA

Undoubtedly philosophers are right when they tell us that nothing is great or little except by comparison.

Gulliver's Travels

Unraveling the mystery of physiologic changes with growth intrigues the developmental exercise physiologist. Yet these same changes in body dimensions provide some of the greatest challenges to understanding the child's responses to exercise. Unquestionably body size plays a critical role in determining both anatomic form and physiologic function. Our biologist colleagues have recognized this for over a century, and comparative physiologists have long struggled to identify the best means of describing these relationships. Recognizing the dimensional principles between size and function is a necessary starting point for understanding changes in physiologic responses to exercise in growing children.

This chapter will review the alternative means of "normalizing" physiologic variables to body size. We will pay special attention to (a) concerns regarding the traditional use of body mass (ratio standard) and (b) newer approaches to adjusting for body dimensions.

THE PROBLEM OF SIZE

Consider the plight of the researcher who wishes to investigate the effects of an enhanced physical education program on the aerobic fitness of a group of sixth-grade children. At the beginning of the school year, the mean value of maximal O_2 uptake for the class is, say, 1.83 L/min; 9 months later the average $\dot{V}O_2$max is found to have increased to 2.15 L/min. The significant rise in aerobic fitness is clear-cut, but the interpretation is not: was the improvement a physiologic adaptation to the increased activities in the physical education class? Or was the change in the group's maximal aerobic power simply a reflection of the growing heart, lungs, red cell mass, and muscle size that contribute to $\dot{V}O_2$max?

A similar problem arises when one compares physiologic variables between groups. Knowing that the average resting stroke volume of a set of 10-year-old children is 52 ml, whereas that of a group of young adults is 85 ml, is not necessarily enlightening. What we need to know is, would these two groups have different stroke volumes if their body dimensions were the same? Likewise, the parents of a 12-year-old girl want to know whether the $\dot{V}O_2$max of 2.1 L/min you just determined on their daughter's treadmill test indicates that she has normal cardiovascular fitness. How can you determine whether or not this value is what it "should be for her size"?

In these examples of longitudinal measurements, cross-sectional comparisons, and definitions of normative data, it is clear that some method must be devised to "normalize" measurements to account for changes in size during the childhood years. Indeed, the matter is of critical importance for the developmental physiologist, whose subjects are in a state of continuous dimensional change. If we are to have insight into the physiologic changes that accompany the growth of children, we must possess an accurate means of comparing subjects of different sizes. It follows, too, that erroneous methods of comparison will lead only to confusion and obfuscate a true understanding of developmental exercise physiology.

The critical importance of factoring size to physiologic measurements notwithstanding, the solution to this problem is not simple. A number of issues preclude an easy answer:

1. The relationship between body size and a particular physiologic variable may change with age. Resting metabolic rate (y), for instance, is related to body mass (x) by the equation $y = ax^{1.02}$ in humans up to a mass of 10-12 kg, but in the range of 12-35 kg the equation is $y = ax^{.58}$ (12).

2. The most appropriate means of standardizing a physiologic variable to body size may depend on the question being addressed. Expressing maximal O_2 uptake relative to body mass has appeal when one is seeking a marker of endurance fitness in weight-bearing activities (e.g., 1-mile run), since it is, in fact, the body mass that has to be transported around the high school track. But using $\dot{V}O_2$max per kg would not seem to be an appropriate tactic for normalizing cardiac functional reserve. That's because even though maximal cardiac output is a major determinant of O_2 uptake, "per kg" introduces the prominent influence of variability of body composition (e.g., body fat) into the denominator (15).

3. Methods for standardizing physiologic measures to body size are empiric. They are descriptive and may have served well for making intra- and interindividual comparisons. But they typically provide no insight into the physiological basis for the observed relationship. For instance, we might be able to establish that performance on a vertical jump relates to body mass by the equation $y = ax^{.80}$. But *why?* The observed mathematical relationship provides no answer. For this reason, it is difficult to ascertain whether or not the method for relating a physiologic variable to a particular marker of body size is a proper one beyond the level of criticism of statistical methodology.

4. Physiologic changes that occur as children age may reflect alterations in function as well as size. Maximal cardiac output should be expected to rise during the childhood years as the heart increases in size, but changes in myocardial contractility might also occur. If so, we would be in error if we used "per kg" to normalize maximal cardiac output simply because we know that heart size correlates closely to body mass.

Heusner made the important observation that animals (and children) can differ by both quantitative and qualitative properties (11). The former, which are dependent on body size, he termed *extensive properties*. These include variables such as O_2 uptake, leg muscle strength,

and lung volumes. *Intensive properties*, on the other hand, include size-independent factors such as temperature, pressures, enzyme concentrations, and muscle contraction efficiency. Heusner emphasized that when we consider the statistical relationship of a physiologic measure to any size marker (such as body mass), we cannot ignore the possibility that the observed association may reflect intensive as well as extensive properties. That is, physiologic variations in children may be attributable to qualitative, functional differences as well as to size.

Muscle strength, for instance, increases during childhood at a greater rate than would be expected for body size (4). The strength of a muscle is related to its cross-sectional area, and this in turn (by dimensionality theory, to be described further on) can be expected to be predicted by the square of body height. But studies in children reveal that strength actually relates to height by exponents considerably greater than 2.0. It has been hypothesized that alterations in neural or biochemical influences on the strength of muscular contraction may be responsible.

Returning to our researcher faced with the difficulties of adjusting physiologic data among children of different sizes, what are the options? If data were available on physiologic variables in large numbers of children, it might be possible to create normal curves of such measures according to height or mass. Individuals could then be evaluated serially to determine whether or not they followed the expected patterns as they grew. Alternatively, the physiologic measures could be related directly to body mass, height, or some other dimensional index, the so-called *ratio standard*. This traditional means of adjusting physiologic variables to size has come under increasing criticism (14, 22, 24), leading to a consideration of several alternative methods of standardizing for differing body dimensions.

Dimensionality theory has its roots in simple geometric principles, relating physiologic variables to body stature. Scaling by *allometric equations* has a long tradition in the biologic sciences, although most available information deals with interspecies differences in size-related functions among adult animals. Use of *regression analysis* with analysis of covariance may provide insights that differ from those offered by the traditional use of ratio standards.

This chapter will review the various approaches to normalization of physiologic data based on markers of body size. The optimal denominator would (a) be easily and accurately measured and (b) adequately reflect differences in biologic variables relative to body size and function across a wide age range. It is clear that no such universal standardizing factor, critical to an understanding of developmental exercise physiology, has yet been identified.

Longitudinal Comparisons With Normative Data

The pediatrician assessing the growth of a child is not as much interested in the patient's current height and weight as in the rate of change of these measurements with time. To ascertain the rate of change, one plots the child's values at each office visit on graphs that show normative data on height and weight relative to age, expressed as percentile lines. The patient's values are expected to track on a given percentile with time; a deviation from the expected pattern of growth may signal illness and need for diagnostic and therapeutic intervention.

Would it be possible to create such charts for exercise physiologic variables? If so, deviations from expected rates of improvement with age in muscle strength or aerobic fitness, for instance, could be identified by serial testing and comparison with normative data.

In fact, Jokl produced just such percentile grids in the 1930s for field performance (distance run, shot put) for children between the ages of 6 and 18 years, based on testing of 27,000 South African subjects (13). Similar charts that could be used for longitudinal evaluation could be easily created from the data of more contemporary testing programs (see fig. 2.1).

While this is an attractive concept for assessing intrasubject changes with time, translating the idea into the exercise testing laboratory is fraught with obvious logistical difficulties. Creating normative data for variables such as $\dot{V}O_2max$ would require a prohibitive number of subjects. Unlike values for easily measured and reproduced variables such as height and weight, values

for physiologic measurements during exercise are recognized to vary significantly between laboratories, presumably because of differences in equipment, testing conditions, and supervising staff.

Importantly, too, the creation of normative grids for age would be of limited use for comparing physiologic variables between groups of subjects of different size. But if such charts were available, they could be put to valuable clinical use. For example, knowing that a patient with significant aortic valve insufficiency was not improving as expected with age in treadmill endurance time or absolute $\dot{V}O_2max$ might signal a need for surgical intervention.

Ratio Standards

Many physiologic variables, particularly O_2 uptake, have traditionally been related to body mass (kg) as a means of comparing raw data on individuals of different size. There are several arguments for the use of this *ratio standard*. Body mass is easily and accurately measured. Use of body mass as a denominator often makes good physiologic sense; for example, one would expect body mass to closely reflect cardiac output, since the heart has to perfuse the total body volume. And in some cases, body mass would appear to be an appropriate normalizing factor because it represents the actual exercise workload (e.g., expressing O_2 uptake per kg body mass when comparing treadmill running economy between individuals of different size).

The use of body mass as a ratio standard, however, is not without its difficulties. For instance, does relating

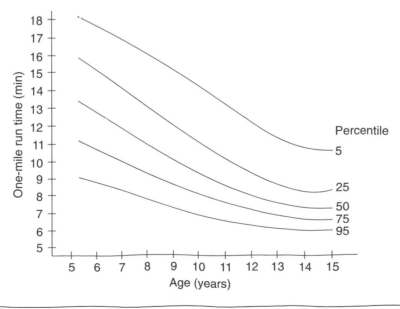

Figure 2.1   Example of how longitudinal grids can be created from normative data by percentiles. Data are from 1-mile run times in boys reported by the American Alliance for Health, Physical Education, Recreation and Dance (1).

O_2 uptake to body mass carry the same meaning when we compare physiologic variables during weight-bearing and non-weight-bearing exercise? That is, does $\dot{V}O_2$max per kg on the treadmill provide the same physiologic information as $\dot{V}O_2$max during cycle testing? In the first instance, we are saying that this is the highest O_2 uptake a subject can demonstrate when moving a given mass (his or her own) up a treadmill slope at a given speed. In the latter case, the workload is provided by the wheel resistance rather than the subject's body and is mass-independent; $\dot{V}O_2$max per kg is used here in an attempt to normalize aerobic fitness to body size. Do the two ratio standards have different physiologic implications? The answer is not altogether clear.

A more obvious pitfall to the use of body mass as a ratio standard surrounds the observation that people with the same body mass may have very different body composition. It would be folly to attempt to relate upper body strength measures to body mass as a means of comparing a 60 kg adolescent who has 40% body fat to a 35 kg child with 12% body fat.

Another concern is the way ratio standards can distort data. In 1949, Tanner published an article entitled "Fallacy of Per-Weight and Per-Surface Area Standards, and Their Relation to Spurious Correlation" that challenged the validity of the ratio standard (22). Others have subsequently echoed these concerns (14, 23). The basic issue is that in the use of ratio standards there is no assurance that the physiologic variable in question (the numerator) changes proportionally in the subject population to body mass (the denominator). In fact, many variables do not change at the same relative rate as body mass, and O_2 uptake is one of them. As will be discussed in detail later, as subjects increase in size, resting metabolic rate rises at a disproportionately slower rate than does body mass. That is, $\dot{V}O_2$ per kg is negatively related to body mass. The larger the subject, the lower the resting O_2 uptake per kg body mass.

Assume that we want to collect data to establish a normal value for resting O_2 uptake relative to body mass. We take all the absolute values determined for $\dot{V}O_2$ in a group of subjects, divide by individual body mass, and then take an average (say 5.0 ml $\cdot$ kg^{-1} $\cdot$ min^{-1}). Subjects who have a higher value than this will be considered "hypermetabolic," while those with a lower $\dot{V}O_2$ per kg will be labeled "hypometabolic."

With use of this standard approach, it has been assumed that O_2 uptake relates to body weight by the equation $Y = k(wt)$. This line, illustrated as A in figure 2.2, necessarily passes through the origin, and values for the hypermetabolic subjects lie above the line whereas those for the hypometabolic will lie below. However, if we plot the actual absolute O_2 uptake values against the body mass of our subjects, we will find that the empirically derived regression equation will be in the form $Y = bx + a$ (line B of figure 2.2). This regression line, which expresses the true relationship between body weight and resting O_2 uptake in our subject population, is very different from that predicted by the ratio standard.

It is easy to see the error introduced in this case by use of the ratio standard. When "per kg" is used as the de-

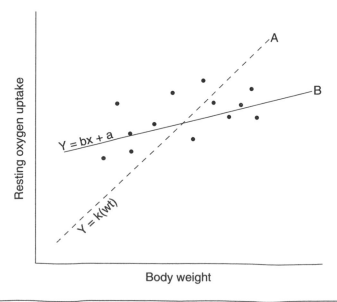

Figure 2.2   Theoretical values of resting O_2 uptake in a group of subjects actually relate to body weight by equation B, the regression standard. If equation A, the ratio standard, is utilized, misinterpretation of the data is likely. Adapted from Katch 1973.

nominator, light-weight individuals have artifactually high values and many will be falsely labeled as hypermetabolic. Large subjects are given values that are falsely low, and many will be erroneously considered hypometabolic.

The only time that ratio standard values will appropriately reflect those obtained from an empirically derived regression line is when the two regression coefficients k and b are equal and when a equals 0. In the case presented, this situation would exist only if $\dot{V}O_2$ and body mass changed proportionately in the subject population, which is not the observed relationship.

How much error is introduced by use of ratio standards? The actual difference in the value of Y obtained by the regression equation and by the ratio standard equation can be determined with the equation

$$Y_{regr} - Y_{ratio} = (b - k)X + a.$$

If b and k are different, the difference in values for Y by the two methods is dependent on X and becomes larger as X becomes farther from the mean value. It follows that the risk of error introduced by use of the ratio standard becomes greater (a) the more heterogeneous the population is in terms of the measure X, and (b) the greater the extent to which changes in X depart from proportionality with changes in Y. As will be demonstrated in examples later in this chapter, these factors may be of sufficient magnitude to produce fallacious comparisons between subject populations when the ratio standard is used.

Other ratio standards besides body mass have been utilized in developmental exercise physiology. Lean body mass, lean leg volume, and body surface area have each served as denominators to standardize particular physiologic variables in children. But besides the potential pitfall already described, each possesses the additional disadvantage of being difficult to measure accurately.

Boys typically have a higher $\dot{V}O_2$max expressed per kg body mass than girls, but Davies et al. reported that these differences essentially disappeared when absolute $\dot{V}O_2$max was related to lean leg volume (8). This makes intuitive sense, since the denominator in this case reflects the actual size of the working motor that is consuming chemical energy. Measurements of body strength relative to muscle size are of interest by the same reasoning.

Similar arguments have been made concerning the use of lean body mass (LBM) to reflect muscle mass as a denominator for physiologic measures involving muscle work. Indeed, many have contended that LBM is the preferred expression for examining O_2 uptake during exercise (7). Gitin et al. noted, however, that $\dot{V}O_2$max per LBM was meaningless as a measure of exercise fitness (at least in weight-bearing activities) because this "mathematical adiposectomy" ignored the weight load imposed by body fat (10, p. 757). The same issue arises in Davies' conclusions, which were based on findings during non-weight-bearing (cycle ergometer) exercise. Lean body mass might, however, be an appropriate denominator for considering size in certain forms of fitness. There is some evidence, for example, that an association exists between heart and peripheral muscle mass, suggesting that $\dot{V}O_2$max per LBM might serve as a useful indicator of cardiac functional reserve.

Body surface area (BSA) has been used to standardize physiologic measurements that are considered to be related to surface functions (skin heat loss, gastrointestinal absorption, drug metabolism). The accuracy of this approach has long been suspect (5). Metabolic rate, for instance, does not rise proportionately with BSA during childhood as might be expected. However, this argument is overshadowed by the greater concern that BSA in a subject is never actually measured, but only calculated, and that the methods of calculation might induce significant error. Burch and Giles (5) noted that BSA is often estimated from height and weight by the formula of DuBois and DuBois, originally derived in 1916 from body molds of inflexible paper on nine subjects (9). Areas such as nose, ears, and gluteal folds were not actually measured, and in most subjects, areas of only one leg and arm were estimated.

Dimensionality Theory

Certainly Jonathan Swift was not a physiologist. But in *Gulliver's Travels* he presented the Ministers of the King of Lilliput with an essential problem in relating body size to metabolic rate by dimensionality theory (21). Their captive Man Mountain needed to be fed, but how much? Finding that Gulliver exceeded the Lilliputians' 6 in. height by a factor of 12, and that their body proportions were similar, the Ministers of Lilliput concluded that his dietary requirement would be 1728 (12^3) times theirs.

Their analysis of the situation, frequently cited in the biologic literature, follows classic mathematical principles dating back at least as far as Archimedes: if figures are geometrically similar (have the same proportions), surface area relates to the square, and volume to the cube, of linear dimensions (23). That is,

$$SA = kL^2 \quad and \quad V = kL^3$$

where SA is surface area, V is volume, L is length, and k is factor of proportion. If a fish doubles its length, its mass (essentially interchangeable with volume in animals) will increase by a factor of 8. The sage Lilliputians, figuring that food requirement should be proportionate to body mass, arrived at Gulliver's food allotment by determining the difference in the cube of their linear dimensions.

These principles of *dimensionality* have a crucial influence on both biologic and nonbiologic forms. Supporting structures (e.g., columns, legs) vary in strength by their cross-sectional area, which is proportional to the square of the height of the structure. But the load (mass) these structures must support increases with the cube of the structure's height. That's why ants have spindly legs while elephants have proportionately thick legs. An ant the size of an elephant would not be able to support its weight. Similarly, as noted by Thompson, "it follows at once that if we build bridges that are geometrically similar, the larger is the weaker of the two" (23, p. 18).

Asmussen and Heeboll-Nielsen proposed that dimensionality theory could be useful in normalizing anatomic and physiologic variables to body size (2). They reasoned that anatomic measures such as stride length should be directly related to body linear dimension (L), while those associated with area (respiratory area of the lungs, cross-sectional area of muscle) should increase by the square of body height. The maximal tension produced by a muscle, for instance, is related to its cross-sectional area and should therefore be proportionate to L^2. Volumes and weights (blood volume, heart weight) would be expected to vary with L^3. Time can be considered related to L. Oxygen uptake is $\dot{V}O_2$ per unit time, or L^3/L, and therefore by dimensionality theory would be proportionate to L^2 (3). By this method, then, physiologic variables in individuals of different sizes can be related to various powers of body height.

When Asmussen and Heeboll-Nielsen examined actual exponents of height relative to various anatomic and physiologic factors in 400 Danish boys, however, they found considerable variation from the numbers predicted by dimensionality theory. The authors concluded that these discrepancies were caused by functional changes during childhood independent of size; they suggested that comparing actual versus predicted exponent values might provide a means for distinguishing qualitative versus quantitative changes in physiologic variables during the growing years.

It should be noted that dimensionality theory requires that the bodies being compared be geometrically proportional. In fact, body segment proportions are not entirely similar during childhood, as on a relative basis the head becomes progressively smaller and the legs become longer. But by the age of 7 years, these differences are sufficiently small in relation to the mature adult as to have little impact on dimensionality analysis (2).

Scaling by Allometric Equations

Scaling, or the means of evaluating the structural and functional consequences of changes in size of animals, has long captured the attention of comparative biologists (6, 17, 23). As early as the mid-1800s it was recognized that the resting metabolic rate of animals measured relative to body weight became greater as the size of the animal diminished. In 1883 Rubner touched off a century of controversy and experimental investigation by suggesting that differences in animal metabolism disappeared when values were related to BSA (16). In contemporary times, Calder noted that between 1977 and 1981, an average of 78 articles appeared *yearly* on the subject of animal scaling (6).

This intense interest in the relationship of size to function and structure has been necessarily prompted by the dramatic range of body dimensions observed in the animal kingdom. Among the land-living mammals, for instance, the giant rhinoceros may weigh up to 30,000 kg, varying in weight from the smallest mammal, the 2 g shrew, by a factor of 10^7. Carrying the illustration further, the smallest free-living organism, the *Mycoplasma*, varies in weight from the largest animal, the 100-ton blue whale, by a factor of 10^{21}! It is not difficult to understand why identifying a valid means of comparing physiologic and anatomic variables within this mismatch of sizes is a critical issue for comparative biologists (6, 17).

Such variations in body dimensions, of course, are not nearly as extensive in the field of human developmental exercise physiology. The 5-year-old boy weighing 20 kg varies from the 90 kg college subject by a factor of only $10^{.65}$. But the principles and methods developed by our biologist colleagues to account for size in their physiologic measurements may prove highly useful even through this relatively narrow size range.

Body mass is the dimensional measure adopted by comparative biologists as the usual standard for physiologic comparisons—assumed in this discussion to be equivalent to (a) body weight when subjects are in the same gravitational condition and (b) body volume, since the density of all animals is close to 1.0. While height might conceptually serve equally well, the use of stature poses some interesting problems. As Schmidt-Nielsen asked (17), for instance, how would one compare the metabolic rate of a giraffe with that of a rhinoceros using body height as the denominator? (Is it height above the ground? Or body length? Should the neck be included?—and so on.) Weight, as discussed previously, is an attractive normalizing factor for size because it can be measured simply and accurately and often plays an important role in exercise function (such as the energy demands placed on the exercising muscle during weight-bearing locomotion).

In 1891 Snell introduced the use of allometric equations to relate the mental capacities of various animals to brain size (20). The use of these equations has since become the standard approach to relating anatomic and physiologic function to body size in the animal kingdom. With this approach, a physiological variable (Y) is scaled to body mass (X) according to the allometric equation

$$Y = a(X^b)$$

where a is the proportionality coefficient and b is the scaling factor.

If b = 1.0, the physiologic variable increases linearly in direct proportion with body mass. If b > 1.0, the physiologic variable increases at a proportionately greater rate in the subject population than does body mass; and if b < 1.0, the converse is true. If there is no relationship between changes in the variable with body mass, b = 0 (as would be the case for blood hemoglobin concentration, which is similar among all mammals). If b < 0, an increase in body mass is associated with a decrease in the variable (heart rate or stride frequency, for example). The exponent b, then, is a scaling factor that describes the influence of size (in this case, body mass) on the physiologic variable in question. That is, if within any population of subjects, or in serial measurements of the same subjects, both X and Y of the allometric equation are changing, the value of the exponent b describes the relationship between these changes.

Insights into a great number of physiologic relationships have been gained through allometric analysis in animals, ranging from the size of eggs to the O_2 affinity of blood (see fig. 2.3). It has been suggested, for instance, that the life span of animals is limited by a certain allotment of a common number of heartbeats. Is this true? It is well recognized that smaller animals have a shorter life span, as expressed by the equation t_{life} = 11.8 $M^{.20}$. Smaller animals also have faster heart rates, with the time for a single beat (t_h) empirically related to body mass by the equation t_h = .259 $M^{.25}$ (17). Although one cannot conclude that a fixed allowance of heartbeats limits life expectancy, the similar scaling factors suggest that the two may somehow be associated.

The allometric equation can be identified through logarithmic transformation of raw data for Y and X into the linear regression equation

$$\log Y = \log a + b(\log X)$$

which is a straight line whose slope is b. In the logarithmic transformation the relationship between the physiologic variable and mass is more easily visualized, and intersubject comparisons are facilitated.

Winter reviewed the ways in which allometric equations can be utilized to compare physiologic variables

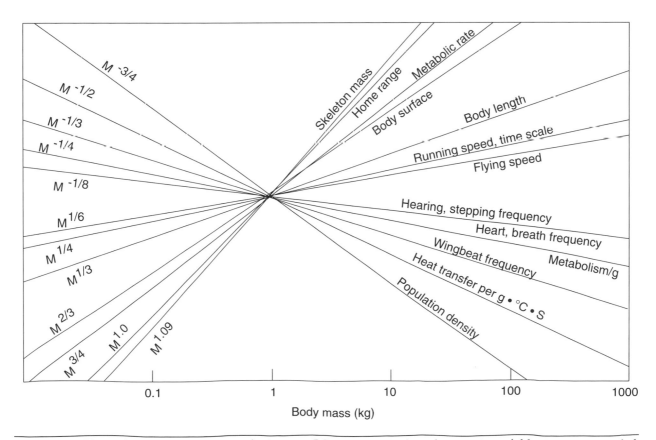

Figure 2.3 Examples of scaling factors to body mass (M) for physiologic and anatomic variables in warm-blooded mammals. Reprinted from Calder 1984.

between groups (24). After logarithmic transformation to a linear model, intergroup comparisons are possible with use of analysis of covariance (ANCOVA), which adjusts the data for body mass. Alternatively, raw values of X can be raised to the power b, the scaling factor, and values for this power function ratio can be compared using appropriate standard t or ANOVA tests.

Allometric analysis allows us the opportunity to uncover new relationships through manipulation of scaling exponents. For example, as noted by Calder (6), resting metabolic rate in animals is related to $M^{.75}$, while life span is almost proportional to $M^{.25}$. Through allometric cancellation, $(M^{.75})(M^{.25})/M^{1.0} = M^0$, telling us that the total energy metabolism per kg body mass during a lifetime is independent of body size.

Allometric equations and other alternatives to the ratio standard have only begun to be utilized in the evaluation of physiologic changes during childhood. It will be of interest to see whether these approaches upset traditional concepts based on the ratio standard.

It is worthwhile at this point to reiterate certain caveats outlined in the introduction of this chapter as they relate to allometric equations. First, the scaling factor b expresses an empirically derived association but makes no inferences regarding causality. *Why* does resting metabolism relate to $M^{.75}$ in animals? Why is the wingbeat frequency of a bird associated to body mass by a scaling factor of .33? The answers are not forthcoming through allometric analysis. Instead, allometry is limited to defining relationships that enable anatomic and physiologic comparisons between animals of different sizes (or the same animal at different stages of growth).

It is important to remember, too, that identifying a scaling factor of body mass that permits comparison of a physiologic variable in different subjects does not necessarily imply that size is the only contributor to the relationship. Qualitative changes in function need be considered in any search for the physiologic bases for scaling factors, particularly in the growing organism.

Many questions remain to be answered regarding the use of allometric equations and scaling factors in developmental exercise physiology. For instance, scaling to body mass implies that the components of mass have the same physiologic importance and that the composition of mass is similar between individuals. We know, of course, that this is not true. The impact of variations in body fat content, for instance, might be expected to affect scaling factors for endurance performance in a population of subjects heterogeneous for body composition (17).

Regression Standards

Individual values for physiologic variables can be appropriately compared to normative data expressed by regression equations. Silverman and Anderson used this approach when presenting information on the metabolic cost of walking in children (albeit in only four subjects) (19). They described walking economy by the multiple regression equation log $\dot{V}O_2$ per kg = .0969(speed) + .021(gradient) + .75, where speed is in km/hr and gradient is sin (slope in degrees). Considerations in relating exercise data by linear regression equations have been discussed by Katch (14). Calder noted that once factors other than mass are incorporated into multiple regression equations, the ability to evaluate relationships by allometric cancellation is lost (6).

If the relationship between a variable and body mass is linear, intergroup comparisons can be conducted by ANCOVA (24). With this technique, one can assess differences in means of the variable in two or more groups with a covariate (such as body mass, height, or surface area) partitioned out.

Winter and Maughan showed how ANCOVA can reveal relationships that are obscured by use of the ratio standard (25). They examined muscle strength of the quadriceps versus muscle cross-sectional area (by computed tomography scan) in young men and women, using both ratio and regression standards. Comparison by ratio standard indicated that strength per cross-sectional area was not significantly different in the two groups (mean of 9.49 and 8.95 N/cm^2, respectively, p >. 05). Examination by ANCOVA revealed, however, that muscle strength per cross-sectional area was gender-dependent; quadriceps strength was greater in the males (adjusted means 688 vs. 541 N in the females, p < .001).

Tanner pointed out that the linear regression standard and allometrically derived scaling factors cannot necessarily be used interchangeably (22). The reader is referred to Tanner's discussion of how distribution of data may affect one's decision about which technique to use. Whether the statistical considerations he reviews will significantly influence biologic results is problematic.

SUMMARY

It is obvious from the preceding discussion that there exists no single means of optimally normalizing physiologic data for size. The proper denominator may vary according to the physiologic question being addressed, or by the distribution of the data, or by the ease of measurement.

Throughout the subsequent chapters of this book, we will focus attention on the various methods that have been used to standardize body dimensions with respect to specific physiologic issues. There is growing suspicion that many of the concepts of physiologic change with growth that are based on the traditional ratio standard may be challenged by use of alternative methods of factoring out body size in children. On the other hand, differences in statistical approach may ultimately offer no particular advantages or insights. For instance, Shephard labeled the controversy over which exponent of height should be used to standardize measurements of $\dot{V}O_2$max "rather sterile," since height, the square of height, and the cube of height all provide similar results. He contended that "given the long tradition of body mass standardization, there are no strong reasons for abandoning this approach in the routine interpretation of such data as maximum O_2 intake, physical working capacity, and muscle force" (18, p. 85).

Likewise, true biologic changes in growth that might be accurately predicted by an allometric scaling factor could be obscured by imprecision of measurement techniques or by variability in test-retest reproducibility.

Difficult-to-measure variables such as maximal cardiac output and ventilatory anaerobic threshold (as will be discussed in a later chapter) are good examples.

As a final note, it is worth repeating a caution regarding the search for the ideal scaling factor for physiologic variables. It is likely that such a factor would provide a tool for intra- and intersubject comparisons only, without implications for causality. Finding that O_2 uptake at a given submaximal running speed scales to $M^{.75}$ would provide no answer as to *why*. Consideration of differences in biomechanical factors, substrate utilization, ventilatory efficiency, stride frequency, elastic recoil, or the host of other influences that could covary with body mass should in no way be diminished even if a means of standardizing running economy for body size were known.

References

1. American Alliance for Health, Physical Education, Recreation and Dance. Youth fitness testing manual. Washington, DC; 1980.
2. Asmussen, E.; Heeboll-Nielsen, K. A dimensional analysis of physical performance and growth in boys. J. Appl. Physiol. 7:593-603; 1955.
3. Bar-Or, O. Pediatric sports medicine for the practitioner. New York: Springer-Verlag; 1983.
4. Blimkie, C.J.R. Age- and sex-associated variation in strength during childhood: anthropometric, morphologic, neurologic, biomechanical, endocrinologic, geometric, and physical activity correlates. In: Perspectives in sports medicine and physical fitness. Vol. 2, Gisolfi, C.V; Lamb, D.R., eds. Youth, exercise, and sport. Indianapolis: Benchmark Press; 1989:p. 99-164.
5. Burch, G.E.; Giles, T.D. A critique of the cardiac index. Am. Heart J. 32:425-426; 1971.
6. Calder, W.A. Size, function, and life history. Cambridge, MA: Harvard University Press; 1984.
7. Cooper, K.H. A means of assessing maximal oxygen intake. Correlation between field and treadmill testing. J. Am. Med. Assoc. 203:201-204; 1968.
8. Davies, C.T.M.; Barnes, C.; Godfrey, S. Body composition and maximal exercise performance in children. Hum. Biol. 44:195-214; 1972.
9. DuBois, D.; DuBois, E.F. Clinical calorimetry, tenth paper. A formula to estimate approximate surface area if height and weight be known. Arch. Intern. Med. 17:863-866; 1916.
10. Gitin, E.L.; Olerud, J.E.; Carroll, H.W. Maximal oxygen uptake based on lean body mass: a meaningful measure of physical fitness? J. Appl. Physiol. 36:757-760; 1974.
11. Heusner, A.A. Body size, energy metabolism, and the lungs. J. Appl. Physiol. 54:867-873; 1983.
12. Holliday, M.A.; Potter, D.; Jarrah, A.; Bearg, S. The relation of metabolic rate to body weight and organ size. Pediat. Res. 1:185-195; 1967.
13. Jokl, E. Introduction. Med. Sport 11:1-28; 1978.
14. Katch, V.L. Use of the oxygen/body weight ratio in correlational analysis: spurious correlations and statistical considerations. Med. Sci. Sports 5:252-257; 1973.
15. Rowland, T.W. Jack Sprat had it right. Pediatr. Exerc. Sci. 4:283-286; 1992.
16. Rubner M. Ueber den Einfluss der Korpergrosse auf Stoffund Kraftwechsel. Z. Biol. 19:535-562; 1883.
17. Schmidt-Nielsen, K. Scaling. Why is animal size so important? Cambridge: Cambridge University Press; 1984.
18. Shephard, R.J. Physical activity and growth. Chicago: Year Book Medical; 1982.
19. Silverman, M.; Anderson, S.D. Metabolic cost of treadmill exercise in children. J. Appl. Physiol. 33:696-698; 1972.
20. Snell, O. Das Gewicht des Gehirnes und des Hirnmantels der Saugethiere in Beziehung zu deren geisten Fahigkeiten. Sitzungsberichte der Gesellschaft fur Morphologie und Physiologie in Munchen 7:90-94; 1891.
21. Swift, J. Gulliver's Travels. New York: Doubleday; 1954.
22. Tanner, J.M. Fallacy of per-weight and per-surface area standards, and their relation to spurious correlation. J. Appl. Physiol. 2:1-15; 1949.
23. Thompson, D. On growth and form. Cambridge: Cambridge University Press; 1961.
24. Winter, E.M. Scaling: partitioning out differences in size. Pediatr. Exerc. Sci. 4:296-301; 1992.
25. Winter, E.M.; Maughan, R.J. Strength and cross-sectional area of the quadriceps in men and women. J. Physiol. 435:175P; 1991.

CHAPTER 3

EXERCISE TESTING

The well-planned laboratory exercise test is fundamental to the study of developmental exercise physiology. Insight into physiological responses to exercise can be acquired only with a structured exercise protocol conducted in a controlled, monitored setting. Clearly, information about the evolution of exercise responses in children is only as good as the methods utilized in obtaining it. It is essential, then, that proper testing techniques receive careful attention.

The basic approach to exercise testing of children is no different from that for adults; it should include a valid study design, appropriate testing protocol for the question being addressed, and proper monitoring of physiological variables. However, special considerations are important in testing children. Young subjects are both emotionally and physically immature. Working with children demands more time and personal attention to prevent fear, inadequate understanding, and lack of motivation that can limit exercise responses. Exercise protocols and testing equipment must be scaled down to match the child's size, and the influence of smaller body dimensions on monitoring techniques (e.g., dead space in breathing valves) needs to be considered.

The child's safety becomes a primary issue. This applies particularly during treadmill testing, when precautions need to be taken to prevent accidental falling. Children do not always communicate with staff well during testing, and special attention to both the subject's well-being and the proper functioning of equipment is necessary.

Most importantly, effective exercise testing requires a warm, supportive staff, sensitive to the child's concerns and limitations. We can expect the inexperienced child to be intimidated by the complexity of testing and monitoring equipment. With care and encouragement, however, even children as young as 3 to 5 years will cooperate to provide a good exercise effort. Failure to recognize these important aspects of testing children may seriously interfere with the study's success.

This chapter will address the proper techniques for exercise testing of children in the laboratory setting. As noted previously, the central focus will be on the healthy child. While many of the aspects of exercise testing and protocol design covered in this chapter are applicable to children with chronic disease, other specific testing methods may be appropriate for such subjects. The chapter will treat testing methods that address aerobic fitness and those that address anaerobic fitness separately—a division that will be retained in subsequent sections of this book. Techniques for strength testing will be addressed separately in chapter 13.

PREPARING FOR EXERCISE TESTING

A number of considerations are important before subjects arrive in the laboratory for the first testing session. These will make up a pretesting checklist:

1. Is a pilot study important to "work out the bugs"? Unforeseen problems with new testing methods are typical, often surfacing in the first few subjects, invalidating early data, and causing delays in the study. This may be particularly true when techniques previously used with adults are being applied to children. One can often avoid this pitfall by planning on testing a small group of subjects initially to specifically pinpoint problems and modify protocols before formal testing begins.

2. Has the study been approved by the appropriate human research committee? In the current legal climate, such approval is obligatory for all studies in children. Early application is wise, to prevent delays in the start of the project if the committee requires modifications (such as changes in the permission form).

3. Is a parents' informational meeting important? Children's participation in research is fully dependent

upon the cooperation of the parents, and parents are much more likely to cooperate if they are fully informed about the intent and methods of the study. While each parent should receive this information at the time of signing the permission form, an initial evening group meeting is sometimes helpful in avoiding misconceptions and assuring enthusiastic participation.

4. Should an initial laboratory orientation/habituation visit for the subjects be scheduled? Considering the importance of avoiding apprehension in testing subjects, it is generally considered wise to have children make a visit to the laboratory before the first testing session to become familiar with the testing equipment and procedures. During this time the investigator can develop a personal rapport with the child and answer questions. This also provides an opportunity for the child to learn how to run on the treadmill or pedal a cycle ergometer at a constant pace. Besides allaying anxiety, the visit saves time for the investigator during subsequent testing sessions.

5. Has the appropriate research literature been reviewed? This is the best way to devise exercise testing protocols for questions new to the laboratory. A comprehensive knowledge of the methods and results of previous studies will prevent having to "reinvent the wheel."

6. Have an adequate number of subjects been enrolled in the study? One of the most common errors in study design is an insufficient "n" to answer the question being addressed. Consultation with a statistician before the study begins will help assure that the number of children participating as subjects will provide sufficient "power" for subsequent statistical analysis.

7. If the study is designed to address findings in normal healthy subjects, what form of medical screening is necessary? Children who have chronic conditions such as asthma, anemia, congenital heart disease, or musculoskeletal problems are usually not appropriate subjects for such studies. Likewise, a study of normal children should not include those who are taking medications that would influence exercise performance (e.g., beta-blockers such as propranolol for migraine headaches). Most investigators feel comfortable obtaining such information from the parents. In certain cases, however, consultation with the child's physician may be appropriate.

8. Have the child and parents received instructions regarding diet and activity prior to testing? When information about date, time, and location of testing is sent to the child and family, other details are important. The child should be advised not to exercise vigorously or participate in sports on the day of testing.

No solid food should be consumed within 3-4 hr of the testing session. Usual exercise clothing should be worn (shorts, T-shirt, sneakers). Single-piece outfits (such as swimsuits for girls) should be avoided, since they make applying electrocardiograph leads to the chest difficult. Also, the child should sleep well the night before testing. Only once does a subject have to appear for testing on the day after a sleep-over, wearing hiking boots, having just finished a soccer game, and munching a candy bar ("for energy"), for the investigator to learn the importance of these details.

The Testing Environment

The types of equipment and number of personnel necessary for exercise testing depend, of course, on the nature of the study. Several general considerations are important, however.

Testing is best conducted in a well-lit, air-conditioned laboratory where (for most studies) temperature can be maintained between 20 and 22 °C (68-72 °F) with comfortable, stable humidity. Adequate space is important to prevent crowding created by testing equipment, monitoring devices, and staff. A minimum of 400 ft^2 has been suggested (105).

Knowledge of the proper operation and calibration of treadmill or cycle, as well as of monitoring equipment, is the responsibility of the testing staff. Periodic safety checks of electrical equipment are necessary. Comprehensive reviews of equipment for exercise testing are available (37, 51, 55).

The appropriate number of staff necessary to conduct the test varies with the complexity of the study. For most testing protocols, three to four people are involved: one greets subjects on their arrival at the laboratory, providing initial orientation information, obtaining informed permission, and determining anthropometric measurements (height, weight, skinfold thicknesses). Two staff members operate the equipment, usually one to control the treadmill/cycle and the other to obtain heart rate and other physiologic data. The attention of an additional staff member should be fully directed to the child, assuring the subject's safety and compliance with the testing protocol.

Conducting the Exercise Test

Upon arriving at the exercise laboratory, subjects are told in understandable terms why the research study is being conducted and why their participation is important. Expectations are outlined clearly and completely. For most tests, children can be reassured that there will be no pain but that they will be asked to "work hard." If the test is a maximal one, they should understand that they need to exercise to the point at which they are giving their very top effort. They also need to realize that they are in charge of when the test will stop; that is, it is expected that in a maximal test a child will give her very best effort before signaling the end. Relating the exercise test to life experiences may be helpful (e.g., "At the end it will feel like you're running up a steep hill").

After anthropometric measures have been made, the child is instructed on the use of the exercise testing apparatus, and a short "warm-up" exercise follows. This pretest exercise may influence subsequently measured submaximal physiologic variables. Inbar and Bar-Or showed that boys 7 to 9 years old who warmed up had about 8% greater O_2 uptake during the early minutes of cycling than subjects who did not warm up (54).

For treadmill testing, the child is told (1) how to straddle the belt before the treadmill is started and to step on the slowly moving belt while holding on to the handrails, (2) to concentrate by focusing straight ahead rather than looking around, (3) to learn to walk or run without holding the handrails, and (4) how to grab the handrails (without stepping off the treadmill) at the point of maximal effort.

It is generally held that except in special circumstances (when subjects are very young, disabled, or unfit), the child should not grasp the handrails during treadmill testing. Holding on to handrails diminishes metabolic cost of exercise, decreasing heart rate and O_2 uptake and prolonging the test. Ragg et al. reported that adults lasted 15 min walking unassisted on a treadmill protocol but 25 min when holding on to handrails (80). Maximal values of O_2 uptake and heart rate were not affected, however. Likewise, Sheehan et al. found no significant differences in $\dot{V}O_2$max or peak heart rate when the same boys performed a running treadmill protocol with and without holding on to the handrails (97). Green and Foster suggested that the effect of decreasing metabolic cost depends on how tightly subjects grasp the handrails (47).

In the typical progressive cycle test it is explained that the child's job is to maintain a steady pedaling rate, identified by the speedometer or metronome. The optimal pedaling rate is 50-60 rpm, and the saddle height should be adjusted to create a knee angle of approximately 160° with the leg extended. Differences in crank length may cause small changes in mechanical efficiency (60), but Elias et al. contended that a standard 17.5 cm crank arm could be used with children weighing between 26 and 47 kg without significant differences in efficiency (36).

Children appear to be motivated to greater exercise efforts if testing is conducted in a friendly, informal manner, with plenty of verbal support. Here is a chance for the staff to express some latent cheerleading talents: "Doing super! You're getting a great score! That's the way to keep those legs moving!"

Testing that requires a maximal exercise effort calls for particular encouragement from the staff. Children who are not trained athletes have never experienced a situation in which they are called upon to "go until you can't go any more." It is therefore difficult for many to identify that point in time when they have given their "best." Some will say they have reached their limit when exertion first becomes uncomfortable, far short of true exhaustion. Subjects need continued verbal encouragement to persevere when physiologic cues (heart rate below expected target maximum) and observational cues (lack of rapid breathing or unsteadiness of gait) indicate that they have not reached a true maximal effort. Statements such as "I know you're getting tired, but you're doing great! Let's see if you can keep going for another 30 seconds!" will often stimulate greater efforts. It is not often wise to ask a child during the later stages of a progressive test, "How are you feeling?" This may remind the child that he is getting uncomfortable and cause him to stop.

There is no clear-cut agreement about whether parents should be allowed in the exercise laboratory during testing. Some investigators feel that the parents' presence may distract the child and add to anxiety. On the other hand, for some children the supportive encouragement of the parents might contribute to a greater exercise effort. This author usually tells parents that many children seem to do better with testing if the parents are not present but that they may observe if they feel it would help the child. If parents or siblings are present, they are asked to sit out of the child's line of vision.

MEASUREMENT OF AEROBIC FITNESS

The energy for physical activities involving prolonged sustained exercise is derived from aerobic metabolism. Performance in endurance activities such as running, swimming, and cycling is thus dependent upon the functional capacity of the O_2 delivery chain—lungs, heart, and vascular supply—as well as on the aerobic capacity of the exercising muscle. In the laboratory, we evaluate the integrative function of these systems, or aerobic fitness, by mimicking the field condition—the performance of sustained exercise involving repetitive contraction of large muscle groups—while monitoring aerobic physiologic variables.

Although aerobic activity may take diverse forms (cross-country skiing, swimming, skating), practical considerations have largely limited testing in the laboratory setting to treadmill running/walking or the cycle ergometer. Each has its advantages and drawbacks, and the selection of testing modality is often governed by the goals of the research study. Testing protocols may be *intermittent*, with subjects being allowed to rest between work stages, or may be *continuous*. Information can be obtained at maximal exercise, defined as the point in a test of progressively increasing workload when the subject can no longer sustain the exercise, or at submaximal effort, during which steady state physiologic data are measured in response to a standard work condition.

These principles are no different for children than for adults. Obviously, however, size differences dictate the need to carefully consider the appropriateness of testing protocols for young subjects. This section will review the considerations that influence aerobic testing methods in children.

"Maximal" Aerobic Testing

Defining a test as "maximal" implies that a child has given his or her very best effort before being stopped by fatigue. The use of this term, however, can lead to confusion. Maximal O_2 uptake, the hallmark of aerobic fitness, is a clearly defined physiological condition in which the limits of the O_2 delivery/uptake systems have been met. Certain criteria have been established to identify $\dot{V}O_2$max in children, and these will be reviewed later in this chapter. It is possible to exercise at workloads above $\dot{V}O_2$max (albeit for only a short time) relying on alternative anaerobic energy sources. A test in which the subject exercises to exhaustion, then, may be of longer duration than that needed to elicit $\dot{V}O_2$max.

On the other hand, it may not be clear on the basis of physiologic and subjective criteria whether a subject actually reached a true $\dot{V}O_2$max during a progressive exercise test. For this reason, many investigators prefer to identify a child's performance on such tests as indicative of "peak" rather than "maximal" values. In this case, "peak" refers to a measure of endurance performance on the test without implying that maximal O_2 uptake was recorded. The present author favors use of the terms "exhaustive" or "peak" exercise to indicate the best effort the child is willing to provide, reserving "maximal" to signify those results for which criteria for $\dot{V}O_2$max were met.

Cycle Versus Treadmill Testing

Choice of testing modality is affected by both practical and physiologic considerations. Experience in a particular laboratory may also influence the type of testing approach.

Practical Issues.   Testing with the cycle ergometer offers several advantages over the use of the treadmill. The cycle is relatively inexpensive, quieter, and more easily calibrated, and the testing poses very little risk of injury. The cycle can be easily transported for studies involving multiple testing sites. Not all testing populations, however, are familiar with cycle exercise. More-

over, cycle testing with mechanically braked ergometers requires the subject to pedal at a constant rate, and this may be difficult for young or unfit subjects. Electronically braked ergometers that adjust workload to pedaling frequency help alleviate this difficulty. Peak performance on the cycle can be limited by local muscle fatigue as much as by the extent of aerobic function. Bar-Or suggested that this concern may be particularly important in testing of children, who have a relatively undeveloped knee extensor muscle mass (10).

Walking or running on the treadmill is a natural form of locomotion for all healthy children, and speed and slope, rather than the motivation or compliance of the subject, dictate the work rate. The latter advantage makes treadmill testing more appropriate for younger subjects. A risk of falling exists during treadmill testing, creating a need for greater diligence on the part of the testing staff.

Besides the advantages and disadvantages already outlined, selection of treadmill versus cycle ergometer may be dictated by the goals of the study. Investigations of *mechanical efficiency*, or the energy required to perform a given amount of work, require cycle ergometry because the workload (i.e., resistance applied to the wheel) can be easily quantitated. On the other hand, exercise on the treadmill is weight-bearing, and the work demands placed on the subject are influenced by biomechanical factors (such as efficiency of gait) and body mass; therefore, the precise workload cannot be easily determined. Metabolic cost of submaximal exercise on the treadmill is consequently expressed as exercise *economy*, defined as the O_2 uptake per kg body weight at a given treadmill speed and elevation.

The relative quiet and subject stability during cycle testing are more amenable to measurement of variables such as blood pressure, pulse oximetry, and cardiac output (by indirect Fick or thoracic bioimpedance). Withdrawal of blood specimens from indwelling catheters is facilitated during cycle testing, as is measurement of aortic flow by Doppler ultrasound.

Physiologic Differences.   Patterns of physiological responses during exercise are similar for treadmill and cycle testing, but the magnitudes of these values at maximal exercise differ. Peak heart rate (HRmax) and $\dot{V}O_2$max are typically greater during treadmill testing, whereas respiratory exchange ratio (RER) at exhaustive exercise is usually higher on the cycle. These differences, which mimic those observed in adults (49), may reflect a greater anaerobic component and local muscle fatigue at high workloads with cycle exercise.

In testing the same children using different protocols, Cumming and Langford reported average HRmax (SD) for the Godfrey and James cycle protocols (to be discussed later) of 195 (5) and 197 (7) beats per minute (bpm), respectively, while values during the Bruce (treadmill running) and Balke (treadmill walking) were 204 (5) and 198 (5) bpm (27). In their study of a large group of 7-12-year-old children who exercised using the James cycle protocol, Washington et al. reported mean HRmax values of 191-196 bpm (117). Cumming et al. observed an average HRmax of 196-204 in 327 children tested with the Bruce treadmill protocol (24).

Most studies in children indicate higher RERmax values with cycle compared to treadmill exercise. In a direct comparison of the same 11-14-year-old boys, Boileau et al. found a mean RERmax of 1.04 (.04) during treadmill walking and 1.11 (.05) during cycle testing (16). Typically RERmax in cycling protocols with children ranges from 1.02 to 1.11, while treadmill exercise usually produces values of .98-1.04 (84). The RERmax on treadmill testing may be dependent on slope at peak exercise.

Reports comparing $\dot{V}O_2$max during cycle and treadmill testing have consistently described differences of 7-12%. The higher values on the treadmill presumably reflect the recruitment of a greater exercising muscle mass. In the study of Cumming and Langford, mean $\dot{V}O_2$ values were 48.2 ml · kg^{-1} · min^{-1} on both the cycle and treadmill walking protocols and 54 ml · kg^{-1} · min^{-1} on the Bruce treadmill running protocol (27). Close similarities in the rank order of $\dot{V}O_2$max were seen between the tests.

Boileau et al. reported average $\dot{V}O_2$max of 48.7 and 44.9 ml · kg^{-1} · min^{-1} for the same boys on maximal treadmill walking and cycle protocols, respectively (16). Correlation coefficients between the two tests were .95 for absolute $\dot{V}O_2$max and .84 for weight-relative $\dot{V}O_2$max. Mácek et al. described similar findings when comparing $\dot{V}O_2$max between treadmill and cycle testing in 11-14-year-old boys (54.1 vs. 50.3 ml · kg^{-1} · min^{-1}) (65). These differences were substantiated by Turley et al., who reported an average 10.6% greater $\dot{V}O_2$max on the treadmill in 9-year-old children, with individual differences ranging from 0.0% to 20.0% (106).

Reliability of cycle and treadmill values for $\dot{V}O_2$max on repeated testing appears to be similar. Turley et al. observed test-retest correlations of .95 and .94 for weight-relative $\dot{V}O_2$max on the two tests, respectively (106). Boileau et al. reported r = .97 and .95 for repeated absolute $\dot{V}O_2$ with treadmill and cycle, respectively, but r = .87 and .88 for weight-relative $\dot{V}O_2$max (16).

TESTING PROTOCOLS

There exists no standard exercise testing protocol for children. Testing methodology has varied widely and has often been modified to fit the specific needs of the research question as well as the population of subjects being tested. A number of factors bear consideration in selection of the testing protocol:

1. The nature and intensity of the exercise should be consistent with the fitness level of the subjects. A cycle or treadmill walking protocol, for instance, would hardly be suitable for an investigation involving child distance runners. These subjects require a treadmill running protocol with speeds of 6-9 mph (29).

2. Workload increments need to conform to the size of the subjects. Eight-year-old children might be expected to have difficulty adapting to speed increases of 2 mph during flat treadmill running.

3. Measurement of submaximal variables usually necessitates a period of steady state exercise. A study that includes an assessment of walking economy, for instance, requires a protocol containing a submaximal stage of at least 3 min to permit steady state measurements of O_2 uptake (see section on measurement of $\dot{V}O_2$max later in this chapter).

4. A sufficient period of time must be available for any desired submaximal determinations. A protocol with 1 min stages will not provide adequate time for estimation of submaximal cardiac output by CO_2 rebreathing techniques.

5. Intensity should be selected for proper test duration. Protocols for progressive tests should bring a child to exhaustion in approximately 8-12 min. Tests of longer duration may cause boredom and loss of concentration; if tests are shorter, the more intense exercise may intimidate the novice testing subject.

Cycle Protocols

Most cycle protocols call for a pedal cadence of 50-60 rpm and vary in stage duration (1-3 min), initial workload, and load increments according to body size. The James, Godfrey, and McMaster protocols have been used most extensively in children (see table 3.1).

The James protocol involves 3 min stages and groups subjects by body surface area (56). Normative data for this protocol have been published by James et al. (56) and Washington et al. (117).

The Godfrey protocol is similar, but work stages are 1 min in duration, and subjects are grouped by height. Godfrey et al. have provided normative values (46). The McMaster protocol involves 2 min stages but can be modified to 3 min stages for submaximal steady state measurements (10, 91).

Tanner et al. suggested that cycle protocols with appropriate work increments for children could be custom-designed for a given subject population (103). The average maximal work on the cycle ergometer is reportedly 3.5 W/kg for boys and 3.0 W/kg for girls during the childhood years (22), and an optimal test duration is 10

Table 3.1   Cycle ergometer protocols

	Rate (rpm)	Body measure	Initial load	Increment	Stage duration (min)
James	60–70	Surface area (m²)	(kg · m/min)	(kg · m/min × 2)	
		< 1.0	200	100	3
		1.0–1.2	200	200	3
		> 1.2	200	300	3

If more than 3 levels of exercise are necessary, add 100–200 kg · m/min until exhaustion.

	Rate (rpm)	Body measure	Initial load	Increment	Stage duration (min)
Godfrey	60	Height (cm)	(W)	(W)	
		< 120	10	10	1
		120–150	15	15	1
		> 150	20	20	1
McMaster	50	Height (cm)	(W)	(W)	
		< 120	12.5	12.5	2
		120–140	12.5	25	2
		140–160	25	25	2
		> 160	25	50 (male)	2
				25 (female)	

Reprinted from Rowland 1993.

min. It follows, then, that for boys, work increments should be 0.35, 0.70, and 1.05 W/kg when stages of 1, 2, and 3 min, respectively, are used. For girls, the values are 0.30, 0.60, and 0.90 W/kg.

Another alternative for cycle testing is the ramp protocol, in which workload is increased continuously or in rapid small increments. This protocol may be useful for small children or those with particularly low levels of fitness, who may tolerate the step increments in more traditional protocols poorly. Tanner et al. compared findings on a ramp protocol in which workload was increased by 0.025 W/kg every 6 s (by a computer-ergometer interface) to findings obtained with the James protocol (103). They observed no significant differences in peak O_2 uptake, minute ventilation, or cardiac index. Exercise time and peak heart rate were greater with the ramp protocol, consistent with the suggested advantage of this protocol: at high-intensity exercise the subject may tolerate small increases in workload but will be unable to sustain the full step increase of a traditional protocol. However, the ramp protocol's lack of submaximal steady state may serve as a drawback for some studies.

Treadmill Protocols

Many variations on the theme of increasing treadmill speed and/or slope have been utilized in exercise testing of children. These protocols are generally selected (1) to avoid overly steep gradients, which cause subject insecurity, a need to hold on to handrails, risk of falling, altered biomechanical factors, and increased anaerobic work; (2) to avoid high speeds, which may be problematic for children with a short stride length; (3) to increase slope or speed, but not both, to minimize adaptive changes for the young subject; and (4) to limit duration of the test to 8-12 min.

The Balke Protocol and Its Modifications.
Most progressive protocols used for research testing of children have involved a constant belt speed with stepwise increases in treadmill slope. These represent adaptations of the Balke protocol used for adults, in which gradient is increased 1% every minute at a walking speed of 3.3 mph. In modified Balke protocols, then, a constant treadmill speed is selected to allow for the size, age, and fitness level of the subject and as a means of controlling test time (see table 3.2).

Testing of young, nonathletic, or obese children usually is best conducted with a walking protocol, generally at treadmill speeds of 3.0-3.75 mph. Rowland et al., for example, studied physiologic responses to exercise in obese adolescents walking at 3.25 mph with a 2% increase in gradient every 3 min beginning at 6% (94). This protocol resulted in treadmill endurance times of 6 to 9 min with an 8-10% maximal slope.

Walking protocols are generally not as suitable for physically active or athletic children, for whom test du-

Table 3.2   Modified Balke treadmill protocol

Subject	Speed (mph)	Initial grade (%)	Increment (%)	Stage duration (min)
Poorly fit	3.0	6	2	2
Sedentary	3.25	6	2	2
Active	5.00	0	2 1/2	2
Athlete	5.25	0	2 1/2	2

Reprinted from Rowland 1993.

ration becomes overly long and the maximal slope excessively steep. Subjects reported by Paterson et al., who walked at 3.4 mph with a 2.5% increase every 2 min, had an average endurance time of 18 min (at a 20% grade) (79). Starting the test at 6-10% slope will shorten walking tests, but maximal exercise for fit subjects will still be conducted at a very steep slope.

Modified Balke running protocols are appropriate for most active children over age 10 years, who can usually run comfortably on a treadmill without holding on to the handrails. Most investigators have used speeds of approximately 5 mph with a slope increase of 2.5% every 3 min (2, 79, 97). This protocol usually results in a test duration of 8-12 min in the normal 9-15-year-old child. Peak effort is typically reached at a treadmill slope of 10-12.5% during running at a comfortable speed. Higher treadmill speeds can be utilized for subjects who are more athletic.

Some investigators have elected to simply have each subject select a comfortable running speed and then increase slope 2.5% every 2-3 min (67, 118). This approach is appropriate, of course, only if one's interests are limited to measurements at peak exercise (i.e., when there is no need to standardize submaximal data).

Specific protocols have been designed to measure submaximal O_2 cost (economy) and maximal O_2 uptake during the same test. These are particularly useful when one wishes to identify the percentage $\dot{V}O_2$max at which economy is being measured. Cunningham had high school runners run horizontally at 6, 7, 8, and 9 mph in stages of 4 min each before increasing the slope 2.5% every minute to exhaustion (29). In nonathletic children ages 9-12 years, Rowland and Cunningham utilized a 3.25-3.75 mph walking protocol of an initial 4 min at 8% slope, then an increase in gradient of 2% every minute (88).

Bruce Protocol.   The most commonly employed treadmill test in clinical practice, the Bruce protocol, has drawbacks that have limited its use in the research setting (84). This protocol involves increases in both treadmill slope and speed at 3 min intervals, beginning

at 1.7 mph and 10% grade (see table 3.3). The work increments are unequal and were selected simply to simulate light, moderate, and maximal exercise stress. Most adolescents will walk during the first three stages and begin running in the fourth or fifth stage (12-15 min into the test).

Advocates of the Bruce protocol for children have argued that (1) the same protocol can be used for all ages, (2) physiologic responses to submaximal exercise can be measured, (3) maximal O_2 uptake can be estimated from endurance time, (4) longitudinal data can be obtained in a given subject by using the same protocol as he or she grows, and (5) the protocol starts slowly and gives the subject a chance to acclimate to treadmill exercise (24). Results of testing with children using the Bruce protocol have been published, but the authors cautioned that normative data should be created by each individual laboratory (24).

Others, critical of this protocol, have contended that the work increments between successive stages are too large, that 3 min stages are too long for small children, that the increments are unequal, that it is difficult to test highly fit subjects (such as distance runners) who must wait 12 min into the test before beginning a slow run (at an 18% slope), and that the protocol changes speed and slope at the same time (53, 84).

Table 3.3   The Bruce treadmill protocol

Stage	Speed (mph)	Grade (%)	Time (min)
1	1.7	10	3
2	2.5	12	3
3	3.4	14	3
4	4.2	16	3
5	5.0	18	3
6	5.5	20	3
7	6.0	22	3

Reprinted from Rowland 1993.

Treadmill Testing of Small Children.   Successful maximal treadmill testing in small children requires particular motivational skills. Shuleva et al. were able to urge children 3-6 years to exhaustive efforts using a protocol of 4 km/hr walking at a 10% slope (increasing 2.5% every 2 min up to 22.5%, when the speed was increased 1 km/hr) (98). Average test duration was 9-10 min. Three aspects of this study were important in motivating subjects to a peak effort: the children were thoroughly oriented and acclimated to treadmill walking, they were acquainted with several of the testing staff, and cash prizes were offered. Maximal treadmill testing in children 4-6 years old has also been reported by Robinson (83) and Åstrand (4).

Step Tests

Exercise testing using a stepping protocol to estimate aerobic fitness has been carried out principally for field testing or for studies evaluating large numbers of subjects. Step tests are based on the premise that the heart rate measured during or immediately after a standard stepping exercise is inversely related to the subject's maximal aerobic power.

The Harvard step test, developed to measure fitness in adults during World War II, is the prototype of these protocols. Subjects exercise to fatigue stepping up and down on a 50 cm (20 in.) bench, 30 steps/min; heart rate is counted as they sit during recovery (5). Using a somewhat different approach, McArdle et al. found good correlations between recovery heart rate and measured $\dot{V}O_2$max in college men and women (71). In that study, subjects performed stepping on a 16 in. bleacher to a four-step cadence (up-up-down-down) at a rate of 22 and 24 steps/min for the females and males, respectively. Pulse rates measured for a 15 s period at 5-20 s into recovery were converted into equations that allowed predictability for true $\dot{V}O_2$max of ±16% (95% confidence limits).

Similar protocols have been employed for estimating aerobic fitness in children. Jette et al. described step-testing methodology for children 7-14 years of age (57). They found that double 20 cm steps were the most feasible; shorter steps failed to trigger an adequate heart rate, and taller ones (as used in the Harvard test) were difficult for shorter children to negotiate. The children performed three 3 min stages of increasing cadence and number of ascents, with 30 s between each stage. Intensity was selected at each stage to elicit approximately 60%, 65%, and 70% of $\dot{V}O_2$max. Heart rates were recorded electrocardiographically between 5 and 15 s into recovery. Multiple regression equations utilizing weight, sum of four skinfolds, and postexercise heart rate closely predicted the directly measured treadmill $\dot{V}O_2$max (r = .96).

Bailey and Mirwald used the same step design but had children step for a 6 min period at 114 steps/min (8). An additional 3 min stage was added at 120 steps/min for subjects whose heart rate was below 162 bpm. Those whose heart rate exceeded 162 bpm were felt to exhibit low aerobic fitness.

Yoshinaga et al. reported the use of a simplified Master two-step test for preschool children ages 4-6 years (123). They employed a 20 cm stair with 72 steps up and down over 3 min. A similar protocol has been used to evaluate older children (116) as well as to test those with heart disease (102) and arrhythmias (75).

The feasibility, validity, and reproducibility of step tests in children have not been well examined. Step tests have been criticized for being poorly standardized and offering little variability of workloads (5). Certainly in children this technique is confounded by the normal developmental decline in submaximal heart rate (i.e., a lower step test heart rate could reflect higher fitness and/or advanced biological age). The published data, however, suggest that further investigation into the value of these tests appears warranted.

Rowing Ergometers

Use of the rowing ergometer as a testing modality in children has received little attention. Rowing devices require a certain level of skill, and the workload is controlled by the subject through two separate variables, the strength and rate of pulling. Rowing does offer potential value in exercise testing, however. It is safe, it engages muscles of both the upper and lower extremity, and it permits accurate measurement of the work accomplished.

Wilson and Chishlom described the feasibility of the rowing ergometer in measuring $\dot{V}O_2$max in 12-14-year-old boys (121). Subjects were asked to generate load increments of 0.5 W/kg at 2 min intervals, disregarding pulling rate. Power output over time was recorded by computer. Maximal O_2 uptake averaged 47.6 ml $\cdot$ kg^{-1} $\cdot$ min^{-1}, while mean peak heart rate was only 88% of that predicted.

MEASUREMENT OF $\dot{V}O_2$MAX

The principles surrounding the measurement of maximal O_2 uptake during exercise testing of children are not different from those for adults, and these methods will not be reviewed here. It is important, however, to examine the influence of small body size on measuring techniques, means of identifying a maximal test, reproducibility, and influence of testing protocol on $\dot{V}O_2$max in young subjects.

Equipment

In most laboratories, measurement of gas exchange parameters by computerized metabolic systems has replaced Douglas bag techniques. This technology was designed for use in adults, and scaling down the size of components of these systems may be important for retaining accuracy in testing small subjects. However, the extent to which differences in factors such as mouthpiece size, valve dead space, tubing diameter, and mixing chamber dimensions influence physiologic measurements in children has not yet been established.

Use of adult-sized valves with large dead space may cause children to inspire significant volumes of expired gas. On the other hand, if the valve is too small, resistance to breathing will increase at high-intensity exercise. Staats et al. suggested that valves with a dead space of 115 ml should be used only with large adults who are expected to have a maximal minute ventilation of over 160 L/min (100). These authors considered a commercially available valve with 59 ml dead space appropriate for smaller adults and children with a body surface area over 1.0 m^2, but indicated that smaller children should use valves with a dead space of 35 ml.

Many metabolic systems utilize a mixing chamber for measurement of expired O_2 and CO_2 concentrations. Staats et al. recommended that the size of this chamber be tailored to the size of the subject. Because children have smaller tidal volumes, an overly large mixing chamber may cause error in measurement of gas exchange variables. The authors suggested a 6 L chamber for adults and children with body surface area over 1.0 m^2 and a 4 L box for those with surface area less than 1.0 m^2 (100).

Reproducibility

Maximal O_2 uptake is highly reproducible in children with use of a given testing method. Test-retest correlation coefficients for $\dot{V}O_2$max of .88-.94 have been consistently reported in tests using the cycle ergometer (7, 16, 106, 107, 120). Similar reliability has been observed with treadmill protocols. Boileau et al. found correlation coefficients of r = .87 and .88 for weight-relative $\dot{V}O_2$max when they retested the same 11-14-year-old boys on treadmill walking and cycle protocols, respectively (16). In a similar study of 13-14-year-old boys, Miyamura et al. obtained a test-retest correlation of r = .90 (74).

Paterson et al. reported that reliability for $\dot{V}O_2$max on a treadmill running protocol was greater than for walking (79). Eight boys ages 10-12 years were tested three times over a 4-week period. Reliability coefficients were r = .47 for walking and r = .95 for running. Intraindividual variability was greater with treadmill walking (10-14%) than with running (3-6%).

Influence of Testing Modality

As noted above, the means of testing affects values for maximal O_2 uptake in children. In evaluations of the same subjects, average $\dot{V}O_2$max values obtained with treadmill protocols are approximately 7-10% greater than with the cycle ergometer (16, 27, 106), and treadmill running protocols typically elicit 6-10% greater values than treadmill walking (79, 97, 124). These variations presumably reflect differences in extent of muscle mass recruited during cycling, walking, and running exercise.

It appears, however, that testing protocol differences within each of these forms of exercise generally have no significant influence on $\dot{V}O_2$max values. Sheehan et al. compared $\dot{V}O_2$max during a continuous running test (5 mph with 2% grade increments every 3 min) with the values during an intermittent running protocol in which the 10-12-year-old subjects walked at 2.5 mph for 3 min between each running stage (97). Mean $\dot{V}O_2$max values were 47.7 and 48.7 ml $\cdot$ kg^{-1} $\cdot$ min^{-1}, respectively (p > .05). It took double the time, however, to administer the intermittent test. Skinner et al. reported similar results in comparing $\dot{V}O_2$max differences during continuous and intermittent treadmill walking tests in 6-15-year-old boys (99). Tanner et al. demonstrated no significant differences in $\dot{V}O_2$max during a James 3 min stage cycle protocol and a continuous ramp test (1.09 and 1.11 L/min, respectively) (103).

Defining the Maximal Test

Identification of $\dot{V}O_2$max in a progressive exercise test assumes that the limit of O_2 delivery/uptake has been achieved. Since a child may stop exercising because of "fatigue" before or beyond this limit, several criteria have been used to establish that true $\dot{V}O_2$max has been reached. Defining the maximal test by these standards is important in allowing comparison of results between different laboratories. No single criterion alone appears to be valid; the most common approach has been to define a maximal test by a combination of peak heart rate and/or RER, O_2 uptake plateau, and subjective appearance of the child.

Peak Heart Rate. Because heart rate rises linearly with increasing work rate, a target rate has commonly been employed for defining a maximal test. In adults, formulas such as 220 minus age, or 210 minus (0.65 $\times$ age), have been used to define target rates. These are not applicable for children, as maximal exercising heart rate is unchanged with age at least until the late teen years.

As noted earlier, however, peak heart rate does depend on testing modality. In most studies involving treadmill exercise, children reach a mean rate of about 200 bpm, while cycle protocols typically elicit peak rates of approximately 195. While these criteria are often used to define the maximal test, it is important to recognize that maximal heart rate varies significantly among individuals. Most studies of children indicate a standard deviation of 5-10 bpm (27, 97). This variability does not simply reflect differences in effort, since testing of elite child athletes has yielded similar ranges (70).

The difficulty with using these heart criteria becomes obvious when one considers that statistically, two of six subjects will have values either above or below the standard deviation. The subjects reported by Sheehan et al., for instance, had a maximal heart rate when running on the treadmill of 202 bpm with a standard deviation of 9 bpm (97). Among these children, then, 17% would be expected to have a peak heart rate below 193 despite an exhaustive effort, while an equal number would have a value above 211 bpm. If a criterion of 200 (±5%) were used, a significant number in the former group would be excluded. Likewise, at the target heart rate, many of the latter group might be considered to have been well short of an exhaustive effort.

Maximal Respiratory Exchange Ratio.

A similar problem arises with the use of peak RER to define an exercise effort consistent with $\dot{V}O_2$max. The respiratory exchange ratio, the ratio of CO_2 produced to O_2 consumed, rises from a resting value of .70 to peak at 1.0 or above at exhaustive exercise. This reflects increased CO_2 production from buffering of lactate as well as changes in substrate utilization.

Many have used a peak RER of over 1.0 to define a maximal test in children. While this value is typically observed in young subjects, there is, again, an influence of testing modality on RERmax as well as significant intersubject variability. A number of treadmill studies have indicated mean RERmax values of .98-.99 with standard deviations of .07-.09 (79, 86, 97). Thus, an RERmax of .90-.95 is not uncommon during treadmill exercise in children, nor are values of 1.05-1.10. RERmax on the cycle ergometer is higher, with typical values of 1.02-1.11 and standard deviations of .05-.06 (16, 50, 93, 103).

Subjective Observations.

Staff experienced in exercise testing can identify an exhaustive effort by the appearance of the subject; any test that does not produce breathlessness, facial flushing or pallor, sweating, and unsteady gait is unlikely to be maximal. However, it is disconcerting that Riopel et al. (82) and Cumming and Langford (27) reported a 25% to 39% difference in treadmill times in subjects using the same treadmill walking protocol and the same subjective end points of peak effort.

Oxygen Uptake Plateau.

According to the traditional paradigm, a leveling, or plateau, of O_2 uptake with progressively intense exercise is indication that $\dot{V}O_2$max has been achieved. Since an actual flattening of the $\dot{V}O_2$ curve with peak exercise is not commonly observed, less stringent criteria for change in O_2 uptake in the final stage of exercise have been used to define a plateau in $\dot{V}O_2$. In children these have included (a) < 150 ml/min, (b) < 2.1 ml · kg^{-1} · min^{-1}, and (c) less than 2 SD below the average change in submaximal stages.

While a $\dot{V}O_2$ plateau is a reasonable marker of $\dot{V}O_2$max, only about half of children will satisfy these criteria during exercise testing. Table 3.4 outlines studies describing the $\dot{V}O_2$ plateau in the pediatric age group. The overall mean rate of identified plateau is 56%, with intermittent protocols providing the highest frequencies. When maximal heart rate, RER, and lactate levels as well as anaerobic threshold and tests of anaerobic function are examined, there is no indication that failure to demonstrate a plateau in these studies is related to motivation, aerobic fitness, or anaerobic capacity (28, 66, 87).

It is clear, then, that a $\dot{V}O_2$ plateau should not be used as a requirement for defining $\dot{V}O_2$max in children. Conversely, however, the demonstration of such a plateau should be a useful marker that $\dot{V}O_2$max has been achieved. The best definition of $\dot{V}O_2$ plateau is probably an increase of $\dot{V}O_2$ in the last full stage of less than 2 SD below the mean increase of all submaximal stages. The definition necessitates, of course, uniform increments in energy requirements between all stages. (If a full stage is not completed at the end of exercise, $\dot{V}O_2$ values may need to be prorated to the end of that stage.) This definition allows for the considerable individual variation in $\dot{V}O_2$ increase with progressive stages (66). Using this method, Rowland and Cunningham found that the average criterion for defining a $\dot{V}O_2$ plateau in a group of 7-10-year-old children was 1.8 ml · kg^{-1} · min^{-1} (87). While this approximates the 2.0 ml · kg^{-1} · min^{-1} definition, the range was wide (0.2 to 2.8 ml · kg^{-1} · min^{-1}). In this study the work increment was a 2% increase in treadmill slope every minute at a speed of 3.25-3.75 mph.

What evidence is there that the criteria of heart rate, RER, and subjective findings reflect true $\dot{V}O_2$max in the absence of a $\dot{V}O_2$ plateau? Rowland reported peak $\dot{V}O_2$ findings in nine children who underwent three treadmill tests with successively higher supramaximal workloads after a standard progressive modified Balke running protocol (85). Average maximal heart rate on the initial test was 204 bpm, $\dot{V}O_2$max was 53.9 ml · kg^{-1} · min^{-1}, and RERmax was 0.99. Only three of the children satisfied criteria for $\dot{V}O_2$ plateau. No significant changes in maximal heart rate or $\dot{V}O_2$max were observed on the three supramaximal tests (although RERmax rose, pre-

Table 3.4　Reports of oxygen uptake plateau during exercise testing of children

Reference	N	Sex	Age	Mode	Protocol	Criterion[a]	%Plateau
Boileau et al. (16)	21	M	11–14	C	Cont	< 150 ml $\cdot$ min^{-1}	38
	21	M	11–14	T	Cont	< 150	76
Cunningham et al. (28)	66	M	10	T	Cont	< 2.1 ml $\cdot$ kg^{-1} $\cdot$ min^{-1}	38
Gutin et al. (48)	20	M	10–12	T	Cont	< 2 ml $\cdot$ kg^{-1} $\cdot$ min^{-1}	55
Mahon and Marsh (66)	26	M,F	8–11	T	Cont	< 2 ml $\cdot$ kg^{-1} $\cdot$ min^{-1}	54
Palgi et al. (76)	58	M,F	10–14	T	Cont	< 2 ml $\cdot$ kg^{-1} $\cdot$ min^{-1}	51
Paterson et al. (79)	8	M	10–12	T	Cont	< 2.1 ml $\cdot$ kg^{-1} $\cdot$ min^{-1}	38
							21
Sheehan et al. (97)	16	M	10–12	T	Cont	< 2 SD	56
							31
Shuleva et al. (98)	25	M,F	3–6	T	Cont	< 2 ml $\cdot$ kg^{-1} $\cdot$ min^{-1}	59
Rowland and Cunningham (87)	13	M,F	7–10	T	Cont	< 2 SD	38
Cumming and Friesen (25)	20	M	11–15	C	Interm	< 50 ml $\cdot$ min^{-1}	35
Krahenbuhl and Pangrazi (61)	21	M	10	T	Interm	< 2.1 ml $\cdot$ kg^{-1} $\cdot$ min^{-1}	95
Krahenbuhl et al. (62)	20	M	8	T	Interm	< 2.1 ml $\cdot$ kg^{-1} $\cdot$ min^{-1}	95
Maksud and Coutts (68)	17	M	11–14	T	Interm	< 200 ml $\cdot$ min^{-1}	82
Sheehan et al. (97)	16	M	10–12	T	Interm	< 2 SD	69

Note: T = treadmill; C = cycle ergometer; 2 SD = two standard deviations of mean of increases in oxygen uptake during submaximal stages.

[a]Increase in oxygen uptake during final stage.

sumably because of the steeper treadmill gradients). In this study, then, peak $\dot{V}O_2$ on a standard treadmill running protocol to volitional fatigue was indicative of $\dot{V}O_2$max despite the absence of a $\dot{V}O_2$ plateau, and $\dot{V}O_2$max was consistent with typically employed heart rate and RER criteria.

In summary, there is no easy answer to defining achievement of $\dot{V}O_2$max during progressive exercise testing of children. If a maximal test is assumed, the subject should demonstrate subjective findings of fatigue in association with (a) peak heart rate of 200 bpm (treadmill running) or 195 bpm (cycling or walking), and/or (b) RERmax over .99 (treadmill) or 1.02 (cycling), and/or (c) a $\dot{V}O_2$ plateau.

Submaximal Predictors of $\dot{V}O_2$max

Maximal exercise testing to directly measure $\dot{V}O_2$max is not always feasible in children because (a) it may be difficult to motivate nonathletic children to an exhaustive effort, (b) intense exercise may pose a risk to children with cardiopulmonary or musculoskeletal disease, and (c) metabolic measurement systems may not be available, particularly in field settings or when large numbers of subjects are being tested. Consequently,

several methods have been devised to estimate $\dot{V}O_2$max through measurements during submaximal exercise. Unfortunately, the convenience of these testing protocols is paid for by a sacrifice in precision of assessing aerobic fitness. The significance of this reduction in accuracy often depends on the questions being addressed in the study.

The Åstrand-Ryhming Nomogram. The Åstrand-Ryhming nomogram was developed to estimate $\dot{V}O_2$max in adult subjects from heart rate at a given submaximal cycle workload (or measured $\dot{V}O_2$) (6). The nomogram is based on assumptions that the relationship between O_2 uptake and heart rate is essentially linear, that $\dot{V}O_2$ at a given workload is similar between subjects, and that maximal heart rate can be predicted. Establishing the percentage of maximum represented by a heart rate at a particular workload allows extrapolation of workload (and $\dot{V}O_2$) to maximum.

Studies evaluating use of the Åstrand-Ryhming nomogram in children have been disappointing; predicted values have consistently underestimated measured $\dot{V}O_2$max by 15-25% (17, 52, 122). It has thus been appropriately concluded that the nomogram has no value for predicting $\dot{V}O_2$max in children and adolescents (17). People have made efforts, however, to modify the original nomogram for use in the pediatric age group.

Buono et al. developed a multiple regression equation from testing of 10-18-year-old subjects with directly measured $\dot{V}O_2$max as the dependent variable and with age, body weight, and $\dot{V}O_2$max estimated from the Åstrand-Ryhming nomogram as independent variables (17). A cross-validation study indicated no significant difference between mean value of directly measured $\dot{V}O_2$max and that predicted from the regression equation. The correlation coefficient between the two values was 0.89, with a standard error of estimate of 12%.

Physical Working Capacity. The cycle workload at a heart rate of 170 bpm (physical work capacity, PWC_{170}) has also been utilized as a marker of aerobic fitness in children. The predictive power of PWC_{170} in estimating $\dot{V}O_2$max is based on the assumption that different values reflect variations in maximal stroke volume, a major factor influencing individual differences in $\dot{V}O_2$max. Several reports have described normative data for PWC_{170} in children (1, 14, 23, 34). These demonstrate that PWC_{170} values increase with age and that they are closely related to weight, height, and body surface area. Boys have greater PWC_{170} than girls at all ages (42, 101).

Controversy has surrounded the utility of PWC_{170} as a marker of aerobic fitness. Binkhorst et al. reported the association of PWC_{170} with $\dot{V}O_2$max in boys and girls 6-18 years old (15). The average difference between directly measured $\dot{V}O_2$max during cycling and that predicted from regression equations relating PWC_{170} to $\dot{V}O_2$max ranged from –0.18 to +0.25 L/min (depending on age and sex), with an average standard deviation of the error of 0.31 L/min. On the basis of these findings, the authors "strongly advised [investigators] not to use prediction formulas [from PWC_{170}] for the accurate individual $\dot{V}O_2$max determination" (p. 232).

Cumming and Danzinger presented graphic data on 10-11-year-old children that indicated an average error of approximately 6.3% with the use of PWC_{170} to estimate $\dot{V}O_2$max (23). One standard deviation caused the error to increase to 10.7%. The authors concluded that PWC_{170} is a valid method for estimating aerobic fitness but "that the additional time involved in measuring O_2 consumption does not add a great deal of information" (p. 206).

Rowland et al. studied 35 boys and girls ages 9-11 years (92). Physical work capacity and $\dot{V}O_2$max related moderately closely in absolute terms (r = 0.71 and 0.70 for girls and boys, respectively), but the association was weaker when expressed relative to body weight (r = 0.65 and 0.48, respectively). When $\dot{V}O_2$max was calculated from the regression equation of $\dot{V}O_2$max versus

PWC_{170}, the average error for directly measured $\dot{V}O_2$max was 3.4 ml · kg⁻¹ · min⁻¹ (SD 2.5) for the girls and 2.8 ml · kg⁻¹ · min⁻¹ (SD 2.6) for the boys. Thus although mean predictability was good, the variability was wide, with a 10-15% error at 1 SD. These authors considered PWC_{170} to provide "only a crude estimate of $\dot{V}O_2$max [that] should not be used to predict individual maximal aerobic power" (p. 186).

PWC_{170} determined during treadmill testing appears to have even less usefulness as a marker of aerobic fitness. Valentine et al. found that measured $\dot{V}O_2$ was associated with treadmill PWC_{170} in 10-13-year-old boys when expressed in absolute terms (r = 0.60, p < .01), but not when measured relative to body weight (r = 0.34, p > .05) (110).

Anaerobic Threshold. The anaerobic threshold has been defined as that point in a progressive test when the rise in blood lactate level begins to accelerate. Many believe that this change may be identified noninvasively by a disproportionate rise in minute ventilation versus O_2 uptake (the ventilatory anaerobic threshold, or VAT). (The measurement and implications of the anaerobic threshold in children will be discussed in chapter 12.) The VAT has been interpreted as a marker of aerobic fitness, since it may reflect the level of exercise intensity when O_2 delivery mechanisms begin to become limiting. Supporting this concept, studies in adults have indicated a reasonably close correlation (r = 69-.87) between VAT and $\dot{V}O_2$max (81).

Reports of the association between VAT and $\dot{V}O_2$max have been more varied in children. Reybrouck et al., for instance, demonstrated correlation coefficients of only r = .28 and .52 in boys and girls, respectively, during treadmill testing (81)—similar to the r = .47 with treadmill walking reported by Kanaley and Boileau (58). Other studies in children have demonstrated a close relationship between VAT and $\dot{V}O_2$max. Rowland and Green reported a coefficient of r = .85 during treadmill running in girls (90), and Cooper et al. found r = .92 with cycle testing of children (19).

Time to Submaximal Steady State

An increase in exercise intensity triggers a rise in metabolic rate ($\dot{V}O_2$) that rapidly levels off if the workload remains constant. Since submaximal physiologic measurements need to be obtained in this stable condition, it is important that work stages be of sufficient duration to permit attainment of a steady state. Time required for steady state has not been systematically evaluated in children but is presumably influenced by the relative work intensity. In adults, steady state is generally reached by 3 min at low-moderate work intensities (119). At higher workloads, 6 min is required, and at very high exercise intensities, steady state may not be achieved at all (19). Other factors that potentially affect time to steady state include increments of workload, type of exercise, and physiologic variable being measured.

While a 6 min exercise duration has been used in submaximal studies involving children (30, 41, 62), time to steady state appears to be typically much shorter at low-to-moderate intensities, consistent with the findings in adults. The subjects reported by Ebbeling et al. walked for 7 min at each of three treadmill speeds (3.35, 5.03, and 6.70 km/hr) that elicited mean $\dot{V}O_2$ values of 14.3, 19.7, and 30 ml $\cdot$ kg^{-1} $\cdot$ min^{-1}, respectively (35). Statistical analysis of values of $\dot{V}O_2$ for the last 3 min revealed no significant differences, indicating that steady state had been achieved within 4 min for all three exercise levels.

On the basis of his extensive testing experience, Godfrey contended that submaximal heart rate and $\dot{V}O_2$ in children level off after 2-3 min (45). Supporting this, Unnithan reported no differences in mean $\dot{V}O_2$ values at 3 min and 6 min (30.1 and 30.5 ml $\cdot$ kg^{-1} $\cdot$ min^{-1}, respectively; approximately 51% $\dot{V}O_2$max) in a group of 12-year-old boys running on the treadmill at 5 mph (108). On the basis of this information, use of stage durations of 2.5 min (64), 3 min (86, 109), and 4 min (89, 29) has been common in protocols assessing submaximal steady state exercise in children.

MEASURING ANAEROBIC FITNESS

Energy from anaerobic metabolic pathways is utilized for short-burst, high-intensity exercise. Measuring "anaerobic fitness" in the laboratory is difficult because there is no easily determined physiologic marker (such as $\dot{V}O_2$max) to estimate either the anaerobic contribution to a particular activity or a subject's level of anaerobic capabilities. The most direct indices—such as high-energy phosphate turnover and glycolytic activity—require invasive biopsy techniques that are neither feasible nor ethical in standard exercise testing of children.

As a consequence, laboratory testing for anaerobic fitness has relied on performance outcomes during all-out exercise of less than 1-2 min duration. While the metabolic validation of these tests as markers of anaerobic function is limited, results relate closely to performance on short-duration field tests expected to reflect anaerobic fitness (12). Protocols for anaerobic testing have included stair-stepping, cycle, and treadmill exercise. In general, these were initially designed for use in adults and have subsequently been adapted for work with children. Consequently, experience in methods for evaluating anaerobic fitness in the pediatric age group is limited.

In these tests, *peak anaerobic power* is designated as the highest work output achieved, the product of velocity times the applied workload or braking force. *Anaerobic capacity* is defined as the total amount of energy that can be generated in anaerobic exercise conditions (72). By this definition anaerobic capacity must be determined in exercise in which anaerobic energy sources are exhausted.

Sargeant discussed two caveats particularly pertinent to testing of anaerobic function (96). First, anaerobic tests are highly specific to the muscle groups being evaluated. Findings of anaerobic fitness of the leg muscles (as determined on a cycle ergometer, for instance) cannot be assumed to provide information about the capacity of the arm muscles. Second, the anaerobic capability of a muscle group is highly dependent on the velocity as well as the force of its contraction. It follows that maximal power output can be determined only when testing is conducted simultaneously at an optimal velocity and resistive force. This observation creates a particular challenge to designing protocols appropriate for evaluation of anaerobic fitness.

Margaria Stair-Running Test

In 1966 Margaria et al. described a technique for assessing anaerobic fitness during rapid stair climbing (69). In this test, subjects ascend a flight of stairs at maximal speed, two steps at a time. A photoelectric timing device records the time taken to cover the fourth to sixth step. The work output is then calculated on the basis of the size of the steps, subject body mass, and vertical velocity component. This test allows calculation of power in the initial few seconds of exercise before onset of fatigue. Although designed for adults, this method has been utilized in children (31, 32, 69). In a study involving small children, Davies et al. had subjects run up only one step at a time (31).

Wingate Anaerobic Test

While several cycling protocols measure anaerobic fitness (20, 59), the Wingate test has emerged as the most popular means of assessing anaerobic characteristics of children and adolescents. Based on an earlier protocol of Cumming (21), this test involves all-out cycling for 30 s against a fixed resistance selected relative to body weight. Peak and mean power as well as the fatigue rate, or amount of power decline during the 30 s of exercise, are measured.

Bar-Or described the advantages of the Wingate test: (a) it is inexpensive, noninvasive, and easy to administer, and uses commonly available ergometers; (b) direct assessment of anaerobic-dependent exercise performance is made; (c) the test is applicable to a variety of subject populations, including the physically disabled;

and (d) both arm and leg anaerobic function can be studied (11). The methodology, reliability, and validity of this test have been extensively reviewed (11, 12); the reader is referred to these reviews for further details.

Equipment. The Wingate test uses simple equipment; subjects exercise on a standard mechanically braked cycle. Ergometers in which load is applied through hanging weights provide greater precision than those that use a pendulum. The calibration of the cycle ergometer is particularly important in mechanical power testing (113). It is possible to count pedal revolutions by direct visualization, and a stop watch can be used to determine the 30 s exercise period. However, many laboratories utilize photoelectric or electromagnetic devices to count cycle revolutions and on-line computer systems for calculation of indices of power output.

Protocol. A 3-4 min warm-up period followed by a 3 min rest is considered important for optimal performance on the Wingate test. Inbar and Bar-Or found that warming up improved mean power of 7-9-year-old boys by 7% but did not influence peak power (54). During warm-up, subjects should cycle at an intensity that stimulates a heart rate of 145-155 bpm (leg cycling) and 120-130 bpm (arm cranking). They should perform several brief 3-4 s all-out sprints during warm-up.

Knowing that the 30 s test will call for a peak effort, some subjects may attempt to pace themselves by holding back on a maximal effort in the early parts of the test. It is therefore important to instruct subjects to pedal as hard as possible right from the start and throughout the duration of the test.

To begin the test, the subject pedals or arm cranks at maximal effort against zero resistance. The prescribed load (discussed in a later section) is applied 2-3 s later, when the initial inertia of the cycle has been overcome. The 30 s counting of revolutions begins at this point. A short cool-down period of low-resistance pedaling follows the end of the test.

Power is calculated by multiplying the constant braking force by the velocity of the perimeter of the flywheel. Measurements obtained at 3-5 s intervals during the test allow calculation of three power indices (see fig. 3.1). Peak anaerobic power, the greatest power recorded during the specified measurement interval, is usually achieved within the first 5-10 s of the test in adults but may occur later in children. Peak power is considered a marker of muscle "explosive power." Mean power, or the average power generated during the 30 s, is an indicator of muscle endurance. Peak and mean power, then, may provide insight into different forms of anaerobic fitness. The rate of fatigue, or amount of falloff of power during the 30 s, is expressed as a percentage of

peak power. Its relevance to anaerobic fitness is less clear.

The Wingate test is not long enough to exhaust anaerobic energy stores (111), but the short 30 s duration limits aerobic contributions. Still, it has been estimated in adults that between 13% and 28% of the total energy supply for the Wingate test is derived from aerobic metabolism (9). In children, the value may be higher. Van Praagh et al. reported values of 60-70% $\dot{V}O_2$max during Wingate testing of 7-15-year-old boys (112).

Variables. Optimization of power production on the Wingate test is dependent on the force setting. A number of factors including physical fitness, age, gender, and body composition determine the optimal setting for individual subjects, and the best load for children has not been fully resolved. Recommendations for optimal braking force for leg and arm tests have been provided by Bar-Or (12) (see tables 3.5 and 3.6). Bar-Or pointed out that performance on the Wingate test is related to the fat-free mass of the child; values in these tables are therefore not applicable to subjects with an abnormal ratio between muscle and total body mass (as with obesity, anorexia nervosa, motor disabilities) (12). Bar-Or recommended individualizing braking forces in these subjects on the basis of the capabilities they have demonstrated during the sprint portions of the warm-up.

Performance on the Wingate test is contingent upon adequate subject motivation. Encouraging the child to provide a maximal cycling effort is therefore critical. Geron and Inbar found that factors related to emotion, such as competition and rewards, improved peak power output in young adults (44). Bar-Or recommended that

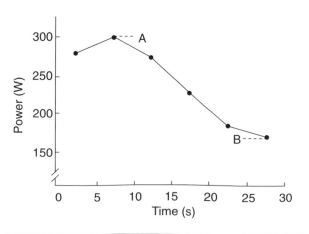

Figure 3.1 Indices of anaerobic fitness during the Wingate test. A = peak power. Average of A and B = mean power. Reprinted from Bar-Or 1987.

Table 3.5   Optimal braking force for the Wingate anaerobic leg test

Body weight (kg)	Monark (kp)		Fleisch (weights)	
	Girls	Boys	Girls	Boys
20–24.9	1.3–1.7	1.4–1.8	13–17	14–18
25–29.9	1.7–2.0	1.8–2.0	17–20	18–20
30–34.9	2.0–2.3	2.1–2.5	20–23	21–25
35–39.9	2.3–2.7	2.5–2.7	23–27	25–27
40–44.9	2.7–3.0	2.8–3.2	27–30	28–32
45–49.9	3.0–3.3	3.2–3.5	30–33	32–35
50–54.9	3.3–3.7	3.5–3.9	33–37	35–39
55–59.9	3.7–4.0	3.9–4.2	37–40	39–42
60–64.9	4.0–4.3	4.2–4.6	40–43	42–46
65–69.9	4.3–4.7	4.6–4.9	43–47	46–49

Reprinted from Rowland 1993.

pending further research, environmental conditions that might affect performance be standardized (12).

Two other factors, pedal crank length and use of toe stirrups, may influence results in Wingate testing. Use of toe stirrups has been found to improve power output by 5-12% (63), presumably by allowing force to be applied throughout the full pedal revolution. If the crank length is not appropriate for a subject's leg length, changes in muscle tension, torque, and muscle energetics could potentially influence power output. Within the usual range of subject size, however, this effect is probably small. Bar-Or observed that a change in optimal crank length of 5 cm will be expected to alter mean power by only 1.24% (11). In children, Klimt and Voight recommended a 13 cm crank length for 6-year-old children and 15 cm for those 8-10 years old (60).

But Elias et al. showed that mechanical efficiency was not compromised when children weighing 26-47 kg used a crank arm shorter than the standard 17.5 cm (36).

Validity and Reliability.   Findings on the Wingate test are highly reproducible in both arm and leg tests. Test-retest reliability coefficients in studies of peak and mean power 1-2 weeks apart have ranged from .89 to .97 (13, 33, 104). Several investigators have compared results on Wingate testing to performance on athletic events considered to reflect anaerobic fitness (25 m swim time, 50 yd dash, skating sprints). Correlation coefficients have indicated a moderately close relationship, with r values of 0.69 to 0.92 (see Bar-Or [12] for references).

Table 3.6   Optimal braking force for the Wingate anaerobic arm test

Body weight (kg)	Monark (kp)		Fleisch (weights)	
	Girls	Boys	Girls	Boys
20–24.9	0.8–1.0	0.8–1.1	8–10	8–11
25–29.9	1.0–1.2	1.1–1.3	10–12	11–13
30–34.9	1.2–1.4	1.3–1.5	12–14	13–15
35–39.9	1.4–1.6	1.5–1.6	14–16	15–16
40–44.9	1.6–1.8	1.7–1.9	16–18	17–19
45–49.9	1.8–2.0	1.9–2.1	18–20	19–21
50–54.9	2.0–2.2	2.1–2.3	20–22	21–23
55–59.9	2.2–2.4	2.3–2.5	22–24	23–25
60–64.9	2.4–2.6	2.5–2.8	24–26	25–28
65–69.9	2.6–2.8	2.8–3.0	26–28	28–30

Reprinted from Rowland 1993.

Force-Velocity Test

In the force-velocity test, pedal revolutions are counted while the subject performs a series of brief all-out sprints (5-8 s) against increasing braking forces. A plot of the product of force and velocity (power) against force describes a parabolic curve, the apex of which identifies the peak power, as well as the optimal braking force and pedaling velocity (see fig. 3.2). In this graphic expression, the maximal power corresponds to the value corresponding to one-half the maximum velocity (obtained by projecting velocity to the point of zero force).

Van Praagh et al. outlined specifics for applying this technique in their study of 12-year-old children (115). Their ergometer was designed for children, with a 13 cm crank length and its frame, handlebars, and saddle height adapted for smaller subjects. As in the Wingate test, a 3 min warm-up that included several short sprints and a subsequent 5 min rest period preceded the test. Subjects wore toe-clips and straps and were not allowed to stand off the seat. The initial braking force was 4.9 N (0.5 kp). After each sprint, subjects rested in the recumbent position for 3 min. Braking forces ranged from 4.9 to 78.5 N (0.5 to 8.0 kp).

In this study the mean optimal velocity was 109 and 114 rpm for the girls and boys, respectively. This corresponds closely to the optimal velocity of 110 rpm reported by Sargeant for maximal instantaneous power of 14-year-old boys on an isokinetic (constant rate) ergometer (96). It also approximates the pedaling velocity typically observed during the Wingate test (11). The optimal braking force in the children studied by Van Praagh et al. was 0.068 kp/kg for the girls and 0.085 kp/kg in the boys (115).

The force-velocity test carries certain advantages over the Wingate test (115). The Wingate test does not provide information on the force and velocity components of muscle power. The optimal force for the Wingate test is selected relative to total body mass, whereas that determined by the force-velocity test is a factor of effective muscle mass. The repeated brief sprints of the force-velocity test are less strenuous than the highly fatiguing Wingate test; performance is therefore less likely to be influenced by motivational factors. The Wingate test, on the other hand, provides information on both peak and mean power and takes less time to administer.

Accumulated Oxygen Deficit

The O_2 deficit has been defined as the O_2 equivalent of the energy that is not supplied by aerobic metabolism during exercise (111). When measured during brief exhaustive exercise, then, O_2 deficit should reflect true anaerobic capacity. In fact, this measure has been considered a more sensitive indicator of anaerobic capacity than the other commonly used anaerobic tests outlined earlier, which (a) do not exhaust anaerobic energy supplies and (b) involve an uncertain amount of aerobic contribution (95, 111).

The concept of the O_2 deficit is an old one, having been applied to the evaluation of anaerobic components of exercise function since the early 1900s (95). As currently used, this technique involves measurement of the total amount of anaerobic energy sources during the course of a test, rather than rate of energy expenditure—thus the term accumulated O_2 deficit. The deficit is indicated by the difference between actual O_2 uptake during supramaximal work and that predicted from the relationship of work and O_2 uptake during submaximal exercise.

The validity of this method in reflecting anaerobic capacity is indicated by the leveling off of accumulated O_2 deficit that occurs with increasing supramaximal work. This plateau has been demonstrated in adults by 120 s of supramaximal running but by a duration as short as 60 s on the cycle ergometer (43, 73). The accumulated O_2 deficit method assumes that mechanical efficiency during supramaximal exercise is similar to that during submaximal work, a conclusion that Saltin has challenged (95). Saltin contended that exercise in supramaximal conditions resulted in a higher rise in O_2 uptake than that predicted from submaximal work. Consequently, any extrapolation of supramaximal energy demands from submaximal exercise would underpredict O_2 cost at supramaximal exercise.

Exercise with this method for assessing anaerobic capacity in children is limited (18, 38). Carlson and

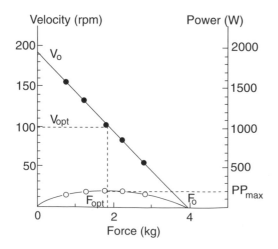

Figure 3.2 An example of a force-velocity test. PP_{max} (peak power) is determined as the apex of the parabolic curve of velocity versus power. This valve corresponds to 1/2 maximal velocity and identifies optimal braking force (F_{opt}) and pedaling velocity (V_{opt}).

Naughton used the accumulated O_2 deficit technique in their study of 18 healthy boys and girls (mean age 10 years) (18). Subjects performed four to five submaximal steady state cycle tests on separate laboratory visits to create individual linear regression equations for work versus O_2 uptake at submaximal intensities. These equations were used to identify work rates that corresponded to 110%, 130%, and 150% of $\dot{V}O_2$max. Supramaximal tests were then conducted at each of these work rates, with subjects pedaling at 90 rpm to exhaustion or until rpm fell below 60-70. Accumulated O_2 deficit was calculated at each of the supramaximal loads as the difference between the predicted and actual O_2 utilization over the test duration.

Both absolute and weight-relative O_2 deficit diminished with increased supramaximal work in the girls but was essentially stable at all loads in the boys. The authors suggested that the girls did not achieve optimal anaerobic performance at the two higher intensities because the exercise intensity was too severe. This conclusion is supported by the decline in peak RER (1.14, 1.11, and 1.02) and heart rate (202, 198, and 190 bpm), respectively, in the three supramaximal tests of increasing work. Carlson and Naughton considered the accumulated O_2 deficit method a potentially valuable tool for quantitating anaerobic capacity in children, but further research is important to define the optimal equipment and protocols for young subjects (18).

Oxygen deficit should not be confused with O_2 debt, which is the O_2 uptake measured during recovery from exercise that exceeds basal $\dot{V}O_2$ levels. Although O_2 debt serves as an indicator of anaerobic capacity (77), it is influenced by non-anaerobic factors (temperature, gluconeogenesis, lactate oxidation) and is not considered a sensitive indicator of the anaerobic energy contribution to exercise (95).

Treadmill Tests

Researchers have used several protocols for estimation of anaerobic fitness by high-intensity treadmill running. Paterson and Cunningham had 10-15-year-old subjects run at a 20% grade at speeds ranging from 4.5 to 7.0 mph (77). Treadmill time to exhaustion (which ranged from means of 80 to 100 s in the different age groups), O_2 debt, and postexercise blood lactate levels served as markers of anaerobic fitness.

More recently, anaerobic fitness in children has been estimated via computer analysis of power output during sprint running on a nonmotorized treadmill (39, 114). Fargeas et al. found correlations of r = .94 and .77 for absolute and body mass-relative power, respectively, on such a treadmill protocol and on the force-velocity cycle test in 8-14-year-old children (40). Values for the cycling test, however, were significantly higher than on the treadmill.

Postexercise Blood Lactate Levels

Since lactic acid is a by-product of anaerobic metabolism, peak levels of blood lactate after short, high-intensity exercise have been used as a means of estimating anaerobic fitness. The validity of this approach has been highly suspect because muscle cell lactate is not necessarily in equilibrium with that in the extracellular fluids, and also because blood lactate levels are an expression of clearance and elimination rates as much as muscle production. Consequently, blood lactate concentrations cannot be assumed to reflect concentrations of muscle lactate (3).

Paterson and Cunningham used postexercise lactate levels as indicators of "anaerobic capacity" in 10-15-year-old children (77). In an earlier study using the same treadmill protocol, the test-retest coefficient for postexercise lactate levels was only r = .53, with wide intraindividual variability (78). Measurement of lactate levels during exercise testing of children has therefore not been embraced as a useful means of evaluating anaerobic fitness; lactate values have been used largely to estimate submaximal anaerobic threshold and to identify maximal testing efforts (3, 26).

Several considerations are important if one uses lactate levels during exercise testing of children. These have been reviewed by Armstrong and Welsman (3). Peak blood lactate levels are reached 1-2 min after a maximal progressive test in children, as compared to 5-7 min postexercise in adults. Lactate levels may vary according to mode of exercise, test protocol, site of blood sampling, and lactate assay methodology. These factors must be considered when one makes comparisons of lactate levels obtained in different studies.

SUMMARY

Effective laboratory exercise testing of children requires close attention to age- and fitness-appropriate protocols. There is no single "best" test for either aerobic or anaerobic fitness, but certain protocols offer advantages depending on the type of information required. The experience and comfort of a testing laboratory and its staff with particular testing procedures are also important.

Children are generally excellent exercise subjects if the staff provides a supportive, encouraging testing environment. The child's safety should remain a paramount consideration in all testing situations; this requires attention to prevention of injury, preparation for emergencies, and safety of equipment.

There is considerable need for an understanding of the ways in which differences in testing protocols in children affect physiologic responses to exercise. Likewise, we have little knowledge of how these responses are influenced by factors such as mouthpiece size, valve dead space, and mixing chamber volume during assessment of gas exchange variables. Considering the varied sizes of subjects in the pediatric exercise laboratory, one must be suspicious that these may alter the results obtained.

References

1. Adams, F.H.; Linde, L.M.; Miyake, H. The physical working capacity of normal school children. I. California. Pediatrics 28:55-64; 1961.
2. Armstrong, N.; Balding, J.; Gentle, P.; Williams, J.; Kirby, B. Peak oxygen uptake and physical capacity in 11- to 16-year olds. Pediatr. Exerc. Sci. 2:349-358; 1990.
3. Armstrong, N.; Welsman, J.R. Assessment and interpretation of aerobic fitness in children and adolescents. Exerc. Sports Sci. Rev. 22:435-476; 1994.
4. Åstrand, P.O. Experimental studies of the physical working capacity in relation to sex and age. Copenhagen: Munksgaard; 1952.
5. Åstrand, P.O.; Rodahl, K. Textbook of work physiology. 2nd ed. New York: McGraw-Hill; 1977:p. 345-347.
6. Åstrand, P.O.; Ryhming, I. A nomogram for calculation of aerobic capacity from pulse rate during submaximal work. J. Appl. Physiol. 7:218-221; 1954.
7. Baggley, G.; Cumming, G.R. Serial measurement of working and aerobic capacity of Winnipeg school children during a school year. In: Cumming, G.R.; Taylor, A.W; Snidal, D., eds. Environmental effects of work performance. Canadian Association of Sport Sciences; 1972:p. 173-186.
8. Bailey, D.A.; Mirwald, R.L. A children's test of fitness. Med. Sport 11:56-64; 1978.
9. Bar-Or, O. A new anaerobic capacity test. Characteristics and applications. 21st World Congress in Sport Medicine; September 1978; Brasilia, Brazil.
10. Bar-Or, O. Pediatric sports medicine for the practitioner. New York: Springer-Verlag; 1983.
11. Bar-Or, O. The Wingate anaerobic test. An uptake on methodology, reliability, and validity. Sports Med. 4:381-394; 1987.
12. Bar-Or, O. Noncardiopulmonary pediatric exercise tests. In: Rowland, T.W., ed. Pediatric laboratory exercise testing. Champaign, IL: Human Kinetics; 1993:p. 165-186.
13. Bar-Or, O.; Dotan, R.; Inbar, O. A 30-second all-out ergometric test: its reliability and validity for anaerobic capacity. Isr. J. Med. Sci. 13:326; 1977.
14. Bengtsson, E. The working capacity in normal children, evaluated by submaximal exercise on the bicycle ergometer and compared with adults. Acta Med. Scand. 154:91-109; 1955.
15. Binkhorst, R.A.; Saris, W.H.M.; Noordeloos, A.M.; Van't Hof, M.A.; de Haan, A.F.J. Maximal oxygen consumption of children (6 to 18 years) predicted from maximal and submaximal values in treadmill and bicycle tests. In: Rutenfranz, R.; Mocellin, R.; Klimt, F., eds. Children and exercise XII. Champaign, IL: Human Kinetics; 1986:p. 227-232.
16. Boileau, R.A.; Bonen, A; Heyward, V.H.; Massey, B.H. Maximal aerobic capacity on the treadmill and bicycle ergometer of boys 11-14 years of age. J. Sports Med. 17:153-162; 1977.
17. Buono, M.J.; Roby, J.J.; Micale, F.G.; Sallis, J.F. Predicting maximum oxygen uptake in children: modification of the Åstrand-Ryhming test. Pediatr. Exerc. Sci. 1:278-283; 1989.
18. Carlson, J.S.; Naughton, G.A. An examination of the anaerobic capacity of children using maximal accumulated oxygen deficit. Pediatr. Exerc. Sci. 5:60-71; 1993.
19. Cooper, D.M.; Weiler-Ravell, D.; Whipp, B.J.; Wasserman, K. Aerobic parameters of exercise as a function of body size during growth in children. J. Appl. Physiol. 56:628-634; 1984.
20. Crielaard, J.M.; Pirnay, F. Anaerobic and aerobic power of top athletes. Eur. J. Appl. Physiol. 47:295-300; 1981.
21. Cumming, G.R. Correlation of athletic performance and aerobic power in 12-17 year old children with bone age, calf muscle, total body potassium, heart volume, and two indices of anaerobic power. In Bar-Or, O., ed. Pediatric work physiology. Natanya, Israel: Wingate Institute; 1973:p. 109-134.
22. Cumming, G.R. Exercise studies in clinical pediatric cardiology. In: Lavallee, H.; Shephard, R.J., eds. Frontiers of activity and child health. Quebec, PQ: Pelican; 1977:p. 17-45.
23. Cumming, G.R.; Danzinger, R. Bicycle ergometer studies in children. II. Correlation of pulse rate with oxygen consumption. Pediatrics 32:202-208; 1963.
24. Cumming, G.R.; Everatt, D.; Hastman, L. Bruce treadmill test in children: normal values in a clinic population. Am. J. Cardiol. 41:69-75; 1978.
25. Cumming, G.R.; Friesen, W. Bicycle ergometer measurement of maximal oxygen uptake in children. Can. J. Physiol. Pharmacol. 45:937-946; 1967.
26. Cumming G.R.; Hastman, J.; McCort, J.; McCullough, S. High serum lactates do occur in young children after maximal work. Int. J. Sports Med. 1:66-69; 1980.
27. Cumming, G.R.; Langford, S. Comparison of nine exercise tests used in pediatric cardiology. In Binkhorst, R.A.; Kemper, H.C.G.; Saris, W.H.M., eds. Children and exercise XI. Champaign, IL: Human Kinetics; 1985:p. 56-68.
28. Cunningham, D.A.; VanWaterschoot, B.M.; Paterson, D.H.; Lefcoe, M.; Sangal, S.P. Reliability and reproducibility of maximal oxygen uptake measurement in children. Med. Sci. Sports 9:104-108; 1977.
29. Cunningham, L. Physiological characteristics and team performance of female high school runners. Pediatr. Exerc. Sci. 1:73-79; 1989.

30. Daniels, J.; Oldridge, N.; Nagle, F.; White, B. Differences and changes in $\dot{V}O_2$ among young runners 10 to 18 years of age. Med. Sci. Sports 10:200-203; 1978.

31. Davies, C.T.M.; Barnes, C.; Godfrey, S. Body composition and maximal exercise performance in children. Hum. Biol. 44:195-214; 1972.

32. diPrampero, P.E.; Cerretelli, P. Maximal muscular power (aerobic and anaerobic) in African natives. Ergonomics 1:51-59; 1969.

33. Dotan, R.; Bar-Or, O. Load optimization for the Wingate anaerobic test. Eur. J. Appl. Physiol. 44:237-243; 1980.

34. DuRant, R.H.; Dover, E.V.; Alpert, B.S. An evaluation of five indices of physical working capacity in children. Med. Sci. Sports Exerc. 15:83-87; 1983.

35. Ebbeling, C.; Hamill, J.; Freedson, P.S.; Rowland, T.W. An examination of efficiency during walking in children and adults. Pediatr. Exerc. Sci. 4:36-49; 1992.

36. Elias, B.; Ryschon, T.; Berg, K.; Hofschire, P. Body size and mechanical efficiency during cycling in children [abstract]. Med. Sci. Sports Exerc. 23 Suppl:189; 1991.

37. Ellestad, M.H.; Blomqvist, C.G.; Naughton, J.P. Standards for adult exercise testing laboratories. Circulation 59:421A-430A; 1979.

38. Eriksson, B.O.; Gollnick, P.D.; Saltin, B. Muscle metabolism and enzyme activities after training in boys 11-13 years old. Acta Physiol. Scand. 87:485-497; 1973.

39. Falk, B.; Weinstein, Y.; Epstein, S.; Karni, Y.; Yarom, Y. Measurement of anaerobic power among young athletes using a new treadmill test [abstract]. Pediatr. Exerc. Sci. 5:414; 1993.

40. Fargeas, M.A.; Van Praagh, E.; Pantelidis, D.; Leger, L.; Fellman, N.; Coudert, J. Comparison of cycling and running power outputs in trained children [abstract]. Pediatr. Exerc. Sci. 5:415; 1993.

41. Freedson, P.S.; Katch, V.L.; Gilliam, T.B.; MacConnie, S. Energy expenditure in prepubescent children: influence of sex and age. Am. J. Clin. Nutr. 34:1827-1830; 1981.

42. Gadhoke, S.; Jones, N.L. The response to exercise in boys aged 9-15 years. Clin. Sci. 37:789-801; 1969.

43. Gastin, P.B. Determination of anaerobic capacity in trained and untrained cyclists [doctoral thesis]. Melbourne, Australia: Victoria University of Technology; 1992.

44. Geron, E.; Inbar, O. Motivation and anaerobic performance. In: Simri, U., ed. The art and science of coaching: proceedings of an international seminar. Natanya, Israel: Wingate Institute; 1980:p. 107-117.

45. Godfrey, S. Exercise testing in children. London: Saunders; 1974.

46. Godfrey, S.; Davies, C.T.M.; Wozniak, E.; Barnes, C.A. Cardiorespiratory response to exercise in normal children. Clin. Sci. 40:419-431; 1971.

47. Green, M.A.; Foster, C. Effect of magnitude of handrail support on prediction of oxygen uptake during treadmill testing [abstract]. Med. Sci. Sports Exerc. 23 Suppl:S166; 1991.

48. Gutin, B.; Fogle, K.R.; Stewart, K. Relationship among submaximal heart rate, aerobic power, and running performance in children. Res. Q. 47:536-539; 1976.

49. Hammond, H.K.; Froelicher, V.F. Exercise testing for cardiorespiratory fitness. Sports Med. 1:234-239; 1984.

50. Hansen, H.S.; Froberg, K.; Nielsen, J.R.; Hyldebrandt, N. A new approach to assessing maximal aerobic power in children: the Odense School Child Study. Eur. J. Appl. Physiol. 58:618-624; 1989.

51. Hellerstein, H.K. Specifications for exercise testing equipment. Circulation 59:849A-854A; 1979.

52. Hermansen, L.; Oseid, S. Direct and indirect estimation of maximal oxygen uptake in prepubertal boys. Acta Paediatr. Scand. 217:18-23; 1971.

53. Houlsby, W.T. Functional aerobic capacity and body size. Arch. Dis. Child. 61:388-393; 1986.

54. Inbar, O.; Bar-Or, O. The effects of intermittent warm-up on 7-to-9 year old boys. Eur. J. Appl. Physiol. 34:81-89; 1975.

55. James, F.W.; Blomqvist, G.; Freed, M.D.; Miller, W.W.; Moller, J.H.; Nugent, E.W.; Riopel, D.A.; Strong, W.B.; Wessel, H.U. Standards for exercise testing in the pediatric age group. Circulation 66:1378A-1397A; 1982.

56. James, F.W.; Kaplan, S.; Glueck, C.J.; Tsay, J.Y.; Knight, M.J.S.; Sarwar, C.J. Responses of normal children and young adults to controlled bicycle exercise. Circulation 61:902-912; 1980.

57. Jette, M.; Ashton, N.J.; Sharratt, M.T. Development of a cardiorespiratory step-test of fitness for children 7-14 years of age. Can. J. Pub. Health 75:212-217; 1984.

58. Kanaley, J.A.; Boileau, R.A. The onset of the anaerobic threshold at three stages of physical maturity. J. Sports Med. Phys. Fit. 28:367-374; 1988.

59. Katch, V.L.; Weltman, A.; Martin, R.; Gray, L. Optimal test characteristics for maximal anaerobic work on the bicycle ergometer. Res. Q. 48:319-327; 1977.

60. Klimt, F.; Voight, E.D. Investigations on the standardization of ergometry in children. Acta Paediatr. Scand. 217 Suppl:35-36; 1971.

61. Krahenbuhl, G.S.; Pangrazi, R.P. Characteristics associated with running performance in young boys. Med. Sci. Sports Exerc. 15:486-490; 1983.

62. Krahenbuhl, G.S.; Pangrazi, R.P; Chomokes, E.A. Aerobic responses of young boys to submaximal running. Res. Q. 50:413-421; 1979.

63. Lavoie, N.; Dallaire, J.; Brayne, S.; Barrett, D. Anaerobic testing using the Wingate and the Evans-Quinney protocols with and without toe stirrups. Can. J. Appl. Sport Sci. 9:1-5; 1984.

64. Lussier, L.; Buskirk, E.R. Effects of an endurance training regimen on assessment of work capacity in prepubertal children. Ann. NY Acad. Sci. 301:734-747; 1971.

65. Mácek, M.; Vavra, J.; Novosadova, J. Prolonged exercise in prepubertal boys: I. Cardiovascular and metabolic adjustment. Eur. J. Appl. Physiol. 35:291-298; 1976.

66. Mahon, A.D.; Marsh, M.L. Ventilatory threshold and $\dot{V}O_2$ plateau at maximal exercise in 8- to 11-year old children. Pediatr. Exerc. Sci. 5:332-338; 1993.

67. Mahon, A.D.; Vaccaro, P. Ventilatory threshold and $\dot{V}O_2$max changes in children following endurance training. Med. Sci. Sports Exerc. 21:425-431; 1989.

68. Maksud, M.G.; Coutts, K.D. Application of the Cooper twelve-minute run-walk test to young males. Res. Q. 42:54-59; 1971.

69. Margaria, R.; Aghemo, P.; Rovelli, E. Measurement of muscular power (anaerobic) in man. J. Appl. Physiol. 21:1662-1664; 1966.

70. Mayers, N.; Gutin, B. Physiologic characteristics of elite prepubertal cross country runners. Med. Sci. Sports 11:172-176; 1979.

71. McArdle, W.D.; Katch, F.I.; Pechar, G.S. Reliability and interrelationships between maximal oxygen intake, physical work capacity, and step-test scores in college women. Med. Sci. Sports 4:182-186; 1972.

72. Medbo, J.I. Quantification of the anaerobic energy release during exercise in man [doctoral thesis]. Oslo: University of Oslo; 1991.

73. Medbo, J.I.; Mohn, A.; Tabata, I.; Bahr, R.; Vaage, O.; Sejersted, O.M. Anaerobic capacity determined by maximal accumulated oxygen deficit. J. Appl. Physiol. 64:50-60; 1988.

74. Miyamura, M.; Kuroda, H.; Hirata, K.; Honda, Y. Evaluations of the step test scores based on the measurements of maximal aerobic power. J. Sports Med. 15:316-322; 1975.

75. Okuni, M. Revised guidance for the management of children with arrhythmia. Acta Cardiol. Paediatr. Jpn. 4:307-309; 1988.

76. Palgi, Y.; Gutin, B.; Young, J.; Alejandro, D. Physiologic and anthropometric factors underlying endurance performance in children. Int. J. Sports Med. 5:67-73; 1984.

77. Paterson, D.H.; Cunningham, D.A. Development of anaerobic capacity in early and late maturing boys. In: Binkhorst, R.A.; Kemper, H.C.G.; Saris, W.H.M., eds. Children and Exercise XI. Champaign, IL: Human Kinetics; 1985:p. 119-128.

78. Paterson, D.H.; Cunningham, D.A.; Bonk, J.M. Anaerobic capacity of athletic males aged 10, 15, and 21 years. International symposium: growth and development of the child; 1980; Trois-Rivieres, Quebec.

79. Paterson, D.H.; Cunningham, D.A.; Donner, A. The effect of different treadmill speeds on the variability of $\dot{V}O_2$max in children. Eur. J. Appl. Physiol. 47:113-122; 1981.

80. Ragg, K.E.; Murray, T.F.; Karbonit, L.M.; Jump, D.A. Errors in predicting functional capacity from a treadmill exercise stress test. Am. Heart J. 100:581-583; 1980.

81. Reybrouck, T.; Weymans, M.; Stijns, H.; Knops, J; vander Hauwaert, L. Ventilatory anaerobic threshold in healthy children. Eur. J. Appl. Physiol. 54:278-284; 1985.

82. Riopel, D.A.; Taylor, A.B.; Hohn, A.R. Blood pressure, heart rate, pressure-rate product, and electrocardiographic changes in healthy children during treadmill exercise. Am. J. Cardiol. 44:697-704; 1979.

83. Robinson, S. Experimental studies of physical fitness in relation to age. Arbeitsphysiol. 10:251-323; 1938.

84. Rowland, T.W. Aerobic exercise testing protocols. In: Rowland, T.W., ed. Pediatric laboratory exercise testing. Champaign, IL: Human Kinetics; 1993:p. 19-42.

85. Rowland, T.W. Does peak $\dot{V}O_2$ reflect $\dot{V}O_2$max in children? Evidence from supramaximal testing. Med. Sci. Sports Exerc. 25:689-693; 1993.

86. Rowland, T.W.; Auchinachie, J.A.; Keenan, T.J.; Green, G.M. Physiological responses to treadmill running in adult and prepubertal males. Int. J. Sports Med. 8:292-297; 1987.

87. Rowland, T.W.; Cunningham, L.N. Oxygen uptake plateau during maximal treadmill exercise in children. Chest 101:485-489; 1992.

88. Rowland, T.W.; Cunningham, L.N. Walking economy and stride frequency in children: a longitudinal analysis [abstract]. Med. Sci. Sports Exerc.; 27 Suppl. S93: 1995.

89. Rowland, T.W.; Green, G.M. Physiological responses to treadmill exercise in females: adult-child differences. Med. Sci. Sports Exerc. 20:474-478; 1988.

90. Rowland, T.W.; Green, G.M. Anaerobic threshold and the determination of training target heart rates in premenarcheal girls. Pediatr. Cardiol. 10:75-79; 1989.

91. Rowland, T.W.; Martha, P.M.; Reiter, E.O.; Cunningham, L.N. The influence of diabetes mellitus on cardiovascular function in children and adolescents. Int. J. Sports Med. 13:431-435; 1992.

92. Rowland, T.W.; Rambusch, J.M.; Staab, J.S.; Unnithan, V.B.; Siconolfi, S.F. Accuracy of physical working capacity (PWC$_{170}$) in estimating aerobic fitness in children. J. Sports Med. Phys. Fit. 33:184-188; 1993.

93. Rowland, T.W.; Staab, J.S.; Unnithan, V.B.; Rambusch, J.M.; Siconolfi, S.F. Mechanical efficiency during cycling in prepubertal and adult males. Int. J. Sports Med. 11:452-455; 1990.

94. Rowland, T.W.; Varzeus, M.R.; Walsh, C.A. Aerobic responses to walking training in sedentary adolescents. J. Adolesc. Health Care 12:30-34; 1991.

95. Saltin, B. Anaerobic capacity: past, present and prospective. In: Taylor, A.W., ed. Biochemistry of exercise VII. Champaign, IL: Human Kinetics; 1990:p. 387-412.

96. Sargeant, A. Short-term muscle power in children and adolescents. In: Advances in pediatric sport sciences. Vol. 3, Bar-Or, O., ed. Biological issues. Champaign, IL: Human Kinetics; 1989:p. 41-66.

97. Sheehan, J.M.; Rowland, T.W.; Burke, E.J. A comparison of four treadmill protocols for determination of maximal oxygen uptake in 10-12 year old boys. Int. J. Sports Med. 8:31-34; 1987.

98. Shuleva, K.M.; Hunter, G.R.; Hester, D.J.; Dunaway, D.L. Exercise oxygen uptake in 3- through 6-year old children. Pediatr. Exerc. Sci. 2:130-139; 1990.

99. Skinner, J.S.; Bar-Or, O.; Bergsteinova, V.; Bell, C.W.; Royer, D.; Buskirk, E.R. Comparison of continuous and intermittent tests for determining maximal oxygen intake in children. Acta Paediatr. Scand. 217 Suppl:24-28; 1971.

100. Staats, B.A.; Grinton, S.F.; Mottram, C.D.; Driscoll, D.J.; Beck, K.C. Quality control in exercise testing. Progr. Pediatr. Cardiol. 2:11-17; 1993.

101. Strong, W.B.; Spencer, D.; Miller, M.D.; Salehbhai, M. The physical capacity of healthy black children. Am. J. Dis. Child. 132:244-248; 1978.

102. Takarada, M.; Hayashi, T.; Chinen, M. Metabolic rate of Master two-step test: applications for judgement to assess exercise capacity of children with heart diseases. Shonika Rinsho 27:150-155; 1974.

103. Tanner, C.S.; Heise, C.T.; Barber, G. Correlation of the physiologic parameters of a continuous ramp versus an incremental James exercise protocol in normal children. Am. J. Cardiol. 67:309-312; 1991.

104. Tirosch, E.; Bar-Or, O.; Rosenbaum, P. New muscle power test in neuromuscular disease. Am. J. Dis. Child. 144:1083-1087; 1990.

105. Tomassoni, T.L. Conducting the pediatric exercise test. In: Rowland, T.W., ed. Pediatric laboratory exercise testing. Champaign, IL: Human Kinetics; 1993:p. 1-18.

106. Turley, K.R.; Rogers, D.M.; Wilmore, J.H. Maximal testing in prepubescent children: treadmill versus cycle ergometry [abstract]. Med. Sci. Sports Exerc. 25:S9; 1993.

107. Turley, K.R.; Wilmore, J.H.; Simons-Morton, B.; Williston, B.J.; Reeds, J.; Dahlstrom, G. The reliability and validity of the 9-minute run in third grade children. Pediatr. Exerc. Sci. 6:178-187; 1994.

108. Unnithan, V. Factors affecting submaximal running economy in children [doctoral thesis]. Glasgow: University of Glasgow; 1993.

109. Unnithan, V.B.; Eston, R.G. Stride frequency and submaximal running economy in adults and children. Pediatr. Exerc. Sci. 2:149-155; 1990.

110. Valentine, B.G.; Freedson, P.S.; Goodman, T.L. Prediction of maximal oxygen consumption from a one mile walk and PWC_{170} in 10-to 13-year-old boys [abstract]. Pediatr. Exerc. Sci. 4:99; 1992.

111. Vandewalle, H.; Peres, G.; Monod, H. Standard anaerobic exercise tests. Sports Med. 4:268-289; 1987.

112. Van Praagh, E.; Bedu, M.; Falgairette, G.; Fellman, N.; Coudert, J. Oxygen uptake during a 30-s supramaximal exercise in 7 to 15 year old boys. Congress of Pediatric Work Physiology; 1989 Sept. 11-15; Budapest, Hungary.

113. Van Praagh, E.; Bedu, M.; Roddier, P.; Coudert, J. A simple calibration method for mechanically braked cycle ergometers. Int. J. Sports Med. 13:27-30; 1992.

114. Van Praagh, E.; Fargeas, M.A.; Leger, L.; Fellman, N.; Coudert, J. Short-term power output in children measured on a computerized treadmill ergometer [abstract]. Pediatr. Exerc. Sci. 5:482; 1993.

115. Van Praagh, E.; Fellman, N.; Bedu, M.; Falgairette, G.; Coudert, J. Gender difference in the relationship of anaerobic power output to body composition in children. Pediatr. Exerc. Sci. 2:336-348; 1990.

116. Wakabayashi, R.; Osano, M. Simple exercise test for infants and children. Shoni Naika 15:1651-1655; 1983.

117. Washington, R.L.; van Gundy, J.C.; Cohen, C.; Sondheimer, H.M.; Wolfe, R.R. Normal aerobic and anaerobic exercise data for North American school-age children. J. Pediatr. 112:223-233; 1988.

118. Webber, L.M.; Byrnes, W.C.; Rowland, T.W.; Foster, V.L. Serum creatinine kinase activity and delayed onset muscle soreness in prepubertal children. Pediatr. Exerc. Sci. 1:351-359; 1989.

119. Whipp, B.J.; Wasserman, K. Oxygen uptake kinetics for various intensities of constant-load work. J. Appl Physiol. 33:351-356; 1972.

120. Wilmore, J.H.; Sigerseth, P.O. Physical work capacity of young girls, 7-13 years of age. J. Appl. Physiol. 22:923-928; 1967.

121. Wilson, B.A.; Chishlom, D. Total body maximal aerobic power in children as measured by Concept II rowing ergometer [abstract]. Pediatr. Exerc. Sci. 5:487; 1993.

122. Woynarowska, B. The validity of indirect estimations of maximal oxygen uptake in children 11-12 years of age. Eur. J. Appl. Physiol. 43:19-23; 1980.

123. Yoshinaga, M.; Oku, S.; Aihoshi, S.; Nomura, Y.; Haraguchi, T.; Mizumoto, Y.; Inoue, H. A simplified Master's two-step test for pre-school children. Acta Paediatr. Jpn. 31:578-586; 1989.

124. Zanner, C.W.; Benson, N.Y. Continuous treadmill walking versus intermittent treadmill running as maximal exercise tests for young competitive swimmers. J. Sports Med. 21:173–178; 1981.

CHAPTER 4

BODY COMPOSITION

Body composition has a significant influence on the physiological responses to exercise. The exercise scientist is most particularly interested in the relationship between the size of the body "motor" (i.e., exercising muscle mass) and the "baggage" (body fat) it is obliged to carry about. In growing subjects, this issue has special relevance because the relationship between these two variables changes both with age and between genders. A knowledge of maturational differences in body composition is therefore important if we are to accurately interpret the physiological trends during the pediatric years.

This chapter will explore these differences. The major impediment to understanding body composition changes during childhood has been uncertainty regarding the validity of measurement techniques in immature subjects. Specifically, the accuracy of methods and equations used for estimating body composition in adults appears to be seriously weakened when these methods are applied to children. It is important, then, to begin this discussion by reviewing methods of estimating body composition and the ways in which these are influenced by the process of body growth. Our current understanding of the normal pattern of development of the body's components during the childhood and adolescent years will then be reviewed. Finally we will examine the influence of body composition on measures of physical fitness.

IMPORTANCE OF BODY COMPOSITION

The concepts this chapter addresses—those surrounding the maturation of body composition—have a profound impact not only on the measurement and expression of physical fitness but also on the future health of children. The important issues include the following:

- *Effect on field and laboratory exercise performance.* Body fat has a major influence on exercise performance in both field and laboratory settings. Endurance tests such as the 1-mile run have been used as indicators of "cardiovascular fitness" without regard to the potentially important influence of body fat on performance times. Indeed, from the studies examining this question, it is not difficult to conclude that the major health risk indicated by poor performance on weight-bearing endurance tests is most likely that of obesity itself (30). The importance of this influence of body fat on performance, and the ways in which it affects the interpretation of test results in children, will be discussed later in this chapter.

- *Gender differences in physiological measures.* Differences in body composition between boys and girls may help explain gender-related variations in physiological responses to exercise. Numerous examples will appear in the chapters that follow. The most obvious is the accumulation of body fat that females experience at puberty—a change that occurs at the time males are increasing their muscle bulk. Such changes must be considered, for instance, when one attempts to understand patterns of maximal O_2 uptake that separate adolescent boys from girls. Can the decline in $\dot{V}O_2$max per kg at puberty in girls be explained by their greater body fat? If one expresses strength relative to muscle size, do gender differences disappear? Such questions can be addressed only if we accurately assess body composition changes in children and adolescents.

- *Effect of obesity on cardiopulmonary fitness.* Does obesity depress cardiovascular and pulmonary fitness, as the poor endurance performance of overweight subjects might suggest? If so, exercise treatment programs should be designed to satisfy criteria of duration, intensity, and frequency that have been recommended for improving aerobic fitness. If not, such programs might be better constructed to include low-level exercise to burn off calories and at the same time be more easily tolerated by obese subjects. This question will be addressed later in this chapter.

• *Adverse health outcomes.* Although this book focuses on physiological rather than health issues, the importance of body composition in relation to the health of children cannot be ignored. For wrestling coaches establishing minimum body fat levels for their teams and physicians managing adolescents with anorexia nervosa, the critical issue becomes undernutrition and inadequate body fat stores. At the other extreme, excess body fat in children often serves as an antecedent for lifelong obesity. And the obese adult suffers from excessive morbidity and mortality from coronary artery disease, hypertension, diabetes mellitus, and orthopedic disease. Identification, treatment, and prevention of childhood obesity is therefore a primary goal for health providers in the pediatric years.

Even during childhood, a strong relationship exists between obesity and risk factors for adult chronic disease. Excess body fat in children is linked to adverse serum lipoprotein profiles and systemic hypertension. Body fat has a major influence on the connection between physical fitness and coronary risk factors during childhood as well. Studies describing a negative correlation between physical fitness and blood pressure in children, for instance, often indicate that this relationship disappears when body fat is taken into account (1, 18).

MEASUREMENT OF BODY COMPOSITION

Unfortunately, short of cadaver analysis, there is no means of directly measuring fat and muscle mass. Most techniques for indirectly assessing body composition have divided the body into *fat mass* (FM) and *fat-free, or lean, body mass* (FFM)—the so-called *two-compartment model.* In this model, FFM consists of all components of the body except body fat, including muscle, bone, viscera, and connective tissue. Methods for estimating body composition with the two-compartment model typically assess either FFM or FM and then obtain a value for the other compartment by subtraction from total body weight.

Body composition measurement techniques can be divided into those utilized in the laboratory setting, such as underwater weighing densitometry and determination of total body water or potassium, and those employed in the field, including measurement of skinfold thicknesses, body mass index, and bioelectric imped-

ance. The former are more accurate but expensive and time- and labor-intensive, and these procedures are generally used as criterion measures for the field methods. The critical research issues, then, have involved several questions: (a) how precisely do the criterion measures indicate body composition? (b) how accurately do the field techniques estimate the criterion methods? (c) how do age, gender, and subject population (such as athletes vs. nonathletes) influence the validity of both laboratory and field estimates of body composition?

Considerable evidence indicates that growing subjects represent a unique population in the application of methods for estimating body composition. That is, equations for FM and FFM utilized in adults by all these techniques cannot be translated to children without leading to significant error. This section will address maturity-related influences on the estimation of body composition. This issue has been comprehensively reviewed by Lohman (19-22), Malina and Bouchard (24), and Boileau et al. (4), whose publications will supply the reader with additional information.

CRITERION LABORATORY METHODS

Several laboratory-based techniques have been utilized for indirect assessment of FM and FFM. Those most commonly adopted for children have been determinations of body density by underwater weighing, total body water, and body potassium concentration. These methods were initially developed for use in adult subjects; subsequently it was recognized that modifications were necessary for work with children and adolescents.

Body Density by Underwater Weighing

The density of the body, or body mass divided by body volume, reflects the body's fat content. In adults, the density of fat is 0.90 g/cc while that of lean tissues is approximately 1.10 g/cc. Thus, the higher the whole-body density, the less fat the body contains. Body density can be estimated by dividing its mass in air (M_A) by a volume value obtained by weighing the subject both in air and under water. Mass in air minus weight during full submersion (M_W) equals the volume of water displaced by the body under water once the density of the water (D_W) is considered. An additional correction is made for residual air in the lung (RV, measured indirectly) and volume of gas in the gastrointestinal tract (VGI, usually considered to be 100 ml). The formula for body density becomes:

$$D = \frac{M_A}{(M_A - M_W) - (RV + VGI)} D_W.$$

Equations have been developed that allow estimation of percent body fat from calculated density, with the differences in densities of fat and FFM taken into account. According to the Siri equation (31), for instance,

$$\text{Percent body fat} = \left(\frac{4.95}{D} - 4.50\right) \cdot 100$$

Such equations have been developed for adults, and they assume that density of FFM (about 1.10) is relatively constant among individuals. During childhood, however, progressive changes occur in the chemical composition of FFM; this results in differences in its density compared to that for adults. Use of such equations in children, therefore, will result in inaccuracies in estimation of FM and, by subtraction, of FFM.

In 1923 Moulton suggested from animal and limited human data that chemical maturity—a stable body density—was achieved in children by the age of 3 to 4 years (25). Subsequent estimates of body fat content from density measurements were therefore assumed to be the same for children as for adults. More recent research, however, indicates that chemical maturity of the FFM is not reached until late adolescence (24).

During growth, in fact, the protein and mineral content of FFM increases while that of water progressively declines. Water content of the FFM falls from about 81% at birth to 72% in adulthood (see fig. 4.1a), while the contribution of mineral—an expression principally of bone growth—increases from approximately 5.0% to 6.2% between the ages of 8 and 18 years (see fig. 4.1b). As a result of these changes in water, mineral, and protein content, the density of the FFM increases throughout childhood, accelerating particularly during the pubertal years (see fig. 4.1c). (The density of fat, on the other hand, remains relatively stable at approximately 0.900 g/cc.) Consequently, the use of adult-based equations for relating body density to fat content in children results in an overestimation of percent body fat, typically by about 7-13% (4).

Because of the chemical changes that increase the density of the FFM during childhood, no single equation is applicable for calculating percent body fat from body density in growing children. To account for this chemical immaturity, Lohman developed an equation for percent body fat that included not only body density (D_b) but also water content (w) and bone mineral content (b) (20):

$$\text{Percent fat} = (2.749/D_b - 7.14w + 1.146b - 2.053) \times 100.$$

While such a multicomponent model is preferable in the childhood age groups, Lohman recognized that practical considerations (i.e., lack of equipment to measure body water or mineral content) might make such an approach infeasible. He therefore utilized the Siri equation model to provide a series of equations for estimating body fat from density measurements at different ages, based on average age-specific values for FFM density (20). These are outlined in table 4.1. Lohman cautioned:

> Use of these equations enables one to use densitometry as a criterion method in children; however, the following limitations of this approach are important to consider. First children at a given age vary in their water and mineral content to some extent, and this leads to errors in estimation when one equation is used for all children. Second, various populations of children with a particular physical activity history (e.g., different athletic groups), or particular physique (e.g., mesomorphic), or from a particular ethnic group (i.e., Hispanic), or with a history of a particular disease (i.e., congestive heart failure) may differ in their fat free body density and these equations may not provide exact estimates for various populations. (20, p. 20-21)

Total Body Water (Hydrometry)

Most of the body water content resides in the FFM. In a normal adult 72-74% of the FFM is water, while fat tissue contains little water, generally about 20%. By measurement of total water (TBW), then, FFM has been estimated in adults by the equation FFM = TBW/0.732. Total water is typically determined through dilution techniques, usually with deuterium water.

The accuracy of this approach, of course, is predicated on a constant percentage of water within the FFM among different individuals. As we just saw, this is not the case in children, who exhibit a progressive decline in hydration of FFM during growth. As a result, estimation of FFM by measurement of TBW in children by this last equation will cause an underestimate of body fat, usually by 3-6%. Substituting age-specific values for water content of the FFM, listed in table 4.2, will reduce this error (12, 19, 24).

Body Potassium

In an approach similar to the one that uses TBW, the concentration of potassium in the body is assumed to represent a relatively constant proportion of the FFM. Potassium concentration is measured by the amount of the naturally occurring radioisotope potassium-40 (^{40}K) detected by gamma counter. The equation for adult males is FFM = mEqK/68.1 and that for adult females, FFM = mEqK/64.2. As with TBW, these equations

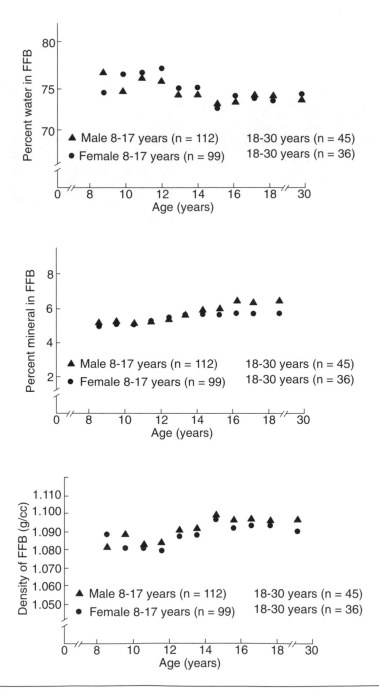

Figure 4.1   a) Average percent water content of the fat-free mass in children and adolescents. b) Percent mineral content of the fat-free mass in children and adolescents. c) Values of density of fat-free mass during childhood and adolescence in males and females. Reprinted from Boileau 1988.

suppose a relatively constant concentration of potassium within the FFM. And, similarly, this is not the case in children. Potassium concentration in the FFM steadily rises during childhood, and values are about 35% greater at age 17-20 than at birth (see table 4.2). Use of the adult equation will therefore overestimate body fatness in children by 7% to 13%. Values for potassium content of the FFM at the various childhood

ages listed in table 4.2 can be used to provide a more accurate estimate of FFM in children and adolescents.

Newer Techniques

New laboratory methodologies for estimating body composition, such as dual energy radiography and magnetic resonance imaging, may provide more accurate

Table 4.1   Equations for estimating % fat from body density based on age and gender

Age (years)	Male C$_1$	Male C$_2$	Female C$_1$	Female C$_2$
1	5.72	5.36	5.69	5.33
1–2	5.64	5.26	5.65	5.26
3–4	5.53	5.14	5.58	5.20
5–6	5.43	5.03	5.53	5.14
7–8	5.38	4.97	5.43	5.03
9–10	5.30	4.89	5.35	4.95
11–12	5.23	4.81	5.25	4.84
13–14	5.07	4.64	5.12	4.69
15–16	5.03	4.59	5.07	4.64
Young adult	4.95	4.50	5.05	4.62

Note: C$_1$ and C$_2$ are the terms in percent fat equation to substitute for the Siri equation of percent fat = [4.95/Db – 4.50] × 100 using the general equation:

$$\% \text{ Fat} = \frac{1}{\text{Db}} \left[\frac{(d_1 d_2)}{d_1 - d_2} \right] \frac{-d_2}{d_1 - d_2} \times 100$$

where Db = body density, d$_1$ = density of fat-free body, and d$_2$ = density of fat = 0.90 gm/cc for all ages.

Reprinted from Lohman 1989.

criterion measures (21). Information in normal children has yet to be accumulated with these techniques.

FIELD MEASURES OF BODY COMPOSITION

The criterion techniques surveyed so far are not feasible for large groups of subjects or in testing situations outside of the laboratory. Methods such as determination of skinfold thicknesses, body mass index, and bioelectric impedance have proven useful for estimating body composition in such settings. In general, they provide a reasonable estimate of composition but suffer from some loss of accuracy versus the criterion methods. These techniques are performed in children in the same manner as in adults. However, equations relating results to body fat content are open to the same sources of error as the criterion methods. It is important, then, to understand the results of field tests as they relate to differences in biochemical immaturity in growing subjects.

Measurement of Skinfold Thicknesses

Because it is easy and inexpensive, measurement of skinfold thicknesses has become popular in field,

Table 4.2   Estimated composition of fat-free mass during growth

Age (years)	Water	Protein	Mineral	Potassium (g/kg)	Density (g/ccm)
Males					
Birth	80.6	15.0	3.7	1.92	1.063
1	79.0	16.6	3.7	2.21	1.068
3	77.5	17.8	4.0	2.39	1.074
5	76.6	18.5	4.3	2.49	1.078
7–9	76.8	18.1	5.1	2.40	1.081
9–11	76.2	18.4	5.4	2.45	1.084
11–13	75.4	18.9	5.7	2.52	1.087
13–15	74.7	19.1	6.2	2.56	1.094
15–17	74.2	19.3	6.5	2.61	1.096
17–20	74.0	19.4	6.6	2.63	1.099
Females					
Birth	80.6	15.0	3.7	1.92	1.064
1	78.8	16.9	3.7	2.24	1.069
3	77.9	17.7	3.7	2.38	1.071
5	77.6	18.0	3.7	2.42	1.073
7–9	77.6	17.5	4.9	2.32	1.079
9–11	77.0	17.8	5.2	2.34	1.082
11–13	76.6	17.9	5.5	2.36	1.086
13–15	75.5	18.6	5.9	2.38	1.092
15–17	75.0	18.9	6.1	2.40	1.094
17–20	74.8	19.2	6.0	2.41	1.095

Header spanning columns Water, Protein, Mineral: Compartments of the FFM (%)

Reprinted from Malina and Bouchard 1991.

school, and clinical settings in children and adults alike. The premise that a relationship exists between body fat content and the sum of any of a number of combinations of standardized skinfold thickness measurements (usually determined by underwater weighing densitometry) generally holds true at all ages. The principal sources of error within any given subject population include (a) individual differences in distribution of body fat, (b) substantial standard errors of estimating body density, and (c) often-significant inter- and intratester variability in skinfold measurements (4).

In addition to these generic sources of error, other problems lead to inaccuracy when equations relating skinfold sums to percent body fat in adults are applied to children. Boileau et al. (3) and Lohman (21) outlined several issues that influence the accuracy and interpretation of skinfold measurements in pediatric subjects:

1. Equations relating skinfold sums to body fat content frequently include prepubescent, pubescent, and postpubescent subjects. The relationship between skinfold sum and body density changes with level of biological maturity—with density increasing at a given skinfold sum as maturity increases (see fig. 4.2).
2. Equations based on the two-component model ignore the influence of biochemical immaturity on FFM density in children, causing erroneous estimates of fat content.
3. Equations used to relate skinfold sums to fat content in children have not been sufficiently cross-validated, and the effect of specific subject sub-

populations (e.g., athletes, those of differing racial backgrounds) on the accuracy of these equations is unknown. That is, it is not clear how widely such equations can be applied outside of the group initially used to create the equation.
4. Different equations have been developed with varying selection of measurement sites and techniques.

Slaughter and her colleagues sought to develop equations that would accurately relate skinfold sums to percent body fat in children taking into account the chemical immaturity of the FFM and the changing relationship between density and skinfold sum with increasing maturity. They constructed such equations, based on the multicomponent approach described previously in this chapter, in a population of subjects ranging from age 7 years to young adulthood (32). These are outlined in table 4.3, which shows different intercepts for maturational level and gender. Notice that these equations are modified for subjects with triceps and subscapular skinfold sum exceeding 35 mm.

The Slaughter equations have been cross-validated in subjects 8-17 years of age and found to be reliable (17). The standard error of estimate with use of these equations is generally between 3% and 4% (17, 21). Equations for children below the age of 7 years have not been developed, and Lohman suggested that "at the present time skinfold measures in young children are best interpreted in relation to national norms" (20, p. 24).

Body Mass Index

The body mass index (BMI) is the mass divided by the square of height (kg/m^2) and is considered to relate directly to body fatness. Because it is easy to measure, BMI has been used predominantly as a marker of body fat content in epidemiological studies, often those involving large numbers of subjects. The basic weakness of BMI as an index of fatness is that it ignores the possibility that muscle tissue rather than fat may contribute to excessive body weight relative to height. That is, many subjects with an elevated BMI have a greater musculoskeletal mass rather than excessive adiposity in relation to body height. The issue is confounded in the childhood years because obese youngsters tend to be tall (13).

Not unexpectedly, then, BMI has not been found to be a particularly sensitive indicator of body composition in children. Correlation coefficients have ranged from .40 to .70 when BMI values are related to skinfold thickness measurements in children (28). Houtkooper found a standard error of estimate of 5.7% when using BMI to predict body fat estimated by underwater weighing in boys and girls (14). Roche et al. reported that skinfold

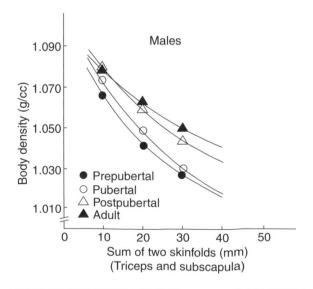

Figure 4.2 Relationship of triceps and subscapular skinfold sum to body density in males of different maturational stages. Reprinted from Boileau 1988.

Table 4.3 Prediction equations of percent fat from triceps and calf and from triceps and subscapular skinfolds in children and youth for males and females

Triceps and calf skinfolds
  % Fat = 0.735 ΣSF + 1.0 males, all ages
  % Fat = 0.610 ΣSF + 5.0 females, all ages

Triceps and subscapular skinfolds (> 35 mm)
  % Fat = 0.783 ΣSF + I males
  % Fat = 0.546 ΣSF + 9.7 females

Triceps and subscapular skinfolds (< 35 mm)[a]
  % Fat = 1.21 (ΣSF) – 0.008 (ΣSF)^2 + I males
  % Fat = 1.33 (ΣSF) – 0.013 (ΣSF)^2 + 2.5 females (2.0 blacks, 3.0 whites)

I = Intercept varies with maturation level and racial group for males as follows:

Age	Black	White
Prepubescent	–3.5	–1.7
Pubescent	–5.2	–3.4
Postpubescent	–6.8	–5.5
Adult	–6.8	–5.5

Note: Calculations were derived using Slaughter et al. (1988) equation.

[a]Thus for a white pubescent male with a triceps of 15 and a subscapular of 12, the % fat would be:

% Fat = 1.21 (27) – 0.008 (27)^2 – 3.4
    = 23.4%

Reprinted from Lohman 1992.

thicknesses bore a closer relationship than BMI to body density in children (27). Lohman concluded that "the widespread use of BMI by itself as a measure of fatness is given a fair rating in children and youth and should only be encouraged when other methods are unavailable or not practical for the particular situation" (20, p. 23).

Bioelectric Impedance

Measurement of bioelectric impedance for estimating body composition also has appeal for work with children because of its testing simplicity. Underlying this technique is the concept that the electrical impedance of an object is influenced by the volume of its conducting tissue. In the human, TBW is the principal conductor, and as noted previously, TBW reflects the FFM. In adults, values for FFM have been shown to be associated with the resistance index (height squared divided by body resistance) (21). Measurement of bioelectric impedance has the potential to serve as a useful field method for estimating percent body fat.

Studies in children with this technique are limited. Houtkooper et al. compared body composition findings obtained by densitometry with those for bioelectric impedance in 9-15-year-old children (15). With use of re-

sistance index and body weight, FFM was predicted with a standard error of estimate of 2.1 kg, and percent body fat with a standard error of estimate of 4.2%. DeLozier et al. studied the relationship of the resistance index to TBW in 96 boys and girls ages 4 to 8 years (11). The correlation coefficient was 0.75, lower than values of .92-.99 previously described in adults. The authors suggested that the low coefficient in this study might be attributable to the small range of values for resistance index and TBW.

Covington et al. found that bioelectric impedance, compared to skinfold measurements, overestimated body fat content in a group of black children; the difference in percentages was greater in the younger subjects (6). An explanation for these findings may be that the bioelectric impedance analysis used the Siri equation to determine body fat and thus the relative biochemical immaturity of the younger subjects was ignored. More information will be needed before the usefulness of bioelectric impedance technique in children can be fully assessed.

A summary of the validity of these testing methods for estimating body fat has been provided by Lohman (20) (see table 4.4).

Table 4.4   Validity of body composition methods for estimating percent fat

Method	Age, years Infancy 0–2	Preschool 3–5	Child 6–11	Youth 12–17
Densitometry	Not applic.	Not applic.	G to VG 1.085†	G 1.092 ± .005†
Body water	G to VG	VG	VG	VG
Body mass index	F,U	F,U	F	F
Triceps skinfold	G (%)	G (%)	G	G
Sum, skinfolds	G (%)	G (%)	G	G
Circumferences	U	U	G*	G*
Impedance	U	U	G*	G*

VG = very good (2%); G = good (3%); F = fair (4–5%); P = poor (6%);
U = uncertain (?). *Need new equations; †vary fat-free body density with age;
% use percentiles from national norms.

Reprinted from Lohman 1989.

THE EVOLUTION OF BODY COMPOSITION DURING CHILDHOOD

On the basis of the methods reviewed, we can draw a picture of changes in body composition during the normal course of childhood. The patterns that emerge are clearly influenced by gender. Additional effects of factors such as race, culture, habitual activity, and athleticism remain to be clarified.

Growth curves for FFM, FM, and percent body fat during childhood and adolescence are depicted in figure 4.3. These were derived by Malina and Bouchard from multiple sources and are based on measurements of TBW using age-specific estimates of body water content (24). Fat-free mass rises throughout childhood similarly in boys and girls until the age of puberty. The acceleration in FFM at this time in males reflects their augmented muscle mass at the adolescent growth spurt. The absence of an increase in FFM at puberty in females means that girls reach adult levels approximately 5 years before males, whose FFM matures at age 19-20 years.

Average fat mass in females is greater than in males from mid-childhood on. This difference becomes more obvious in the pubertal years as girls accumulate greater adipose tissue. Percent body fat slowly declines during early childhood in both sexes after an early jump in infancy. As puberty approaches, females demonstrate a progressive rise that continues throughout adolescence. Males, on the other hand, show a slight increase in relative fatness in the late prepubertal years; percent body fat then slowly declines, reflecting the development of

FFM at puberty. Consequently, females have greater percent body fat than males throughout childhood after age 3-4 years. In the late teen years, the average female has twice the relative fatness of her male counterpart.

Table 4.5 provides age-specific normative data for skinfold thickness sum (triceps plus subscapular) and BMI in United States children (21). Reflecting the relative fatness data described earlier relative to TBW, median skinfold sum changes little in males from age 9 through the teen years. During the same age span, the

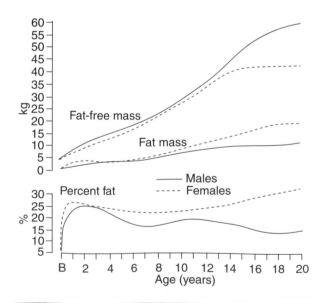

Figure 4.3   Changes in fat-free mass, fat mass, and relative fatness with growth. Data derived from measurements of total body water by various sources. Reprinted from Malina and Bouchard 1991.

Table 4.5 Body mass index (BMI) and sum of two skinfolds by age and gender for selected percentiles

| | BMI | | | | | | Sum of two skinfolds | | | | | |
| | 50th | | 85th | | 95th | | 50th | | 85th | | 95th | |
Age, years	M	F	M	F	M	F	M	F	M	F	M	F
6	15.4	15.2	16.8	17.1	18.2	18.5	12	14	16	19	20	27
7	15.6	15.4	17.1	17.6	18.9	19.6	12	15	17	22	24	28
8	16.0	15.9	18.1	18.6	20.2	21.1	13	16	19	25	28	36
9	16.2	16.3	19.0	19.5	22.4	22.9	14	17	23	29	34	41
10	16.5	16.9	19.2	20.6	21.8	23.6	14	18	24	32	33	43
11	17.2	17.5	20.9	21.7	24.2	24.8	15	19	28	31	39	43
12	17.8	18.6	21.4	22.6	24.1	26.2	15	20	24	34	44	47
13	18.7	19.4	22.6	23.4	26.6	26.8	15	21	28	39	46	52
14	19.6	20.2	23.2	24.1	26.7	26.5	14	24	27	37	39	53
15	20.4	20.7	24.0	24.7	27.8	29.4	14	25	25	41	40	56
16	20.8	20.9	24.0	24.9	26.9	29.6	14	26	24	42	39	58
17	21.5	21.0	24.9	24.3	28.5	29.3	15	27	26	42	41	59

Note: Calculations were derived using National Health Examination Survey norms (1963–1968).
Reprinted from Lohman 1992.

median skinfold sum increases by more than 50% in females. At age 17 the average sum in females is almost twice that of males.

The problems with use of BMI as a marker of fatness in children are highlighted if one examines the age-related norms in table 4.5 as compared to the trends identified by TBW and skinfold indices. Between ages 9 and 17 years the median BMI rises from 16.2 to 21.5 in males; this increase is almost identical to that in females (16.3 to 21.0). These data would lead one to the false conclusion that changes in fatness during adolescence are independent of gender.

INFLUENCE OF BODY COMPOSITION ON PHYSICAL FITNESS

Research data confirm the common observation that overly fat individuals perform poorly on exercise tasks, particularly weight-bearing activities. Watson described an average 46 yd decrement in distance covered in a 12 min walk/run test for each 1% increase in body fat in a group of adolescent boys (35). Boileau and Lohman reported that an increase in body fat from 15% to 30% in children resulted in a fall from the 10th to the 35th percentile in performance times in the 1-mile run (2). Slaughter et al. found that the zero-order coefficient between percent body fat and 1-mile run time in 7-12-

year-old girls (r = 0.55) was greater than that for weight, height, or age (34).

This prominent effect of body fat on physical performance may serve to confound the interpretation of exercise tests. For example, pull-ups, flexed arm hangs, and push-ups are considered tests of upper body muscle strength and endurance. But in a study of 9-11-year-old children, Woods et al. found that percent body fat accounted for a greater variance of performance on these tests than laboratory measures of muscle strength (i.e., one-repetition scores) (36).

In endurance tests, the 1-mile run has been considered an indicator of "cardiorespiratory fitness." However, Cureton suggested that body fatness and cardiorespiratory capacity each accounted for about 25% of the variance on mile run performance (8). That is, finish time in this test may be just as valid an indicator of body fatness as of cardiopulmonary function. This conclusion was supported by the finding of Cureton et al. of similar zero-order correlations between percent body fat and $\dot{V}O_2$max per FFM (considered an indicator of cardiac fitness) with mile run times of .45 and −.40, respectively, in a group of 7-12-year-old healthy children (10).

In a more recent study, Cureton et al. assessed the effect of accounting for body fat on performance on a 1-mile run/walk test in 12-year-old children (9). When finish scores were adjusted for percent body fat, percentile rank changed by more than 10 in 29% of girls and 39% of boys, and 11-14% of the subjects were placed in different pass/fail categories on criterion-referenced standards. As might be expected, the influence of body composition was greatest at the extremes of percent body fat. In a similar study, however, Pate et al. concluded that the degree of influence of body fat on mile run times was not sufficiently great to warrant adjustment of scores for percent fat (26). The reasons for the different results in these studies are uncertain.

Body fat may also significantly influence the results of laboratory exercise tests. Treadmill endurance times on the Bruce protocol published by Cumming et al. have been utilized as norms for aerobic fitness in children (7). In that study, though, the authors described a negative correlation between the ratio of weight to cube of body height (an indicator of "heaviness") and treadmill exercise time (r = .20-.47), suggesting that body fatness contributed significantly to endurance fitness in these subjects.

A consideration of the impact of body fat on fitness is also important in the design of therapeutic exercise programs for children with obesity. Obese youngsters are poorly "fit" in that they cannot perform as well as lean children in weight-bearing activities and have a lower $\dot{V}O_2$max per kg. But why? Several possible explanations have been suggested: (a) extra adipose tissue may simply act as an inert load, excess "baggage" that needs to be transported; (b) obesity might impair normal cardiac or ventilatory function; and (c) the obese child may have depressed aerobic fitness as the result of having adopted a sedentary life style.

Studies of mild-to-moderately obese children and adolescents have failed to indicate any evidence of physiological impairment during exercise. Absolute $\dot{V}O_2$max values are the same or even greater in obese compared to non-obese children (matched for height) (5, 16, 23, 29, 37), and submaximal economy ($\dot{V}O_2$ per kg) is unaffected (29). This evidence supports the conclusion that endurance performance and $\dot{V}O_2$max per kg are depressed in obese subjects because of the inert load created by excessive body fat rather than because of inferior cardiopulmonary functional capacity.

It is important from a therapeutic standpoint to make this distinction, since the means of improving cardiopulmonary fitness (i.e., aerobic training) and those of diminishing body fat (diet and increased physical activity) are very different. As Cureton et al. have pointed out, "It is misleading and may be physically and psychologically harmful to inform overfat children that they have poor cardiorespiratory capacity, based on poor running performance, if the primary problem is overfatness" (8, p. 153).

SUMMARY

The physiological responses to exercise in children must be understood in the context of the alterations in body composition during growth. Composition influences not only performance on physical tasks but also the means of relating physiological processes to changes in body size.

Information about the relative growth of the different body tissues during growth of the child is far from complete. Nonetheless, the understanding that children are different from adults, and that equations for relating various measurement techniques to body composition in mature individuals are not equally applicable to those who are growing, has been a major step. Children are not biochemically mature; specifically, changes in water and mineral content influence the density of the FFM during the process of growth. A two-compartment model therefore appears to be inappropriate for assessing body composition in children. A consideration of multiple components that alter body density is necessary in the construction of both laboratory and field measures of body composition during the pediatric years.

It has become clear, too, that equations for body composition by various measurement techniques often have a narrow applicability to the characteristics of the group under investigation. Further research in children is needed to determine the influence of factors such as race, gender, and athleticism on measures of body composition.

References

1. Armstrong, N.; Williams, J.; Balding, J.; Gentle, P.; Kirby, B. Cardiopulmonary fitness, physical activity patterns, and selected coronary risk factor variables in 11-to 16-year olds. Pediatr. Exerc. Science 3:219-228; 1991.
2. Boileau, R.A.; Lohman, T.G. The measurement of human physique and its effect on physical performance. Orthop. Clin. North Am. 8:563-572; 1977.
3. Boileau, R.A.; Lohman, T.G.; Slaughter, M.H.; Ball, T.E.; Going, S.B.; Hendrix, M.K. Hydration of the fat-free body in children during maturation. Hum. Biol. 56:651-666; 1984.
4. Boileau, R.A.; Lohman, T.G.; Slaughter, M.H.; Horswill, C.A.; Stillman, R.J. Problems associated with determining body composition in maturing youngsters. In: Brown, E.W.; Branta, C.F., eds. Competitive sports for children and youth. Champaign, IL: Human Kinetics; 1988:p. 3-16.
5. Cooper, D.M.; Poage, J.; Barstow, T.J.; Springer, C. Are obese children truly unfit? Minimizing the confounding effect of body size on the exercise response. J. Pediatr. 116:223-230; 1990.

6. Covington, N.K.; Kluka, D.A.; Love, P.A. Relationship between bioelectrical impedance and anthropometric techniques to determine body fat in a black pediatric population. Pediatr. Exerc. Science 2:140-148; 1990.

7. Cumming, G.R.; Everatt, D.; Hastman, L. Bruce treadmill test in children: normal values in a clinic population. Am. J. Cardiol. 41:69-75; 1978.

8. Cureton, K.J. Distance running performance tests in children. What do they mean? JOPERD 53:64-66; 1982.

9. Cureton, K.J.; Baumgartner, T.A.; McManis, B.G. Adjustment of 1-mile run/walk test scores for skinfold thickness in youth. Pediatr. Exerc. Science 3:152-167; 1991.

10. Cureton, K.J.; Boileau, R.A.; Lohman, T.G.; Misner, J.E. Determinants of distance running performance in children: analysis of a path model. Res. Q. 48:270-279; 1977.

11. DeLozier, M.G.; Gutin, B.; Wang, J.; Basch, C.E.; Contento, I.; Shea, S.; Irigoyen, M.; Zybert, P.; Rips, J.; Pierson, R. Validity of anthropometry and bioimpedance with 4- to 8-year olds using total body water as the criterion. Pediatr. Exerc. Science 3:238-249; 1991.

12. Fomon, S.J.; Haschke, F.; Ziegler, E.E.; Nelson, S.E. Body composition of reference children from birth to age 10 years. Am. J. Clin. Nutr. 35:1169-1175; 1982.

13. Hampton, M.C.; Huenemann, R.L.; Shapiro, L.R.; Mitchell, B.W.; Behnke, A.R. A longitudinal study of gross body composition and body conformation and their association with food and activity in a teen-age population. Am. J. Clin. Nutr. 19:422-435; 1966.

14. Houtkooper, L.B. Validity of whole-body impedance analysis for body composition assessment in non-obese and obese children and youth [dissertation]. Tucson, AZ: University of Arizona; 1986.

15. Houtkooper, L.B.; Lohman, T.G.; Going, S.B.; Hall, M.C. Validity of bioelectric impedance for body composition in children. J. Appl. Physiol. 66:814-821; 1989.

16. Huttunen, N.P.; Knip, M.; and Paavilainen, T. Physical activity and fitness in obese children. Int. J. Obesity 10:519-525; 1986.

17. Janz, K.F.; Nielsen, D.H.; Cassady, S.L.; Cook, J.S.; Wu, Y.; Hansen, J.R. Cross-validation of the Slaughter skinfold equations for children and adolescents. Med. Sci. Sports Exerc. 25:1070-1076; 1993.

18. Kwee, A.; Wilmore, J.H. Cardiorespiratory fitness and risk factors for coronary artery disease in 8- to 15-year old boys. Pediatr. Exerc. Science 2:372-383; 1990.

19. Lohman, T.G. Applicability of body composition techniques and constants for children and youths. Exerc. Sport Sci. Rev. 14:325-357; 1986.

20. Lohman, T.G. Assessment of body composition in children. Pediatr. Exerc. Science 1:19-30; 1989.

21. Lohman, T.G. Advances in body composition assessment. Champaign, IL: Human Kinetics; 1992.

22. Lohman, T.G.; Boileau, R.A.; Slaughter, M.H. Body composition in children and youth. In: Advances in pediatric sports sciences. Vol. 1, Boileau, R.A., ed. Biological issues. Champaign, IL: Human Kinetics; 1984:p. 29-57.

23. Maffeis, C.; Schena, F.; Zaffanello, M.; Zoccante, L.; Schutz, Y.; Pinelli, L. Maximal aerobic power during running and cycling in obese and non-obese children. Acta Paediatr. 83:113-116; 1994.

24. Malina, R.M.; Bouchard, C. Growth, maturation, and physical activity. Champaign, IL: Human Kinetics; 1991:p. 87-150.

25. Moulton, C.R. Age and chemical development in mammals. J. Biol Chem. 57:79-97; 1923.

26. Pate, R.; Slentz, C.; Katz, D. Relationships between skinfold thickness and performance on health-related fitness test items. Res. Q. Exerc. Sport 60:183-189; 1989.

27. Roche, A.F.; Siervogel, R.M.; Chumlea, W.C.; Webb, P. Grading fatness from limited anthropometric data. Am. J. Clin. Nutr. 34:2831-2838; 1981.

28. Rolland-Cachera, M.F.; Sempe, M.; Guilland-Bataille, M.; Patois, E.; Pequignot-Guggenbuhl, F.; Fautrod, V. Adiposity indices in children. Am. J. Clin. Nutr. 36:178-184; 1982.

29. Rowland, T.W. Effects of obesity on aerobic fitness in adolescent females. Am. J. Dis. Child. 145:764-768; 1991.

30. Rowland, T.W. Jack Sprat had it right. Pediatr. Exerc. Science 4:283-286; 1992.

31. Siri, W.E. The gross composition of the body. Adv. Biol. Med. Physics 4:239-280; 1956.

32. Slaughter, M.H.; Lohman, T.G.; Boileau, R.A.; Horswill, C.A.; Stillman, R.H.; Van Loan, M.D.; Bemben, D.A. Skinfold equations for estimation of body fatness in children and youth. Hum. Biol. 60:709-723; 1988.

33. Slaughter, M.H.; Lohman, T.G.; Boileau. R.A.; Stillman, R.J.; Van Loan, M.; Horswill, C.A.; Wilmore, J.H. Influence of maturation on relationship of skinfolds to body density: a cross-sectional study. Hum. Biol. 56:681-689; 1984.

34. Slaughter, M.H.; Lohman, T.G.; Misner, J.E. Association of somatotype and body composition to physical performance in 7-12 year-old girls. J. Sports Med. 20:189-198; 1980.

35. Watson, A.W.S. Quantification of the influence of the body fat content on selected physical performance variables in adolescent boys. Ir. J. Med. Sci. 157:383-384; 1988.

36. Woods, J.A.; Pate, R.R.; Burgess, M.L. Correlates to performance on field tests of muscular strength. Pediatr. Exerc. Science 4:302-311; 1992.

37. Zanconato, S.; Baraldi, E.; Santuz, P. Gas exchange during exercise in obese children. Eur. J. Pediatr. 148:614-617; 1989.

CHAPTER 5

ETHICAL ASPECTS OF RESEARCH WITH CHILDREN

It would be most useful if the developmental physiologist could place cardiac catheters in the pulmonary arteries of children, or obtain serial muscle biopsies with exercise, or have young subjects cycle in extreme climatic conditions. If this were so, we would be far ahead in our knowledge of the influences of maturation on cardiac output, glycogen utilization, and thermoregulation during exercise. But ethical considerations say "no"— these procedures are inappropriate in healthy children.

Such limitations create serious constraints on progress in our understanding of developmental exercise physiology, but there is little argument about their importance (2, 36, 37, 38). Children are recognized as a special group of research subjects, characterized by vulnerability and a limited capacity to comprehend. Most importantly, minors are not legally able to consent in their own right to serve as study participants. While it is accepted that the rights and well-being of children as experimental subjects must be assured, there is also a keen awareness of the vital need for continued research efforts in the pediatric age group. Attempts to appropriately balance these two considerations in the exercise testing laboratory have raised many difficult questions:

1. How can we ethically justify the use of children as subjects in research from which they receive no direct benefit (nontherapeutic research)? In such a case, how can the rights of the child, who cannot legally agree to serve as a research subject, be reconciled with the potential benefits of research to the well-being of the general childhood society?

2. Most published guidelines accept that children can legitimately serve as research subjects in studies involving no significant risk, as will be discussed in a later section of this chapter. But what does this mean? We would have no difficulty with protocols that called for urine collection or the use of physical activity questionnaires. Conversely, there would be no inclination to enroll healthy children in research involving liver biopsies or pulmonary artery balloon catheters. But what about serial venipuncture, interviews regarding sexual habits, or prolonged bed rest? Where does the ethical researcher draw the line?

3. How does research that might prove directly helpful to the child (i.e., therapeutic research such as evaluation of cardiac rehabilitation) alter the ethical issue of the risk:benefit ratio for the subjects?

4. How does one secure from the parent or guardian a truly informed permission for a child's participation in research? At what age is it important that the child's assent also be obtained? Can the child be forced to be a participant in a study if he or she refuses?

5. What are the legal implications (particularly to the investigator) of ethical decisions with respect to a child's participation as a research subject?

These are the questions this chapter will address. They are outgrowths of debates surrounding broader ethical issues about human research that have been in progress for centuries. Predictably, then, the questions have no simple answers, or perhaps no answers at all. Ethical concepts have evolved in response to cultural expectations that have altered dramatically with time; what researchers "ought to do" at the turn of the 21st century is different from what was expected of their counterparts 50 years ago or will be 50 years from now. This fact does not, of course, minimize the fundamental importance of recognizing ethical constraints on human research, and the struggle to come to terms with these issues is essential to conducting sound scientific investigation.

Indeed, such concerns cannot be easily ignored. Developmental exercise physiologists are surrounded by constraints regarding the ethical conduct of their research. Human experimentation committees will not approve ethically questionable studies, and journal editors and reviewers will not agree to publish them. Knowledgeable parents will refuse permission for their children to participate in such projects, and children will not allow themselves to be subjected to inappropriate procedures.

It is the investigator, however, who bears the major responsibility for the ethical conduct of the study. It is unethical to recruit subjects for studies that are poorly planned or that are based on a vague or weak scientific premise. In agreeing to participate as research subjects, children (and parents) place their faith in the investigator and in the scientific importance and soundness of the study. It is presumed that the investigator is competent and that the methodology is appropriate. It is assumed that all efforts will be made to reduce risks and that the subjects will be treated in a humane manner. In other words, the ethical responsibility that the investigator bears toward research subjects, particularly children, begins with "good" science.

HISTORICAL PERSPECTIVE

The roots of our current views of ethical behavior in the conduct of research in human beings can be traced back as far as the first century (16). In his historical review, Claude Bernard cited the comment of Celsius, defending the vivisection of condemned prisoners by the Egyptians Herophilus and Erasistratus: "It is not cruel to inflict on a few criminals sufferings which may benefit multitudes of innocent people throughout all centuries" (3, p. 100). The opposing viewpoint, articulated by Bernard himself 1800 years later, set the stage for the ethical controversy that persists to the present day: "The principle of medical and surgical morality consists in never performing on man an experiment which might be harmful to him to any extent, even though the result might be highly advantageous to science, i.e., to the health of others" (3, p. 101). His was the argument familiar to physicians as that sacred dictum of medical practice, *primum non nocere*—first do no harm.

The potential conflict in the research laboratory between the rights of the individual and the welfare of society became magnified after World War II. On the one hand, the fruits of biomedical research were dramatic: the prevention of polio, antibiotics, open heart surgery, the cracking of the genetic code. The value of scientific research to the well-being of society was indisputable. There followed, however, a series of troubling events that led to increasing distrust by the public of scientific

research, particularly the motives of its investigators and abuses of the rights of subjects. Most prominent among these was the discovery of experiments conducted by German physicians on concentration camp prisoners during World War II. In the war crime trials that followed, the Nuremberg Code was written to establish criteria for judging those physicians, and it subsequently served as a set of guidelines for humane and ethical experimentation as articulated in later documents (such as the Declaration of Helsinki in 1964) (10, 28). Not surprisingly, these codes placed heavy emphasis on the rights of the individual serving as a research subject, most specifically the absolute necessity of the subject's permission to participate. These documents did not specifically address children as research subjects.

In the United States, increasing mistrust of scientific research followed reports that antibiotic treatment of 300 black males with syphilis had been withheld in the Tuskegee Syphilis Study, and that cancer cells had been injected into senile patients at the Jewish Chronic Diseases Hospital without their knowledge. And in the 1960s, it was reported that mentally retarded children at the Willowbrook State Hospital in Staten Island, New York, had been deliberately infected with viral hepatitis (4).

In response to these events, the National Commission for the Protection of Human Subjects of Biomedical and Behavioral Research was created in 1974 as directed by the National Research Act. After extensive deliberations, the commission published a set of proposed guidelines that for the first time specifically examined the ethical issues surrounding the use of children as experimental subjects (26). The commission's report underscored several key concepts that are important in the ethical conduct of research in children:

1. A pivotal role of the institutional review board (IRB) at the research site was identified as a means of critically evaluating the ethical and scientific merits of research. As noted by Pearn, "The ethical obligation is on the individual researcher to take the case to a higher objective authority, and this custom is never more important than in research involving children" (30, p. 510). The proposed guidelines indicated that such authority should exist as a committee of peers, or nonscientific individuals (lawyers, ethicists, chaplains) within the institution, who review the ethical appropriateness of the study proposed. Such a group is "collectively disinterested from the point of view of the proposed research but not from the point of view of the child" (30, p. 510).

2. The commission emphasized examination of the risk:benefit ratio as a means of determining the ethical grounds of research in children. In doing so it sep-

arated out the influences of therapeutic (for the subject's benefit) versus nontherapeutic research on ethical decision-making.

3. The requirement of informed proxy consent by parents for research on minors was reaffirmed. This was termed parental "permission" in order to differentiate it from "consent" (for one's own participation). In addition, the guidelines supported the child's involvement in the permission process by indicating the need to acquire the child's "assent" (nonlegal consent) above a certain age.

The commission's recommendations were subsequently formulated as regulations for projects funded by the Department of Health and Human Services (HHS), and later standards created by the Food and Drug Administration (FDA) essentially mirrored these two prior documents (32, 33). In Europe, the British Paediatric Association in 1978 created a Working Party on Ethics of Research in Children. The published guidelines created by this group were designed to "aid ethical committees considering research involving children" (41). The perspective of this group is evident from its premise that "research which involves a child and is of no benefit to that child is not necessarily either unethical or illegal" (p. 229).

PRINCIPLES OF ETHICAL RESEARCH

While specific research protocols and types of subjects may influence ethical judgements by investigators and IRBs, three basic principles are considered to dictate the appropriateness of research involving human subjects: respect for persons, beneficence, and justice (26).

1. *Respect for persons* includes the concepts that (1) individuals should be respected for their autonomy and (2) those who do not have autonomy (e.g., children, the mentally ill, prisoners) need to be protected. Since the autonomous person is capable of dictating his or her own actions and goals, the choice of that individual to participate (or not) in research activities needs to be recognized. As illustrated particularly in the case of children, lack of autonomy is not absolute but varies from those with no self-determination (babies) to individuals capable of making mature decisions but not legally able to do so (older adolescents). The degree to which these people need to be protected relates to both the extent of their autonomy and the amount of risk and benefit in the research situation.

2. *Beneficence* refers to the humane conduct of research. The ethical investigator goes beyond legal and scientific obligations to the subjects to act in a kind and charitable manner, making all efforts to avoid harm and assuring their well-being. This again reflects the Hippocratic dictum of "first do no harm."

The principles of respect for persons and beneficence are both expressions of the concepts of moral duty as found in the philosophy of Immanuel Kant: "Act so as to treat humanity, whether in your own person, or in that of another, always as an end and never as a means only" (20, p. 47).

According to Kant, then, the investigator has a primary responsibility to respect the research subject as a valuable human being; the subject should never be "used" for the goal of obtaining scientific information (34).

It is important to note, however, that the principle of beneficence is not necessarily restricted to individuals serving in a given research project; it might also be taken to apply to the general concept of the ethical responsibility of research to benefit society. John Stuart Mill contended, "Actions are right in proportion as they tend to promote happiness; wrong as they tend to produce the reverse of happiness" (25, p. 10).

From this utilitarian viewpoint, then, research that causes risk or discomfort to individual subjects could be justified by the benefit that it might offer a larger number of people in the future (as in the trial of a new drug or surgical procedure) (34). This of course directly contradicts Kant's concept that it is unethical to place the individual at risk of harm for the sake of benefit to others.

3. *Justice* dictates that the risks and benefits of research are fairly assumed by the population. Injustice occurs in research when certain populations of people (prisoners, institutionalized persons) are utilized as subjects simply because of their easy availability. Likewise, the benefits of research, particularly that provided by public funding, should not be limited to those who have easy access to these benefits or those who can afford to pay for them. Subjects in research studies should, in general, represent the population that is likely to be benefited. This means that children should serve as subjects only in research studies that address issues pertinent to the pediatric age group.

SHOULD CHILDREN ACT AS RESEARCH SUBJECTS?

The Nuremberg Code states quite unequivocally that "the voluntary consent of the human subject is absolutely essential" and that the subject "should have legal capacity to give consent . . . [and] sufficient knowledge and comprehension [of the research project] to make an understanding and enlightened decision" (28,

p. 229). The Helsinki Declaration reaffirmed that "subjects should be volunteers" and that "in research on man the interest of science and society should never take precedence over considerations related to the well being of the subject" (10, p. 232). The 1963 statement of the Medical Research Council in Great Britain indicates that "investigations that are of no direct benefit to the individual require therefore that his true consent to them shall be explicitly obtained" (24, p. 23).

On a literal interpretation of these guidelines, it is impossible for children to ethically participate as subjects in research that does not hold any promise for their direct benefit. Children have no legal right to provide consent for such participation, and it is assumed that in most cases (depending on age and maturity) children have a limited capacity for fully understanding the nature of the experimental study as well as their personal risks in volunteering—thereby violating both bedrock principles of the ethical use of subjects in scientific research.

Paul Ramsey, a professor of bioethics at Princeton University, has been a strong proponent of this viewpoint and argues against the ethical use of children as exercise subjects, even if the risk is small. He fears this would lead to "accordion morality," with ethical guidelines for research being expanded and contracted to satisfy the goals of the research study without regard for the rights and needs of the experimental subjects (9, p. 322).

Such a position would, of course, prove highly detrimental to the pediatric population. Without such nontherapeutic research we would be deprived of a long list of biomedical advances that have clearly improved the health and well-being of children: early investigations of vaccine efficacy, studies that established normal values for blood lead levels, and work that made it possible to determine expected skeletal development via wrist x-rays, for example. That society needs and desires information obtainable only through nontherapeutic experimentation on children is indisputable. An argument for eliminating human experimentation that involves minimal risk to subjects, thus denying benefits to the whole of a population, would have little popular support.

The involvement of children as subjects in nontherapeutic research has been justified on such philosophical grounds. As members of society, often people are seen as having a moral obligation to contribute to the general welfare when little or no personal sacrifice is involved. McCormick contended, "There are some things that all of us, simply as members of the human community, ought to do for others. . . . We can establish a baseline and discover works that involve no notable disadvantage to individuals yet offer genuine hope for the general benefit. It is good for all of us to share in these . . . and hence we ought to want these benefits for others"

(23, p. 16). According to this premise, people can ethically participate as subjects in research that offers no personal benefit if the research "fulfills an important social need" (21, p. 237). But whether or not children possess this same moral obligation to contribute to the welfare of society is a matter of debate (21). Labeling this idea "forced samaritanism," VanDeVeer argued that "even if a given child may develop into an adult who would readily choose to incur such burdens, we simply lack adequate grounds for assuming that any particular child would welcome such burdens if he were capable of choosing" (40, p. 283).

How can we ethically reconcile these two points of view—that of the vulnerable child needing protection, incapable legally or intellectually of accepting risk for research that offers no personal benefit, versus that of the pediatric population, to whose welfare scientific research is so important? One approach would be to consider, in light of the risks and benefits of the research study, whether the child would be expected to consent to serve as a subject if he or she were an adult. By having a parent give permission for the child to participate, one could reasonably presume this would be the child's wishes (9). In other words, would a "reasonable person" be likely to consent?

Redmon pointed out that it would difficult to determine how altruistic such a "reasonable person" would be in any given moral situation, yet stated that "it does make sense to ask how a person with a particular moral outlook, particular values, virtues and vices, would act. Thus the prediction of how the child would later view his participation must be made by those in the child's family, in particular by his parents" (34, p. 81). As an example Redmon cites the children who participated in the first polio vaccine trials, presumably now as adults are proud of their involvement and pleased that their parents allowed them to serve as subjects.

Beyond future pride, there are certain other potential benefits to children who serve as subjects in nontherapeutic research. They learn how scientific research is conducted; serving as a research subject can be viewed as an educational experience. In the case of exercise physiology research, children may gain information about their levels of physical fitness. Redmon notes that participation by children in research can also be viewed as part of their moral education. "We certainly encourage our children to perform acts of benevolence when there is little chance of harm (walking down the road to take an invalid some food), and if the purposes of the research are understood well enough by the child, her participation might be viewed in the same way" (p. 81).

Another approach to ethical decision-making in recruiting children as research subjects has been termed the "golden rule" guideline (6). As Campbell states, "Though this can be a fallible guide, the investigator should ask himself as honestly as he can if this is an experiment to which he would freely submit his own child if appropriate. Are the risks that small? If he feels hesitant or uncomfortable about this question he should not proceed" (5, p. 336).

The HHS regulations on government-sponsored research in children in the United States occupy an ethical middle road based on two considerations: (a) a balance of the risks of participation as a research subject against the study's potential benefits (to the subject as well as to society as a whole) and (b) the appropriateness of proxy consent by the child's parent or guardian. Since this document contains key guidelines for human research committees, it is appropriate to address these issues within the framework of the HHS regulations.

CONSIDERATION OF THE RISK: BENEFIT RATIO

For the purposes of ethical decision-making, the HHS guidelines define four categories of research based on considerations of relative risk and benefit.

1. **Research involving only minimal risk.** According to the HHS guidelines, it is appropriate for children to participate in such research regardless of whether the subject directly benefits or whether the benefit is to society as a whole. Most research in developmental exercise physiology fits into this category, yet it is the thorny issue of defining "minimal risk" that creates difficulties for assessing the ethical limits of research on children. Minimal risk is defined by the HHS and FDA as the "probability and magnitude of physical or psychological harm that is normally encountered in the daily lives or in the routine medical, dental, or psychological examination of healthy children" (27, p. 123). Examples would include urine collection, physical examinations, venipuncture, standard psychological and educational testing, behavioral observations, echocardiograms, electrocardiograms, electroencephalograms, and allergy scratch tests.

Even this reasonably straightforward definition has its difficulties. For instance, the risk encountered in daily living might be considered different by people of different socioeconomic status and in various geographical environments (e.g., farm vs. inner city) (22). And the distinction between the likelihood of an adverse event's occurring versus its potential magnitude is not recognized. The risk in taking an airplane flight is very small in terms of the statistical chance of a crash, but very high in terms of the probable outcome of such an event. On the other hand, the risk of getting sunburn from lying on the beach for an after-

noon is high, but the dangers of the consequences are small. Whether these situations would conform to the definition of minimal risk in the guidelines is uncertain.

2. **Research involving greater than minimal risk with no prospect of direct benefits to individual subjects.** Research to be approved in this category must comply with the following:

A. "The risk represents only a minor increase over minimal risk" (p. 123). No definition of minor increment above minimal risk is provided, and it is left to the individual IRB to determine whether or not the extent of added risk is justified by the information that might be obtained from the study.

B. "The intervention or procedure presents experiences to subjects that are reasonably commensurate with those inherent in their actual or expected medical, dental, psychological, social or educational institutions" (p. 123). Levine offers an example: "It might be appropriate to invite a child with leukemia who has had several bone marrow examinations to consider having another for research purposes. It would be more difficult to justify extending a similar invitation to normal children. This requirement will make it difficult to develop normal control data for examinations and other procedures that present more than minimal risk" (21, p. 248).

C. "The procedure is likely to yield generalizable knowledge about the subjects' disorder which is of vital importance for the understanding of the disorder" (p. 124). Again, the difficulty of defining the importance of a given research project is left in the hands of the IRB.

3. **Research involving greater than minimal risk but presenting the prospect of direct benefit to the individual subjects.** Medical research involving children with serious illness fits into this category (organ biopsies, use of experimental drugs). Physiologic investigations might include studies such as the direct measurement of left ventricular pressure during exercise using new cardiac catheters in patients with aortic valve disease. Investigational review boards make decisions regarding research in this category by balancing the risks assumed by the subjects against the potential benefits to accrue. Included in this consideration is a recognition of the experience a given institution or group of researchers has with a particular procedure. As in the previous example, experimental cardiac catheterization for the patient's benefit might be readily approved in a large children's hospital that performs this procedure four times daily but not in an institution with little previous experience.

4. **Research beyond greater than minimal risk that presents an opportunity to understand, prevent, or alleviate a serious problem affecting the health and welfare of children.** The guidelines indicate that these projects should be reviewed by governmental agencies at the national level. Few studies have fallen into this category. O'Sullivan noted that if the regulations had been in effect at the time of the Salk vaccine trials, ethical considerations of use of children would have led to lengthy governmental review under this section.

The guidelines created by the British Working Party were also based principally on a consideration of the risk:benefit ratio for any given research procedure (40). Whereas the categories of risk were somewhat different from those in the HHS regulations, the end result of balancing risk and benefit in a continuum is not dissimilar from what follows from the guidelines in the United States.

O'Sullivan contended that the concentration on categories of risk in these guidelines could be unfortunate because such emphasis may cause review boards to focus too much on the risk aspects of the risk:benefit ratio (29). The result could be that some IRBs could become too restrictive in approving research involving children, precluding research to the benefit of future children that can be performed only in the pediatric population.

CONSENT BY PROXY

No federal or state laws exist to determine the age at which children can legally participate as research subjects, and age for consent to medical care (usually 18 years) is commonly used instead. Before this age, the child needs the permission of parent or guardian to serve as a research subject. Under the HHS guidelines, "permission" is considered in this situation rather than "consent," as the latter implies the legal volunteering of oneself for participation. In research on children, then, the young subject participates by the process of "consent by proxy" (12).

As noted previously, this concept has not gained universal acceptance by ethicists. VanDeVeer observed that an action taken by person A "by proxy" for person B (as in casting a vote) implies, first, that B has authorized A to take the action and, second, that the will of B is known to A (40). In the case of a parent's approving participation of a small child as a research subject, neither is true. The child has not authorized the parent to speak on her behalf, and the informed opinion of the child (particularly of an infant) is unknown.

Holder has pointed out, however, that outside the context of medical research, parents are routinely given the power to allow their children to participate in activities that involve minor risk:

> As many child custody cases indicate, a parent who is so neurotic as to forbid a child's participation in normal activities to protect the child from injury or germs is quite likely to lose custody on the ground that such overprotection is harmful to the child. If a parent can consent to a child's participation in Little League football, where statistics show that a variety of serious injuries or even death can occur, it seems unlikely that any court would rule that the same parent has no authority to allow the same child to have a blood sample drawn by a licensed physician because the blood will be used in research of no direct benefit to the child. (15, p. 152)

It is important to recognize that enrolling a child as a research subject on the basis of parent permission assumes that the parent is acting in the best interests of the child (i.e., that the child-parent relationship is a loving one). VanDeVeer points out that this cannot be assumed a priori (40). A parent's permission is necessary for research on children, but obtaining such permission does not necessarily imply that such research can be performed ethically. It falls to the investigator to judge whether or not a parent is capable of providing permission as an appropriate advocate of the child.

The exception to need for parental permission is the case of "emancipated minors," defined in many states as those considered to have reached adult status through such means as marriage, childbearing, or military service. In addition, considerable attention has been focused on the question of the ability of "nonemancipated" older adolescents to provide consent for either their own medical care or participation as research subjects before the age of majority (see discussion in a later section).

The HHS guidelines state that the permission of only one parent is necessary except in the category of research involving more than minimal risk without benefit to the individual subject, in which case the permission of both parents should be obtained. The guidelines also recommend that parents be present when small children are participating in research that involves physical or emotional discomfort.

Permission from the parent assumes that details of the research project, including risks, benefits, and procedures, have been fully explained by the investigator. The appropriate content of the consent form has been outlined elsewhere (21). The parent should not feel intimidated by the investigator and should be given an opportunity to refuse to have the child participate. Pearn suggested that such intimidation is easily conveyed in personal conversation and that it is more appropriate to initiate a request for the child's participation in a letter to the parents (30). After the initial letter it is desirable to have a meeting with parents to allow them to ask questions about the project.

In addition to parental permission, the HHS regulations call for "assent" of the child to participate as a research subject. This is based on the concept that although not legally able to consent, children should be able to express the wish to participate or not. They should be told what will happen during the study, whether there will be any discomfort, and how long it will last; they should also be told that they can stop participating if they wish (29).

It is not clear at what age a child should be capable of giving assent. The original proposal of the national commission indicated that assent should be obtained from all children over the age of 7 years. The later HHS document recommended only that the investigator judge the child's ability to assent on the basis of level of maturity. Giertz noted that in Sweden, no particular age has been identified at which the child should be consulted; instead, this is decided on a case-by-case basis depending on the child's level of maturity and understanding (13).

In any event, the properly constructed permission form for research on children should have two signature lines (besides those for the principal investigator and witness) for the child and parent. It is not necessary that the child sign, but, as Levine emphasizes (21), signing the consent form enhances the child's sense of participation in the study.

What happens if the child refuses to participate even though the parent has given permission? Unless the outcome of the procedure will benefit the child, the recommendation is to yield to the child's wishes. On the other hand, if significant benefit is expected, the assent of the child is not necessary as long as the parent's permission has been obtained. An exception to this recommendation may occur in research involving older adolescents. Legal trends toward permitting minors to consent to medical treatment may allow their wishes to prevail in the research setting as well (15). There is growing consensus that defining the legal age of consent arbitrarily as the 18th birthday is inappropriate; instead, the legal right for self-determination may be influenced by other factors such as the individual's level of maturity, the right to privacy, and financial status. As Levine noted, "These judgements become more complicated as the child gets older or as the stakes get higher" (21, p. 251).

Ackerman argued that considerations of proper assent of the child are irrelevant because children will usually simply follow the course of action dictated by their parents (1). Ackerman thought this appropriate in most cases since it is the obligation of parents to direct their children in responsible conduct:

> We are obligated to encourage, direct, advise, and even sometimes "coerce" children to engage in activities that will contribute to their becoming the right kind of persons. If participation in nontherapeutic clinical research is viewed as something that a good person does, then involvement of a child in it might be similarly directed. . . . Standing back and asking the child to make up his own mind—without an attempt to encourage or discourage—is quite foreign to our duties to guide children. (p. 346)

LEGAL ASPECTS

It would help scientific investigators if they could find recourse in legal guidelines for determining the ethical conduct of research in children. Unfortunately, such law "is unwritten, untested by any relevant cases, and apparently largely dependent on current medical and public opinion of what is reasonable. If the law does not hinder us in carrying out what we have regarded as reasonable research, it does not help us either in deciding what *is* reasonable. The responsibility is back with us" (35, p. 441).

Some have contended that a strict interpretation of the law would hold that all nontherapeutic experimental procedures on minor subjects are illegal (11). This follows from the principle that parents are legally obligated to ensure protection of the child's best interests. For example, Dworkin (11) cites a 1944 decision by the United States Supreme Court (in the context of the right of parents to permit their children to sell religious literature on the street): "Parents may be free to become martyrs themselves. But it does not follow [that] they are free, in identical circumstances, to make martyrs of their children before they have reached the age of full and legal discretion when they can make that choice for themselves" (31, p. 158).

Dworkin argued, however, that there was strong sentiment that the law should take a less strict view of experimentation on children. In a 1972 article entitled "Law as a System of Control," Jaffe wrote:

> Judges are sensitive to the ethos of the times. Our society places a high premium on scientific experimentation and the pursuit of knowledge. . . . We should proceed on the hypothesis . . . that in framing our ethical principles the common law will be

hospitable to procedures that recognize the social value of human experimentation without sacrificing the interests of patients and subjects. (18, p. 207)

Skegg provided illustrations in British and Canadian law that he felt supported the view that parents as well as children themselves can legally give consent to participate as research subjects. He cited a 1970 judgment in the House of Lords that a parent could give legal consent for blood tests on a child for forensic purposes (38). Skegg added, "It would be a mistake to exaggerate the scope of lawful non-therapeutic experimentation which this development opens up. It is, for example, extremely unlikely that a court would accept that a reasonable parent would agree to a liver biopsy or cardiac catheterization where there was no prospect of benefit to the child" (p. 755). It seems likely, in other words, that the courts' rulings on such matters would be similar to the HHS guidelines.

These discussions did, in fact, take place before the creation of any of the federal regulations reviewed earlier in this chapter. The force of such guidelines for ethical conduct of government-sponsored research in formulating the future legal viewpoint of research involving child subjects will presumably be prominent.

Currently, scattered state statutes may affect certain aspects of human research (see Hershey and Miller [14] for a review). But Hershey and Miller point out that a variety of legal concerns beyond these few delineated constraints could potentially affect the conduct of research with child subjects (14). For example, an editorial in *The Lancet* raised the unpleasant specter that until legal rulings are pronounced, research workers dealing with children *could* be acting illegally and even be at risk for charges of assault in carrying out their studies (7). It was emphasized that the actions of IRBs and ethics committees do not have legal force. Thus while researchers and IRBs seek to delineate ethical bounds for studies involving children, there are legal implications to their actions that have not yet been tested in the courts.

SPECIAL CONSIDERATIONS

Three practical questions surrounding appropriate procedures in conducting research in children deserve special discussion. These all concern investigations in which the child cannot be expected to benefit from the study's findings. Obtaining blood specimens is critical to many areas of pediatric research, yet the invasive nature of this procedure has led to concern. Even more reluctance surrounds the use of radiation (x-rays, injection

of radioactive-labeled materials) in nontherapeutic research in children. Finally, whether it is appropriate to offer children rewards for participation as research subjects is controversial—is this an unethical incentive or a reward for good work done?

Venipuncture

The commission proposal of 1974 specifically identified venipuncture as a permissible procedure for research with children under the definition of minimal risk. By these standards, then, obtaining blood samples from pediatric subjects is ethical in nontherapeutic research. Adverse effects of venipuncture are limited to minor discomfort, bruising, and, rarely, syncope; the commission considered such risks compatible with the "probability and magnitude of physical and psychological harm that is normally encountered in the daily lives or in the routine medical, dental, or psychological examination of healthy children" (26, p. 123).

Results of a questionnaire assessment of opinions of pediatric researchers supported the idea that venipuncture is a minimal-risk procedure that can be ethically justified in nontherapeutic research (19). Of the 91 respondents, 98% rated venipuncture at the antecubital fossa as either a no-risk or minimal-risk procedure for children over the age of 5 years.

Smith contended that anxiety created by venipuncture might even prove beneficial to children (39). She assessed possible negative effects through a questionnaire administered to parents after their children had undergone phlebotomy. In most cases, no difficulties were reported. In fact, 83% of the parents felt that the experience would prove beneficial to the child in the event that a blood sample needed to be taken in the future. And 40% felt that their child had a greater sense of confidence about facing subsequent visits to a doctor or dentist.

Radiation

Many investigators assume that the use of x-rays and radioactive materials in nontherapeutic research in children is strictly forbidden. Considering the perceived potential adverse effects of such radiation, IRBs (and parents) would be unlikely to allow these procedures in normal healthy children who would receive no benefit from the research.

However, the International Commission on Radiological Protection has stated, "The irradiation, for the purposes of such studies (that is, of no direct benefit to the subject) of children and other persons regarded as being incapable of giving their true consent should only be undertaken if the expected radiation is low (for example, of the order of one-10th of the dose-equivalent limits applicable to individual members of the public) and if valid approval has been given by those legally responsible for such persons" (17). The Working Party on Ethics of Research in Children interpreted this to mean that exposure to x-rays would be justifiable in such situations if the radiation dosage was "comparable to the normal variation in natural irradiation received by, say, individuals living in two different parts of the British Isles" (41, p. 230).

The typical radiation dose from a single chest x-ray is approximately 30-50 millirems, which is one-third of the annual dose from background natural radiation in most locations. Natural external radiation varies from 41 to 105 millirems annually in the United States depending on geographical site, and the radiation exposure from simply eating food is about 25 millirems a year. It has been estimated that the health risk from an x-ray of the chest is 1/20th that associated with an automobile trip across the United States (8).

Financial Incentives

Do financial rewards and prizes offered to children for research participation constitute unethical conduct? Pearn contended that although perhaps appropriate on some occasions for adult subjects, "[payment] must never be given under any circumstances if children are involved" (30, p. 510). The rationale for this stand was stated in the proposal of the National Commission for the Protection of Human Subjects: "Undue influence . . . occurs through an offer of an excessive, unwarranted, inappropriate or improper reward or other overture in order to obtain compliance. Also, inducements that would ordinarily be acceptable may become undue influences if the subject is particularly vulnerable" (26, p. 6).

In reality, however, such incentives are commonly given to children, and it would be easy to cite multiple references in the contemporary research literature as examples. It is this author's feeling that appropriate payment or prizes are justified to reward the child for hard work and minor discomfort *if* all other ethical considerations of the study are met.

SUMMARY

Considerations regarding the ethical conduct of research are especially pertinent in studies involving children. Child subjects are viewed as particularly vulnerable because they cannot legally consent to participate and also are less likely than adults to understand the ramifications of allowing themselves to serve as experimental subjects.

The principal responsibility of the investigator is to avoid placing the young subject at jeopardy for physical or psychological harm. At the same time, however, there is a pressing obligation to conduct research involving children that can result in the improved health and well-being of the pediatric population. A balancing of these considerations has led to the acceptance of research that poses minimal risk to young participants. Steps to assure an appropriate risk:benefit ratio in experiments with children must include: (1) review of the proposed study by a nonbiased research committee, (2) creation of a scientifically sound investigation by the researcher, and (3) informed permission by responsible parent or guardian.

References

1. Ackerman, T.F. Fooling ourselves with child autonomy and assent in non-therapeutic clinical research. Clin. Res. 27:345-348; 1979.
2. Bar-Or, O. The growth and development of children's physiologic and perceptional responses to exercise. In: Ilmarinen, J.; Valimaki, I., eds. Children and sport. Berlin: Springer-Verlag; 1984:p. 3-17.
3. Bernard, C. An introduction to the study of experimental medicine. New York: Dover; 1957.
4. Brady, J.V.; Jonsen, A.R. The evolution of regulatory influences on research with human subjects. In: Greenwald, R.A.; Ryan, M.K.; Mulvihill, J.E., eds. Human subjects research. New York: Plenum Press; 1982:p. 3-18.
5. Campbell, A.G.M. Infants, children and informed consent. Br. Med. J. 3:334-338; 1974.
6. Clinical research on children. J. Med. Ethics 8:3-4; 1982.
7. Clouds over paediatric research. Lancet 2:771-772; 1978.
8. Cohen, B.L.; Lee, I. A catalog of risks. Health Physics 36:707-722; 1979.
9. Comiskey, R.J. The use of children for medical research: opposite views examined. Child Welfare 57:321-324; 1978.
10. Declaration of Helsinki 1964, The, revised 1975. In: Greenwald, R.A.; Ryan, M.K.; Mulvihill, J.E., eds. Human subjects research. New York: Plenum Press; 1982:p. 231-233.
11. Dworkin, G. Legality of consent to non-therapeutic medical research on infants and young children. Arch. Dis. Child. 53:443-446; 1978.
12. Gaylin, W.; Macklin, R. Who speaks for the child? The problems of proxy consent. New York: Plenum Press; 1982.

13. Giertz, G. Ethical aspects of paediatric research. Acta Paediatr. Scand. 72:641-650; 1983.
14. Hershey, N.; Miller, R.D. Human experimentation and the law. Germantown, MD: Aspen Systems Corporation; 1976.
15. Holder, A.R. Legal issues in pediatrics and adolescent medicine. 2nd ed. New Haven, CT: Yale University Press; 1985.
16. Howard-Jones, N. Human experimentation in historical and ethical perspectives. Soc. Sci. Med. 16:1429-1448; 1982.
17. International Commission on Radiological Protection. Ann. Int. Commis. Radiol. Protect. 1:37; 1977.
18. Jaffe, L.L. Law as a system of control. In: Freund, P.A., ed. Experimentation with human subjects. London: Allen and Unwin; 1972.
19. Janofsky, J.; Starfield, B. Assessment of risk in research on children. J. Pediatr. 98:842-846; 1981.
20. Kant, I. Foundations of the metaphysics of morals. New York: Bobbs-Merrill; 1959. Translated by L.W. Beck.
21. Levine, R.J. Ethics and regulation of clinical research. 2nd ed. Baltimore: Urban & Schwarzenberg; 1986.
22. McCartney, J.J. Research on children: national commission says, "yes, if . . ." Hastings Center Rep. 8:531-540; 1978.
23. McCormick, R. Proxy consent in the experimental situation. Perspec. Biol. Med. 14:16-17; 1974.
24. Medical Research Council. Annual report 1962-63. London: HMSO; 1963:p. 21-25.
25. Mill, J.S. Utilitarianism. New York: Bobbs-Merrill; 1957.
26. National Commission. The Belmont reports: ethical guidelines for the protection of human subjects of research. DHEW publication (OS) 78-0010; 1978.
27. National Commission for the Protection of Human Subjects of Biomedical and Behavioral Research. Report and recommendations: research involving children. DHEW publication (OS) 77-0004; 1977.
28. Nuremberg Code, The. In: Greenwald, R.A.; Ryan, M.K.; Mulvihill, J.E., eds. Human subjects research. New York: Plenum Press; 1982:p. 229-230.
29. O'Sullivan, G. Studies involving children. In: Greenwald, R.A.; Ryan, M.K.; Mulvihill, J.E., eds. Human subjects research. New York: Plenum Press; 1982:p. 139-150.
30. Pearn, J.H. The child and clinical research. Lancet 2:510-512; 1984.
31. *Prince v Massachusetts.* United States Supreme Court reports. 321:158; 1944.
32. Protection of human subjects. Proposed regulations on research involving children. Fed. Register 43:31786-31794; 1978.
33. Protection of human subjects. Proposed establishment of regulations. Fed. Register 44:24106-24111; 1979.
34. Redmon, R.B. How children can be respected as "ends" yet still be used as subjects in non-therapeutic research. J. Med. Ethics 12:77-82; 1986.
35. Research involving children—ethics, the law, and the climate of opinion. Arch. Dis. Child. 53:441-442; 1978.
36. Rowland, T.W. Ethical considerations in pediatric research: how much is too much? Pediatr. Exerc. Sci. 1:93-95; 1989.
37. Rowland, T.W. Exercise and children's health. Champaign, IL: Human Kinetics; 1990.
38. Skegg, P.D.G. English law relating to experimentation on children. Lancet 2:754-755; 1977.
39. Smith, M. Taking blood from children causes no more than minimal harm. J. Med. Ethics 11:127-131; 1985.
40. VanDeVeer, D. Experimentation on children and proxy consent. J. Med Philos. 6:281-293; 1981.
41. Working Party on Ethics of Research in Children. Guidelines to aid ethical committees considering research involving children. Brit. Med. J. 1:229–231; 1980.

PART II

PHYSIOLOGICAL RESPONSES TO EXERCISE

Based on the methodologies and considerations of maturity in the previous section, the following chapters describe our current knowledge of the physiological responses to exercise in growing children. These chapters deal with aerobic, anaerobic, and strength fitness as well as endocrine and thermal responses. The information is largely descriptive in nature and leaves many questions of causality unanswered. Information that is known with reasonable certainty, as well as information which remains to be known, will be highlighted. Identifying these gaps in our understanding will serve to underscore the need for future research efforts.

Particular attention will be focused on several key issues of developmental exercise physiology: (1) the differentiation between size-related and size-independent factors which influence the development of physiological function, (2) the influence of puberty, (3) gender-related differences, (4) the relationship between body size and the changing physiological variables of growth, (5) the relative importance of genetic and environmental influences on normal physiological development, and (6) the relationship between physiological change and physical performance during childhood.

CHAPTER 6

MATURATION OF AEROBIC FITNESS

Energy for skeletal muscle contraction in activities lasting more than several minutes is derived from aerobic metabolism. In response to this need, mammals have developed highly complex mechanisms for transporting O_2 from the ambient air to the metabolic machinery of the muscle cell. Flow of O_2 is driven by a series of pressure gradients that begin at the external gas exchanger (the lungs); it is pumped in a transporting medium (blood) bound to hemoglobin, released at the internal gas exchanger (capillary-cell interface), and then consumed in the O_2 "sink" (the mitochondria) (90).

Endurance exercise cannot be optimally performed unless each of the separate links in this chain of O_2 delivery executes its assigned function. The critical importance of the aerobic "team effort" is made apparent by the consequences of failure of any of its members (see fig. 6.1). A decline in hemoglobin concentration of as little as 1-2 grams percent can decrease treadmill endurance time by 20% (30). Patients with chronic lung disease such as cystic fibrosis may show values of $\dot{V}O_2$max less than 50% those of healthy children. Some children with complete heart block exhibit a similar restriction of aerobic fitness because of inability to effectively raise heart rate with exercise (8).

It follows that an appreciation of changes in each of these factors during growth is important for an understanding of the development of aerobic fitness in children. But should we expect that the components of O_2 uptake evolve in concert as the child grows? Not necessarily. Relative to body mass, for instance, total hemoglobin mass and blood hemoglobin concentration rise during childhood, while heart mass per kg either stays the same or declines (66). Adding to the intricacy, components of the O_2 delivery chain also perform nonaerobic functions that maintain homeostasis during exercise. The heart and the circulatory system, for example, are essential in regulation of body temperature, transport of energy substrate, and metabolic waste removal. Understanding the complexity offered by these multiple functions during endurance exercise is daunting, and deciphering their contributions to the maturation of aerobic fitness serves as a major challenge to the developmental physiologist.

This chapter will consider changes in O_2 uptake in the growing child in the context of the role of O_2 delivery as a determinant of endurance exercise performance. This is done with some apology, since it is worth emphasizing from the start that the validity of this concept remains clouded (56). Whereas any factor that limits O_2 delivery will certainly have a negative impact on 5 km run time, there is no assurance that $\dot{V}O_2$max itself necessarily acts to limit race performance. A broken fuel pump will keep an automobile from running effectively, but it would not be appropriate to conclude that the gas pump determines the functional capacity of the car.

As we will see later, a reasonably close relationship between performance in endurance activities and $\dot{V}O_2$max is generally observed in both children and adults. But the mechanism by which *maximal* O_2 uptake (a level of exercise intensity not observed during endurance sport participation) should act as a determinant of exercise-limiting muscle fatigue is obscure. Alternatively, it is plausible that factors that might covary with $\dot{V}O_2$max (like substrate utilization, submaximal economy, or neuromuscular activation) could more directly limit performance in endurance events. There has been limited research on physiological factors that might determine the development of endurance fitness (e.g., in the 1-mile run) in children independent of changes in $\dot{V}O_2$max.

This chapter, and those that follow, will review our current understanding of the growth of aerobic fitness in

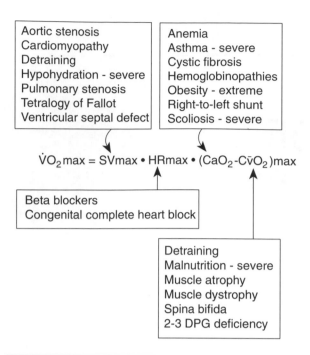

Figure 6.1 Disease processes that impair determinants of $\dot{V}O_2max$. Reprinted from Bar-Or 1986.

children. While much has been learned, it will become apparent from these discussions that many prominent gaps exist in this knowledge. Particular attention will focus on several unanswered questions:

1. What physiologic and anatomic factors are responsible for the development of aerobic fitness during childhood? How much do these changes reflect increases in body size as opposed to maturation of physiologic function?
2. How do changes in maximal aerobic power during childhood become translated into improvements in endurance exercise performance?
3. How does the "plasticity" of aerobic fitness in children compare to that of adults? That is, how much can $\dot{V}O_2max$ be altered either positively (through exercise training) or negatively (by sedentary living) in children? How influential is a child's level of daily physical activity on $\dot{V}O_2max$?
4. What is the explanation for the observation that submaximal running or walking economy (expressed as $\dot{V}O_2$ per kg at a given workload) improves during the course of childhood? How do changes in economy help account for improvements in endurance fitness?
5. How does prolonged aerobic exercise in children affect physiologic function?

RESTING ENERGY EXPENDITURE

It is appropriate to begin this chapter with an examination of O_2 uptake in the resting state, since factors influencing changes in resting metabolic rate as children grow may bear on energy expenditure during exercise. In particular, from the large amount of information available from animal studies one can expect that increase in body size as the child grows will significantly influence rate of O_2 utilization both at rest and with physical activity.

The effect of body size on resting metabolic rate has intrigued comparative biologists since such observations first appeared in the scientific literature of the mid-1800s. In 1883 Rubner observed in his study of seven dogs that the smaller the animal, the greater its resting metabolic rate relative to body weight (69). In fact, relative energy expenditure in the dog weighing 3 kg (88 kcal/kg per day) was more than twice that of the largest 36 kg animal (36 kcal/kg per day). What Rubner found was a close association in his dogs between resting energy expenditure and body surface area.

These findings were consistent with the concepts that Sarrus and Rameaux had set forth more than 40 years earlier (75). Sarrus and Rameaux reasoned that resting metabolic rate expressed per kg body mass should progressively decline with increasing animal size because (1) heat production must equal heat loss to maintain a constant body temperature in homeotherms, (2) the rate of heat lost from the body is related to the body's surface area, and (3) a larger animal possesses a lesser ratio of surface area to body mass than a smaller one. This became recognized as the *surface law:* "The relative rate of heat production is higher in the smaller animal [which] has, relative to its mass, larger body surface area. Heat loss takes place from the surface, and in order to keep warm, an animal must produce heat at a rate equal to the loss" (77, p. 77).

In 1932 Kleiber compiled data on adult animals of several species ranging in mass from 0.15 to 679 kg and found that resting metabolic rate (P_{met}, expressed as kcal per day) varied with mass (M) by the allometric relationship (43):

$$P_{met} = 0.19 \ M^{0.75}.$$

Since then, many have contributed research findings to the pool of data on resting energy expenditure in animals with no change in the conclusion: metabolic rate in the resting adult mammal varies with mass by an exponent of approximately 0.75 (see fig. 6.2). That is, regardless of animal size, resting energy expenditure will be similar when expressed relative to mass to the three-quarters power. This also means that relative resting metabolic rate ($\dot{V}O_2$ per kg) will be expected to vary

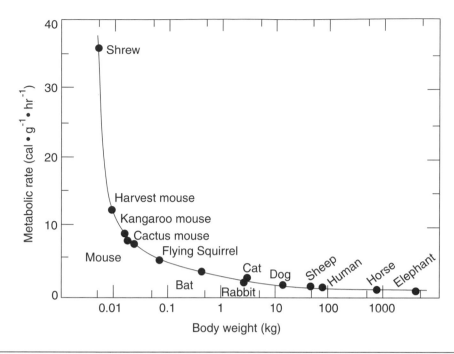

Figure 6.2   Smaller animals have a higher mass-specific resting metabolic rate. Reprinted from McMahon 1984.

with mass by a scaling exponent of –.25 (i.e., the larger the animal the less the relative resting energy expenditure). For example, the resting $\dot{V}O_2$ per kg of a mouse is 10 times that of a whale (43).

It is disconcerting, however, that the .75 scaling exponent does not conform to that expected on the basis of the surface law, which calls for resting energy expenditure to relate to body surface area, or M^{67}. Considerable debate has ensued over the past 50 years in efforts to explain this discrepancy. Perhaps difficulty in assessing the characteristics of heat loss from surface area is the explanation (Is the loss uniform? Does one, for instance, include the ears of a rabbit?). Some have viewed this difference in exponents as evidence against the validity of the surface law. Heusner suggested that the scaling exponent for mass for *intraspecies* comparisons of metabolic rate was actually .67 (36). Blaxter agreed, arguing that "within a species it is common for the relation between minimal metabolism and body weight to vary with a power of weight less than 0.75 [since] the younger and smaller animal has a higher metabolic rate per unit size" (13, p. 134).

Others have attributed the discrepancy between expected and measured exponents to influences of elastic similarity, gravity, and time (77). Calling these arguments "not particularly convincing," Blaxter concluded that the basic concept of the surface law was still opera-

tional. "The metabolic rates of different species represent the problem of maintaining temperature [since] the critical importance of maintaining body temperature between 33 and 39 degrees C. is the one attribute of animals in which they have close similarity" (13, p. 146). In the final analysis, however, it must be concluded that the true explanation for the .75 exponent remains elusive.

The progressive fall in resting $\dot{V}O_2$ per kg as animal size increases could be the result of either a decrease in the relative size of body organs that contribute the most to metabolic rate, or a decline in the metabolic rate of the various body tissues. Evidence suggests a possible role for both these mechanisms.

Most of resting metabolic rate reflects the contribution of only a few organs, particularly the heart, brain, liver, and kidney. It has been estimated that almost three-fourths of the total resting energy expenditure of a 65 kg man can be accounted for by organs that collectively weight no more than 5 kg (37). And many of these organs do decrease in proportion to body size as the size of the animal increases. Schmidt-Nielsen described allometric equations that express these changes: heart and lung weight per kg body mass varies relative to $M^{0.0}$, indicating that the size of these organs does not change relative to body size in animals of different dimensions (77). Scaling exponents for kidney, brain, and liver were

−.15, −.30, and −.13, respectively. Thus, although relative size decreases with increasing body mass for these organs, only brain diminished in accord with the decrease expected for $\dot{V}O_2$ per kg (−.25). Schmidt-Nielsen concluded that change in relative organ size could therefore not fully explain the decline in $\dot{V}O_2$ per kg with increasing animal size (77).

In general, animal studies have demonstrated a decrease in relative rates of O_2 consumption in isolated tissue slices as the size of the animal increases. The conclusion from these observations, that the higher $\dot{V}O_2$ per kg in smaller animals indicates a greater rate of cellular metabolism, is supported by findings that cellular mitochondrial density, cytochrome oxidase concentration, and cytochrome C content are inversely proportional to animal size. Scaling exponents of −.10, −.30, and −.24 have been reported for these factors, respectively, approximating the exponent of −.25 for mass-relative metabolic rate. In animals, total mitochondria in the liver relates to $M^{.72}$, and the surface area of the mitochondrial membranes in summated animal tissue is proportional to $M^{.76}$ (77). The exponents are similar to the value of .75 expected for $\dot{V}O_2$ in respect to mass. All these data support the concept that the "fire" of cellular metabolic machinery burns more intensely at rest in smaller animals than in larger ones.

If differences in resting metabolic rate in children change in relation to size in accord with these adult animal data, the following would be expected: (a) resting metabolic rate should increase relative to mass by an exponent of (or somewhat less than) 0.75; (b) the resulting fall in resting $\dot{V}O_2$ per kg with growth should be partially—but not completely—explainable by a decline in the proportion of body weight accounted for by the major organs of metabolism; and (c) cellular indicators of aerobic metabolism (mitochondrial density, concentration of aerobic enzymes) should become less prominent as the child ages.

How do the findings in children correspond to these theoretical constructs? Relative resting metabolic rate declines during the course of childhood, and this is true whether energy expenditure is related to body mass or surface area (see fig. 6.3). This fall in metabolic rate is not negligible. The basal metabolic rate per kg in an infant is more than twice that of an adult. In the exercise testing age group, the decrease of resting $\dot{V}O_2$ (relative to body surface area) between the ages of 6 and 18 years amounts to 19% in boys and 27% in girls (45).

On the basis of data from several studies, Holliday et al. constructed curves of normal changes in basal metabolic rate (BMR) with increasing body weight in children (37). As can be seen in figure 6.4, this relationship varies during childhood and conforms neither to the curve relating BMR to body surface area nor to $M^{.75}$. In fact, there is no simple mathematical expression that re-

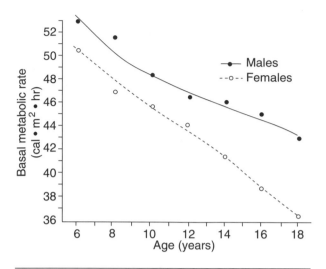

Figure 6.3 Changes in basal metabolic rate with age. Reprinted from Rowland 1990.

lates BMR to weight throughout the course of the growing years. Allometric analysis of these data indicated that BMR relates to mass by the exponent of 1.02 up to a weight of approximately 10 kg; above that weight, the scaling exponent falls to 0.58.

Another issue Holliday et al. addressed was whether the decline in resting $\dot{V}O_2$ per kg during childhood is a consequence of a decrease in the relative weight of the most metabolically active organs or of a fall in tissue O_2 uptake (37). Their conclusion, contrary to the informa-

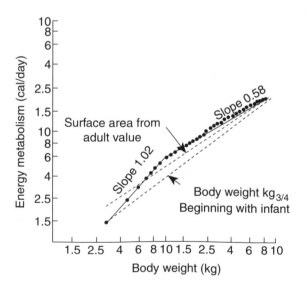

Figure 6.4 Growth of basal metabolic rate with mass in children compared to curves predicted by body surface area ($M^{.67}$) and ($M^{.75}$) (37). Reprinted from Holliday et al. 1967.

tion drawn from adult interspecies comparisons, was that the decline in the combined weights of brain, liver, kidneys, lungs, and heart relative to body weight in growing children directly paralleled the decrease in weight-relative metabolic rate. They described scaling coefficients of 1.0 and 0.53 below and above body weight of 10 kg, respectively, for the metabolic activity of these organs in respect to body mass—values very similar to 1.02 and 0.58 for BMR.

On the other hand, Holliday et al. did not find evidence in the research literature for decreasing resting metabolic activity of tissues with growth as measured either by isolated tissue O_2 uptake in maturing animals or by renal function in children. Using nuclear magnetic spectroscopy, Zanconato et al. showed no differences in the ratio of inorganic phosphate to phosphocreatine at rest between adults and children, suggesting similar basal metabolic activity (92). This is consistent with the findings of Bell et al., who obtained similar values for mitochondrial volume and mitochondrial:myofibrillar volume ratios in vastus lateralis muscle biopsy specimens in 13 6-year-old children compared to adults (10). Eriksson described only a "slight increase" in muscle concentrations of the oxidative enzyme succinate-dehydrogenase with increasing age, and only slightly higher levels in five 11-year-old boys compared to untrained adults (28). However, Haralambie (33) found greater concentrations of aerobic enzymes on skeletal muscle biopsies of children than on those of young adults.

Most data, then, suggest that the decline in the size of the most metabolically active organs with increasing body weight is the major factor in the fall of weight-specific resting metabolic rate during childhood. Evidence that tissues are relatively "hypermetabolic" in younger compared to older children and adults is less convincing.

It is interesting to speculate on the influence of these age-related changes in resting metabolic rate on the assessment of aerobic fitness. First, the smaller the child, the greater will be the "head start" in weight-relative $\dot{V}O_2$ at the onset of exercise. Although these resting differences in $\dot{V}O_2$ with age are small in absolute terms, they may have influence when aerobic power is measured as multiples of resting values. We will return to this issue later in this chapter in the discussion of metabolic scope.

How much will the relatively greater size of highly metabolic organs in children affect energy expenditure during exercise? From an appreciation of changes in tissues contributing to metabolic expenditure at rest compared to those that are most metabolically active during exercise, the answer is, probably little. In adults, the resting blood flow (an indicator of metabolic activity) to the splanchnic organs, brain, and kidney constitutes 25%, 15%, and 20%, respectively, of the total cardiac output, while skeletal muscle receives 18% (5). With intense exercise, increased cardiac output is shunted to the muscle, which then accounts for 80% of flow, while vasoconstriction reduces blood flow to splanchnic organs, brain, and kidney to 5%, 3%, and 4%.

Skeletal muscle mass increases in weight relative to body weight as children grow. It has been estimated, for instance, that the muscles of the lower extremity constitute 40% of total muscle mass at birth but 55% at the time of puberty (51). Changes in the relative size of the most metabolically active tissue during physical activity would then be expected to increase rather than decrease $\dot{V}O_2$ per kg with exercise as the child grows.

In summary, resting metabolic rate in children decreases relative to body size during growth. This relationship is complex and is not uniform during the pediatric years. Most data suggest that this decline in size-related resting $\dot{V}O_2$ can be explained by a decrease in the relative size of the major organs contributing to resting energy metabolic expenditure. Whether the metabolic rate of specific tissues falls with age is less certain.

MAXIMAL AEROBIC POWER

A progressive exercise test to exhaustion on a treadmill or cycle ergometer involves sufficient muscle mass to push the chain of O_2 delivery and consumption to its limits. That O_2 uptake "ceiling" is identified as $\dot{V}O_2$max, or maximal aerobic power—a finite, reproducible value that provides a numerical indicator of a subject's level of aerobic fitness. Exercise at an intensity above that eliciting $\dot{V}O_2$max must draw its energy from anaerobic metabolic sources, with rapidly ensuing lactic acidemia and fatigue. As noted previously, maximal aerobic power also provides a measure of the functional integrity of the components of the O_2 delivery chain. That makes assessment of $\dot{V}O_2$max a useful tool for clinicians, particularly in the management of patients with chronic cardiac or pulmonary disease.

Symmorphosis and Maximal Aerobic Power

Is there a weak link in the O_2 uptake chain that is responsible for delimiting $\dot{V}O_2$max? This issue has occupied hours of debate and volumes of research in adult subjects, but with no clear-cut answer. Strong evidence has been cited for a central (i.e., cardiac) limiting factor, while equally persuasive data have been presented by those convinced that $\dot{V}O_2$max is defined by the muscle cell's capacity to utilize delivered O_2 (74). The question has not been specifically addressed by investigations in children.

The principle of *symmorphosis* described by Taylor and Weibel (82) states that "each element in the chain [of O_2 uptake] should be structured to meet but not exceed the requirements of the others" (77, p. 106). That is, according to this concept there should be *no* weak link in the O_2 uptake chain. If there were, nature would have taken wasteful steps to create unnecessary function in the remaining components. Why build a heart with a maximal cardiac output of 30 L/min if peak ventilation limits $\dot{V}O_2$max when cardiac output is 20 L/min? All the component parts of O_2 delivery and consumption should meet but not exceed functional expectations at $\dot{V}O_2$max. The pediatric corollary holds that "the formation of structural elements that occurs during growth . . . should be regulated to satisfy but not exceed the requirements of the functional system" (90, p. 59).

Intuitively attractive as this concept is, there is evidence to refute it. Besides the previously mentioned research findings in the central (cardiac) versus peripheral (muscle) limitation argument, several observations of ventilatory function appear inconsistent with the principle of symmorphosis. In animals, the maximal diffusing capacity of the lung scales to body mass by the exponent 0.99, not the 0.75 expected according to O_2 uptake (77). In children, maximal minute ventilation during progressive exercise is typically only 60-70% of maximal voluntary ventilation (performed at rest) (57). If these observations debunk symmorphosis, however, one is left with the sticky problem of explaining the reason for the development and maintenance of biologic structures in excess of body need.

Cooper et al. suggested an alternative means of viewing symmorphosis in children (17). They proposed that physiological adaptations to exercise are geared to the rapid changes in intensity typically observed in children rather than to maximal exercise efforts. The dynamics of O_2 uptake have been examined by these authors in a series of studies that will be reviewed later in the chapter.

The "Meaning" of $\dot{V}O_2$max: Caveats

The use of $\dot{V}O_2$max as an indicator of aerobic fitness in children is confounded by the necessity of relating values to increases in body size. The difficulty in selecting a proper denominator to normalize maximal aerobic power in growing children was discussed fully in chapter 2. In this regard there is increasing concern about the appropriateness of using body weight or mass. Nonetheless, most exercise studies in the pediatric research literature have expressed maximal O_2 uptake as $\dot{V}O_2$max ml · kg^{-1} · min^{-1}.

But what does $\dot{V}O_2$max per kg mean? Traditionally, maximal aerobic power has been interpreted as a marker of (a) performance capability in endurance athletic events and (b) cardiovascular functional capacity (cardiovascular fitness). It is important that developmental physiologists critically examine these implications of $\dot{V}O_2$max per kg, which can be significantly influenced by biological maturation as well as body composition.

Caveat #1. **$\dot{V}O_2$max per kg is a valid index of endurance performance only for comparison of children of similar biological age.** In children as in adults, endurance athletes show significantly higher values of maximal aerobic power, and at any given age there is a moderately close association between 1-mile run time, for instance, and $\dot{V}O_2$max per kg. But over a broader range of children's ages this use of $\dot{V}O_2$max becomes problematic, since weight-relative $\dot{V}O_2$max stays relatively stable throughout the course of childhood. Meanwhile, endurance time improves dramatically. A group of typical 5-year-old boys will have a mean $\dot{V}O_2$max of about 50 ml· kg^{-1} · min^{-1}, the same as observed in average 15-year-old adolescents. But the older boys will finish a 1-mile run in half the time the 5-year-olds do (1).

Caveat #2. **Cardiopulmonary fitness is only one of several determinants of endurance exercise performance in children.** The determination of performance capabilities in endurance events is highly complex. Cureton contended that the combination of body fatness and cardiorespiratory capacity accounts for only about one-half of the variance on distance running tests in children (22). The remainder presumably reflects the influences of factors such as running efficiency, skill, motivation, and anaerobic capacity. The role of maximal aerobic power in improvements in endurance fitness as children grow will be addressed further on in this chapter.

Caveat #3. **The influence of body fat content can render $\dot{V}O_2$max per kg useless as a marker of cardiovascular fitness, causing spurious, often misleading conclusions.** Direct measurement of cardiac function during exercise—particularly at exhaustive intensities—is difficult. Since by the Fick principle, maximal aerobic power is the product of cardiac output and arteriovenous O_2 uptake, $\dot{V}O_2$max has often been utilized as an indicator of maximal heart function. When maximal O_2 uptake is related to body mass, however, body fat can profoundly influence values of $\dot{V}O_2$max per kg, rendering them totally inaccurate for assessment of cardiac function. In a large group of subjects ranging from thin to obese, for example, a prominent inverse relationship will be observed between percent body fat and $\dot{V}O_2$max per kg. These findings would falsely imply that fatter individuals have lower levels of cardiovascular fitness. In fact, however, the true message is that obese subjects are simply carrying around a greater load of "baggage." In other words, it is the denominator rather than the numerator of the $\dot{V}O_2$max per kg relationship that has changed.

The absolute maximal O_2 uptake (a good index of maximal cardiac output) will either remain stable or actually rise as obesity increases (65). That is, obesity (within limits) does not appear to impair cardiac fitness but will surely limit endurance performance and lower $\dot{V}O_2$max per kg. It follows that we can use $\dot{V}O_2$max per kg only as an estimate of cardiovascular fitness when comparing individuals of similar body composition.

To summarize, both biological maturity and body composition can profoundly affect the validity of $\dot{V}O_2$max per kg as an indicator of endurance fitness as well as cardiovascular capacity. $\dot{V}O_2$max per kg can be expected to be useful as a marker for these variables only in samples of children that are strictly homogeneous in terms of body fat as well as biological maturity.

NORMAL DEVELOPMENT OF $\dot{V}O_2$MAX

There exist no "normal values" for maximal aerobic power in children. The dozens of studies that have reported $\dot{V}O_2$max in the childhood age group have varied sufficiently in exercise protocol, subject population, and measurement methodology to provide a wide range of values. An examination of both cross-sectional and longitudinal data, however, has provided a picture of the expected levels of $\dot{V}O_2$max in the growing child and the patterns of change in aerobic fitness in both boys and girls.

Cross-Sectional Studies

Not unexpectedly, cross-sectional studies of maximal aerobic power in children demonstrate a progressive increase in absolute $\dot{V}O_2$max with age. This rise is illustrated in the graphs created by Krahenbuhl et al., which include data points for $\dot{V}O_2$max representing a large number of healthy untrained children (5793 males and 3508 females) from 66 studies in the research literature (see fig. 6.5) (49). Values obtained in studies using cycle ergometry were "corrected" by multiplying by a factor of 1.075 to adjust for the higher $\dot{V}O_2$max levels expected during treadmill exercise.

A curvilinear increase in average absolute $\dot{V}O_2$max occurs with increasing age. Mean values for $\dot{V}O_2$max increase from about 1.0 L/min at age 6 years in all children to 2.0 and 2.8 L/min for girls and boys, respectively, at 15 years of age. The mean values for boys exceed those of girls at all ages. The gender difference in $\dot{V}O_2$max is small and the rate of rise similar (about 200 ml/min per year) before age 12. Thereafter, mean values for $\dot{V}O_2$max plateau in girls but continue to rise in boys, and by age 16 years the gender difference is greater than 50%. A similar analysis by Bar-Or of studies in the pediatric literature revealed this same pattern of change in absolute $\dot{V}O_2$max with growth (7).

A considerable disparity of individual values of $\dot{V}O_2$max obtains in children at all ages, as Malina and Bouchard emphasize (52). This suggests that a good

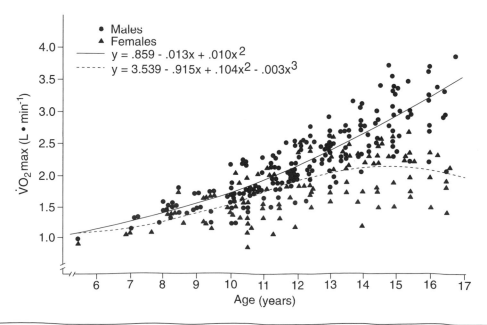

Figure 6.5 $\dot{V}O_2$max related to chronological age (49). Reprinted from Krahenbuhl et al. 1985.

deal of variability may exist around these reported mean rates and patterns of aerobic development. But 4-year longitudinal measurements in Czechoslovakian children by Rutenfranz et al. suggested that interindividual variations in rate of development of $\dot{V}O_2$max are not extreme (71). Maximal O_2 uptake differences between individual subjects ranged from 10% to 20% for all age groups. A Spearman rank order correlation coefficient of 0.8 indicated that the children in this study generally maintained their initial rank of maximal O_2 uptake within the group over time.

The factors responsible for the development of maximal aerobic power in children will be considered in separate sections on the pulmonary, cardiovascular, and peripheral determinants of aerobic fitness. It is sufficient at this point to note that the increase in $\dot{V}O_2$max in the growing child closely parallels the dimensions of these organs. Between the ages of 8 and 12 years, for example, maximal aerobic power in children has been reported to rise from 1.42 to 2.12 L/min (a 49% increase) (55). During this time span the average weight of the lungs increases from 290 to 459 g (58% rise) (63), lung vital capacity grows from 1.890 to 2.800 L (48% increase), and left ventricular volume by echocardiography rises by 52% (34).

When maximal O_2 uptake is expressed relative to body mass, different patterns of change with growth emerge. The analyses of cross-sectional data by Krahenbuhl et al. (49) and Bar-Or (7) indicate that $\dot{V}O_2$max per kg in boys remains stable across the age span of 6 to 16 years, with an average value of approximately 50-53 ml $\cdot$ kg^{-1} $\cdot$ min^{-1} (see fig. 6.6). The expected range in healthy, untrained children is 7-10 ml $\cdot$ kg^{-1} $\cdot$ min^{-1}

above and below this mean. These observations alone suggest that the magnitude of increase in absolute maximal aerobic power in growing boys can be explained solely on the basis of dimensional changes in the O_2 delivery system and peripheral muscle mass, without size-independent functional changes.

The pattern of $\dot{V}O_2$max per kg during growth is different in females. Almost from the age when girls are old enough for exercise testing, a progressive decline occurs in weight-relative maximal O_2 uptake that persists throughout the childhood and teen years (see fig. 6.6). The data complied by Krahenbuhl et al. indicate that the average 8-year-old girl with a $\dot{V}O_2$max of 50 ml $\cdot$ kg^{-1} $\cdot$ min^{-1} can be expected to show a decline to 45 ml $\cdot$ kg^{-1} $\cdot$ min^{-1} by age 12; at age 16 the value will fall to 40 ml $\cdot$ kg^{-1} $\cdot$ min^{-1}.

Differences in body composition may at least partially explain these gender differences in weight-relative $\dot{V}O_2$max, since males exhibit a greater lean body mass (LBM; i.e., less relative body fat) than girls even before puberty. Davies et al. reported, for example, that $\dot{V}O_2$max differences (expressed per kg) between boys and girls essentially disappeared when values were related to leg volume (reflecting the muscle mass engaged in cycle exercise) (25). This does not appear to be the entire answer, however. In the longitudinal data of children 12-17 years reported by Kemper et al., $\dot{V}O_2$max per kg was approximately 20% greater in males at all ages (42). When expressed relative to LBM (estimated by skinfold measurements), gender-related variations were smaller, but a 6% difference remained. Other studies have also demonstrated persistence of gender differences when $\dot{V}O_2$max values are related to LBM (2, 70).

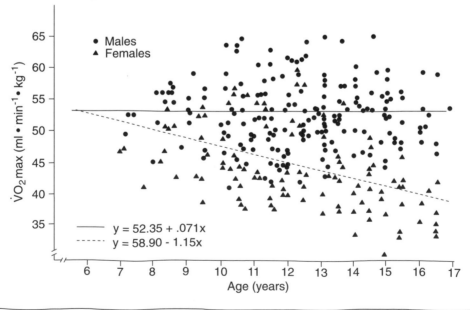

Figure 6.6 $\dot{V}O_2$max relative to body mass related to chronological age (49). Reprinted from Krahenbuhl et al. 1985.

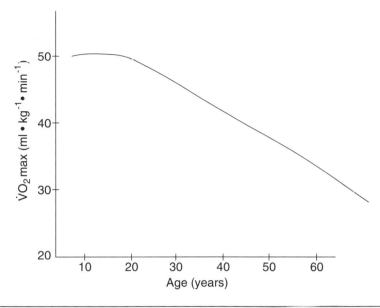

Figure 6.7 Mean values of males for $\dot{V}O_2$max through the life span (from Robinson [60]).

After adolescence, average values for $\dot{V}O_2$max per kg fall progressively throughout the adult years. Robinson's cross-sectional treadmill study of 93 normal males demonstrated this trend in 1938 (60) (see fig. 6.7). Until age 20, $\dot{V}O_2$max levels averaged about 50 ml $\cdot$ kg^{-1} $\cdot$ min^{-1}. Maximal aerobic power fell to 40 ml $\cdot$ kg^{-1} $\cdot$ min^{-1} by age 40, and the average 70-year-old showed a $\dot{V}O_2$max of 30 ml $\cdot$ kg^{-1} $\cdot$ min^{-1}. On the basis simply of values of weight-relative O_2 uptake, then, children are more "aerobic" than people at any other time in life.

Longitudinal Studies

Longitudinal studies of absolute maximal O_2 uptake in children confirm trends suggested by cross-sectional investigations. Figure 6.8 illustrates the findings in four such long-term studies, showing that maximal aerobic power increases approximately 200 ml/min for each year of age before puberty (55). At this point values accelerate in males and plateau in females.

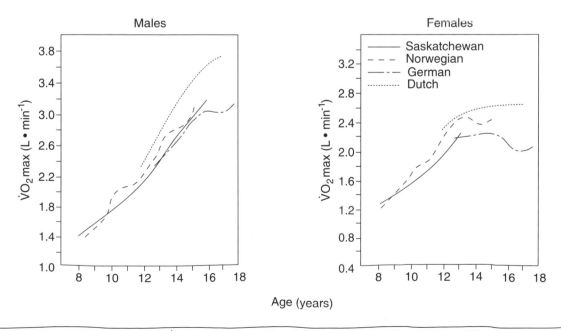

Figure 6.8 Longitudinal studies of $\dot{V}O_2$max with age. Reprinted from Mirwald and Bailey (55).

Table 6.1   Longitudinal studies of $\dot{V}O_2$max in children

Study	N	Sex	Mode	Age span
Hermansen and				
Oseid (35)	20	M	T	11–13
Vanden Eynde et al. (87)	21	M	C	11–13
Binkhorst et al. (12)	17	M	C	11–18
Sprynarova (81)	39	M	T	11–18
Cunningham et al. (20)	62	M	T	10–15
Kemper et al. (42)	93	M	T	13–16
	107	F	T	13–16
Mirwald and Bailey (55)	83	M	T	8–16
	22	F	T	8–16
Rutenfranz et al. (70)	27	M	C	8–15
	32	F	C	8–15
	26	M	C	13–18
	18	F	C	13–18

Note: C = cycle; T = treadmill.

Longitudinal data for $\dot{V}O_2$max per kg are less consistent. Table 6.1 lists the several studies that have provided information about O_2 uptake relative to body weight in serial measurements during childhood and adolescence. Of the studies in males, some have shown $\dot{V}O_2$max per kg to increase (12, 81), others indicate stable values (55), and still others demonstrate a fall in weight-relative maximal aerobic power with age (70). Information from studies in girls indicates a general downward trend in $\dot{V}O_2$max per kg with age.

If one performs the interesting but statistically heretical act of averaging all longitudinal values of $\dot{V}O_2$max per kg at each age, longitudinal curves for boys and girls appear as in figure 6.9. These are remarkably similar to

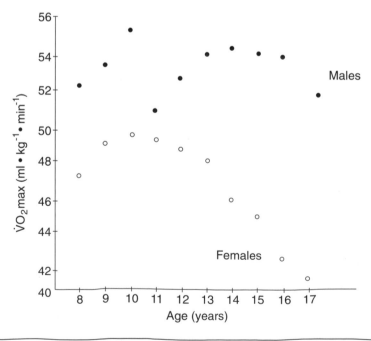

Figure 6.9   Average values of longitudinal studies of $\dot{V}O_2$max per kg with age in boys and girls (from Bar-Or [8]).

those derived from the amassed cross-sectional data of Krahenbuhl et al. (49) and Bar-Or (7) showing stable values in males and a progressive decline in females.

The differences in trends of $\dot{V}O_2$max per kg between individual longitudinal studies could be explained by the variable influences of other factors affecting aerobic fitness. Differences in changes in body composition during growth (particularly adiposity), as well as variations in daily physical activity and sport participation between studies, could easily contribute to these disparities. Ross et al. pointed out that children are not geometrically similar at all ages and that use of a single means of size adjustment (e.g., body weight) is inadequate to express relative O_2 uptake (62).

Allometric Scaling Factors for $\dot{V}O_2$ max

Maximal O_2 uptake in animals, defined as the limit after which there is no further rise in $\dot{V}O_2$ with increased running speed (77), has been examined in relation to body mass in adult species ranging from pygmy mice to horses (83). In these animals, $\dot{V}O_2$max $= 1.92\,M^{.81}$, with average exponents ranging from .79 in wild species to .86 in domesticated animals.

This information interests developmental physiologists because these animals differ in size, not maturity. Identifying a similar scaling exponent for $\dot{V}O_2$max relative to body weight for growing children would therefore suggest that increasing size, rather than qualitative

functional change, is responsible for the rise of maximal aerobic power with age. Moreover, a defined scaling factor for height or weight would provide an answer to the need for an appropriate denominator for normalizing $\dot{V}O_2$max for increasing body dimensions. The means by which allometric scaling exponents are calculated and interpreted were described in chapter 2.

We can determine scaling factors relating maximal O_2 uptake to body mass or height in children by creating allometric equations (1) in a group of subjects of similar biological or chronological age, (2) from cross-sectional values in children of different ages, or (3) in longitudinal data of the same children at different ages. Scaling exponents have been derived by each of these means and are outlined in table 6.2. In this table, scaling factors reported relative to body height have been converted to weight (in parentheses) according to dimensionality theory (i.e., mass relates to the cube of body stature).

Whether or not exponents derived from these different types of analysis can be interpreted similarly is not altogether clear. The influence, for instance, of differences in the heterogeneity of subject size, body composition, and athleticism is problematic. Presumably such factors are responsible for the variety of reported exponents. These scaling exponents resemble those described in animal studies, but are sufficiently dissimilar to preclude conclusions about the relative influences of size and function in the development of maximal

Table 6.2 Scaling factors (b) for maximal oxygen uptake (y) related to height or weight (x) in the equation $y = ax^b$

Study	N	Sex	Age	Mode	Exponent for Weight	Exponent for Height
Cross-sectional						
Cooper et al. (17)	51	F	6–17	C	0.79	
					0.91	
	58	M			1.01	
					1.02	
Åstrand (4)	68	M,F	6–17	T	0.95	
von Dobeln and Eriksson (88)	12	M	11–13	C	(0.66)	1.98
Welsman et al. (91)	29	M	10–11	T	0.92	
	34	F			0.84	
Rogers et al. (61)	21	M	7–9	T	0.37	
	21	F			0.68	
Longitudinal						
Bailey et al. (6)	51	M	8–15	T	(0.82)	2.46

Note: C = cycle; T = treadmill.

aerobic power in children. Likewise, at present no single allometric scaling factor can be identified as a standard for normalizing maximal O_2 uptake in children across studies.

Nevertheless, it is important to note that with the exception of the values for boys in the study by Cooper et al., the reported scaling factors are all less than 1.0. The available data therefore suggest that, contrary to the findings from cross-sectional and longitudinal analyses described earlier, maximal O_2 uptake in both boys and girls increases at a rate slower than that of body mass during growth.

On the other hand, Armstrong and Welsman noted that the constant (a) in the allometric equation ($y = ax^b$) may influence comparisons between groups as much as has the scaling exponent (b) (3). They found similar power function exponents for mass relative to $\dot{V}O_2$max in pre- and postpubertal females (range .65 to .86). The multiplier (a) was significantly less in the prepubertal subjects, however. These findings were suggested to indicate "that there are functional improvements in peak $\dot{V}O_2$ between puberty and young adulthood, [a finding which is] clearly at odds with traditional interpretation of growth-related peak $\dot{V}O_2$ expressed as a simple ratio standard used for growth-related comparisons" (p. 454).

Observations of changes in $\dot{V}O_2$max relative to body height (H) in two longitudinal studies are also of interest. In the children tested serially by Kemper et al., girls showed an increase in $\dot{V}O_2$max between ages 13 and 16 years that was proportional to H^2, while in the boys $\dot{V}O_2$max values related to H^3 (42). Rutenfranz et al. reported that longitudinal changes in maximal aerobic power correlated equally well with $H^{1.0}$ or $H^{2.0}$ in both boys and girls (r = .84-.88) (71). On the basis of these findings the investigators suggested that body height "can be used as a simple, practical measure to provide reference data for $\dot{V}O_2$max, [although] unfortunately it is probable that this relationship is of little value after the individual achieves the height of maturity" (71, p. 286).

In summary, we obviously do not yet have a clear understanding of the relationship between $\dot{V}O_2$max and body size in growing children. As a result, it is uncertain whether aerobic fitness increases during childhood simply because of increasing size or because of improvements in functional capacity that are independent of body dimensions (or both). Newer analytical approaches such as allometric scaling may provide greater insights into this question. We need more information, too, regarding the influence of variables such as body composition, habitual physical activity, gender, and athleticism, which may confound attempts to identify a single factor to "normalize" $\dot{V}O_2$max for increasing body size.

Maximal Aerobic Power and Biological Age

The influence of puberty on the development of $\dot{V}O_2$max has attracted attention in view of the possibility that acceleration of growth might serve to optimize increases in aerobic fitness. We will return to this subject later in the discussion of the effects of endurance training on aerobic fitness of children.

Beunen and Malina reviewed data from six longitudinal and mixed longitudinal studies that examined values of maximal O_2 uptake relative to timing of the adolescent growth spurt (peak height velocity, PHV) (11). The most reliable information indicates that the maximal rate of increase in absolute $\dot{V}O_2$max occurs in boys at or near PHV with a typical velocity of .412 L/min per year (42, 55). The ages of peak velocity for stature, weight, and $\dot{V}O_2$max in the boys studied by Mirwald and Bailey were 14.3, 14.5, and 14.3 years, respectively (55). Data were considered insufficient to allow conclusions in girls.

At least in males, then, a growth spurt is observed in absolute values for maximal aerobic power during adolescence, starting typically at about age 13 and peaking a year later. These changes presumably reflect acceleration in the size of components of O_2 uptake in response to the hormonal changes of puberty. Changes in $\dot{V}O_2$max per kg surrounding puberty are highly variable, with both increase (70) and decrease (55, 70) relative to PHV reported for both boys and girls.

Absolute $\dot{V}O_2$max is observed to rise until the age of menarche but to plateau thereafter (52). Menarche does not appear to influence weight-relative maximal O_2 uptake, which falls progressively from 2 years before to 3 years after age of onset of menses.

The development of $\dot{V}O_2$max closely parallels skeletal maturity. Hollman and Bouchard reported a correlation of r = 0.89 between skeletal age and maximal O_2 uptake in a group of 275 boys 8 to 18 years of age (38). When boys and girls are grouped as early and late maturers on the basis of skeletal age, the early maturers have a greater mean absolute $\dot{V}O_2$max than the late maturers. These differences dissolve at the time of late adolescence (42). When expressed relative to body weight, $\dot{V}O_2$max has been reported to be greater in late maturers (42) and independent of bone age (38, 76, 78).

Absolute $\dot{V}O_2$max bears a moderately close relationship to body weight in pediatric studies. Correlation coefficients of r = 0.60 to 0.80 are typical (49), consistent with findings in adult subjects (41). However, Mayers and Gutin reported r = 0.94 between maximal O_2 uptake and body weight in their study of child distance runners (53), suggesting that the relationship may be closer in homogeneous groups of lean, athletic children.

TEMPORAL TRENDS IN MAXIMAL AEROBIC POWER

Are children becoming less aerobically fit? Despite concern that an increasingly sedentary lifestyle may be impairing the exercise capacity of youth, there is no evidence that levels of maximal aerobic power have declined in children. The question obviously is difficult to answer with certainty. Few studies of $\dot{V}O_2$max in children were performed before the 1960s, and the prominent influence of subject selection and testing methodology on values for $\dot{V}O_2$max lends suspicion to any interlaboratory comparisons.

Nonetheless, an examination of levels of maximal aerobic power in studies of children over the past 50 years shows no obvious overall changes. The early report of treadmill findings by Robinson in the Harvard Fatigue Laboratory in 1938, in 31 male subjects ages 5-19 years, indicated an average $\dot{V}O_2$max of 49.7 ml · kg^{-1} · min^{-1} (60). In 1952, Åstrand described a mean $\dot{V}O_2$max on treadmill testing of 55.6 ml · kg^{-1} · min^{-1} in 64 Swedish boys 4-15 years old (4). Figure 6.10 illustrates data points for mean $\dot{V}O_2$max per kg for boys in treadmill studies since that time as compiled by Freedson and Goodman (29). This analysis fails to reveal any trend for change in weight-relative maximal O_2 uptake in boys over the past half century.

AEROBIC SCOPE

It was previously noted that maximal O_2 uptake relates to body mass in mature animals by $\dot{V}O_2$max = 1.92 M$^{.81}$. The obvious similarity of this equation to that in the resting state, $\dot{V}O_2$ = .19 M$^{.75}$, allows one to conclude that the average animal has an *aerobic scope,* or ratio of maximal to resting O_2 uptake, of approximately 10, and that this value is independent of animal size. (While this is true for the animal kingdom as a whole, considerable variability is observed. Aerobic scope in dogs, for instance, is about 30, and the desert locust reportedly holds the gold medal with a 50-fold increase in metabolic rate during flight!)

Since aerobic scope is not influenced by body size, the ratio of maximal to resting or basal O_2 uptake becomes an attractive means of examining aerobic fitness in growing children. Åstrand introduced this concept in his 1952 monograph (4). He noted that the ratio of measured $\dot{V}O_2$max to basal O_2 uptake (he calculated the latter from reported standard data) rose progressively from 6.8 and 6.6 in boys and girls, respectively, at 4-6 years of age to 13.5 and 12.6, respectively, at ages 16-18 years. These values are similar to those one can calculate from the basal and maximal O_2 uptake data of Robinson (60) (see fig. 6.11).

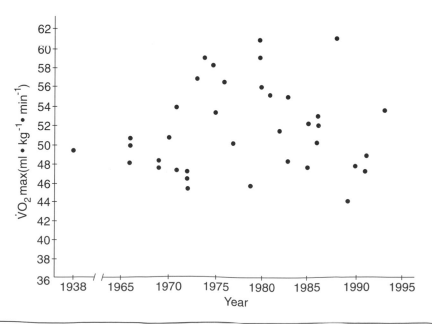

Figure 6.10 Historical values for $\dot{V}O_2$max per kg from studies in children (compiled in Freedson and Goodman [29]).

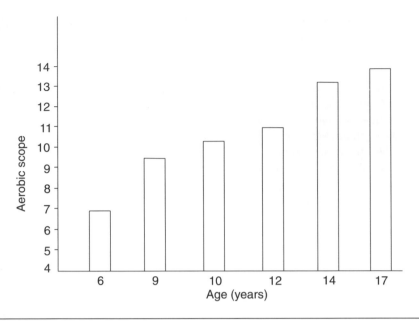

Figure 6.11   Aerobic scope in males (from data of Robinson [60]).

It is not clear how to interpret the observation that between the ages of 6 and 17 years, children double their maximal O_2 uptake in relation to resting values. According to data in mature animals, size itself should not influence aerobic scope. Do the changes in aerobic scope in children indicate functional improvements in O_2 delivery beyond those accounted for by physical growth? Can the increases in aerobic scope observed in children be related to the improvements in endurance performance that occur during childhood? These are intriguing possibilities.

But serious questions arise about the validity of the concept that aerobic scope is an accurate indicator of aerobic reserve during exercise. Most fundamentally, since the determinants of resting metabolic rate are very different from those during physical activities (see p. 77), is it legitimate to use resting O_2 uptake as the multiplier unit for O_2 uptake during exercise? In this regard, reports of both Åstrand and Robinson show clearly that almost all the change in aerobic scope with growth is a result of decreases in basal metabolic rate. Theoretical considerations aside, measurement of aerobic scope is difficult because even small differences in values of basal metabolic rate will profoundly influence aerobic scope.

To summarize, children show a dramatic increase in aerobic scope as they grow, but the significance of this is difficult to interpret. While conceptually aerobic scope is attractive as a means of indicating aerobic reserve independent of body weight, more information is needed concerning its validity and usefulness in children.

$\dot{V}O_2$ MAX AND ENDURANCE PERFORMANCE

Sustained physical exercise is dependent on energy derived from aerobic metabolism. It should follow, then, that changes in maximal aerobic power will parallel those of performance in endurance activities. In general, as children grow, their abilities in aerobic events such as the 1-mile run progressively improve. Examining changes in maximal aerobic power during the childhood years should therefore provide an opportunity to gain insight into the role that $\dot{V}O_2$max plays in determining endurance performance.

Viewed from a broader perspective, the growing child offers an excellent model for dissecting out the principal determinants of endurance fitness. It is not an inappropriate suspicion that the factors responsible for improvements in performance during a child's growth might be similar to those that affect fitness changes related to physical activity or training in adults (see chapter 7). It follows that deciphering fitness determinants as the child grows could provide information regarding physiologic factors responsible for influencing endurance performance at all ages.

Endurance fitness has been evaluated in several performance models. In its purest meaning, endurance should be measured as the time that a particular exercise task can be sustained until subject exhaustion. Evaluation of fitness by this definition is limited, however, by the lack of a clearly defined end point ("fatigue" in this testing setting is principally a psychological rather than a physiologic phenomenon). Alternative models for assessing endurance performance are easier to measure: time required to run (swim, bike, ski, etc.) a given distance, distance run in a specified time, rate of performance decline as fatigue sets in, and time to exhaustion in work of increasing severity. Information is available in children for each of these endurance fitness models.

Time for Distance

Traditionally the most common means of assessing endurance performance has been time for distance. The time required to traverse a particular distance is the challenge created by organized athletic events (track, cross-country) and is the model adopted for most field fitness tests of children in the schools. Thus there is a large amount of cross-sectional time-for-distance data describing normal changes with age for both boys and girls.

One-mile run times for more than 12,000 children, reported by the American Alliance for Health, Physical Education, Recreation and Dance (AAHPERD), show progressive improvement between the ages of 5 and 13 years (see fig. 6.12) (1). In that time span, performance improves almost 100% in boys, with average times falling from 13:46 to 7:27. These data indicate that the typical boy will shorten his 1-mile finish time by about :45 per year. Girls show the same pattern, but the times are slower; and after age 14, average 1-mile run times actually increase in females.

The weights of these subjects are not available. But with use of weights from standard data (63), the allometric equations calculated from the AAHPERD information indicate that for girls, run time = $1.71 M^{-.45}$ and for boys, run time = $1.98 M^{-.67}$.

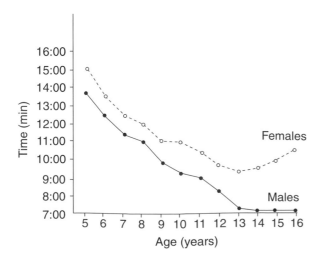

Figure 6.12   One-mile run times in children and adolescents (mean values for over 12,000 subjects). Reprinted from Rowland 1990.

Distance for Time

Cross-sectional data from AAHPERD show similar improvements when children are asked to run as far as possible in 9 min (1). At ages 5, 10, and 15 years the average respective distances run by boys were 1170, 1690, and 1986 yd. Values for girls were 1140, 1460, and 1653 yd. Jackson and Coleman described similar findings (40). Drabik provided 12 min run test results in over 5000 children ages 8-12 years (26). Between these ages the mean distance in boys rose from 2036 to 2405 yd and in the girls from 1759 to 2146 yd.

Performance Decrement

Endurance fitness has been examined as the pattern of decline in pedaling work during a high-resistance cycle test (72). Subjects begin at the same relative work rate (about 100% $\dot{V}O_2max$); the falloff in pedaling rate as the subject fatigues is utilized as an index of endurance fitness. Using this approach, Sady and Katch could find no differences in prepubertal boys and adult men (mean ages 10.2 and 30.0 years) (72). The boys and men were cycling at the same relative intensity (i.e., percentage of $\dot{V}O_2max$) at a load of 543 and 1607 kgm · min^{-1}, respectively. This indicates that absolute endurance fitness, not surprisingly, was clearly greater in the adults.

Time With Increasing Workload

The time to maximal effort during a progressive treadmill or cycle protocol increases as children grow. Cumming et al. combined their cross-sectional data in children (using the Brucc treadmill protocol) with data for adults in order to create curves showing this improvement (19) (see fig. 6.13). Endurance times peaked in the late teen years in males and approximately 5 years earlier in females. Longitudinal data from Kemper et al. demonstrate the same trends (42). At a constant running speed, average maximal treadmill slope increased from 13.5% to 15.5% in males from age 13.5 years to retest at age 16.5 years, whereas maximal slope remained constant during this time in the girls (approximately 10.3%). Improvements in cycle time with increasing age during childhood are indicated in the cross-sectional James protocol data of Washington et al. (89).

These data collectively suggest that (1) endurance fitness by any given model improves during childhood at least until the age of puberty, (2) mean values of endurance performance are consistently greater in males at all ages, and (3) levels of endurance fitness can be expected to peak during adolescence, several years earlier in females than in males.

A number of investigators have reported the relationship between field endurance tests and maximal aerobic power measured in the laboratory. The reader will find

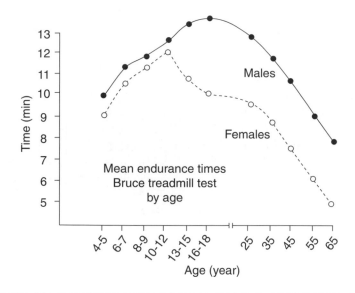

Figure 6.13   Treadmill endurance times in males and females (Bruce protocol) (19). Reprinted from Cumming 1978.

references to these studies in the extensive review by Safrit (73). In these investigations a wide range of correlation coefficients is observed between $\dot{V}O_2$max and run performance on distances from 600 yd to 1600 m (r = .23 to .75), with a mean of r = .57. Correlations were higher in studies of maximal aerobic power and distance run for time (9-15 min), with a range of r = .63 to .90 (mean .77).

It has been argued by Cureton that these correlations may reflect association of body fat content between individuals as much as O_2 uptake (22). On the basis of the assumption that cardiorespiratory function relates best to LBM, he estimated that body fat and cardiorespiratory fitness contribute equally to field performance in endurance events. Moreover, these two factors together account for only half of the variance in endurance performance.

Cumming et al. reported a close relationship between weight-relative $\dot{V}O_2$max and treadmill endurance time in children using the Bruce protocol (19). In a heterogeneous group of 10-20-year-old females ranging from nonathletes to competitive speed skaters, the correlation coefficient was r = .88. Krahenbuhl et al. found similar correlations in young boys (r = .77) and girls (r = .85) using the same protocol (47). Again, the influence of body composition on this relationship is problematic. In a larger group of 327 children, Cumming et al. reported negative correlations between treadmill endurance time and the ratio of weight to the cube of height (an index of obesity), ranging in different age groups from r = 0.20 to 0.47 (p < .05) (19).

It is noteworthy that when child athletes are considered in this analysis, the power of $\dot{V}O_2$max as a predictor of endurance performance is greatly enhanced. Pre-

pubertal male cross-country runners, for instance, typically demonstrate mass-relative $\dot{V}O_2$max values of 65 ml · kg^{-1} · min^{-1}, 30% greater than values for nonathletes (53, 86). Even within a homogeneous group of such runners, $\dot{V}O_2$max per kg correlates closely to race performance. Unnithan reported a correlation coefficient of r = −0.83 between $\dot{V}O_2$max and 3000 m race time in a group of 15 run-trained boys (mean age 11.6 years) (86). Cunningham found that when performance times of high school male and female cross-country runners differed, $\dot{V}O_2$max was the principal determinant associated with running time (21).

A critical appraisal of these data leads necessarily to the conclusion that $\dot{V}O_2$max (a) may be a significant factor separating endurance fitness in highly athletic and nonathletic children but (b) is unlikely to be predominantly responsible for differences in endurance performance as children grow. Viewed from the perspective of the entire childhood age span, this is not surprising. As reviewed previously, maximal O_2 uptake related to body mass appears to change little between the ages of 5 and 15 years in males and shows a progressive decline in girls. During this same time span, endurance performance improves dramatically, with 1-mile run times decreasing by 50% in the boys and 37% in the girls.

How, then, can physiologic/anatomic factors explain the dramatic improvements in endurance fitness in the growing child who has stable values for $\dot{V}O_2$max per kg? Several explanations have been proposed:

Hypothesis #1: **Aerobic functional reserve increases with growth.** Is the relationship of absolute $\dot{V}O_2$max and body size truly constant in boys between ages 6 and 16? The allometric analysis of Armstrong and Welsman, described earlier in this chapter, suggested that maximal aerobic power during childhood and adolescence may improve at a greater rate than can be accounted for by size alone (3). This runs counter to data examined through use of the traditional ratio standard ($\dot{V}O_2$max per kg), which indicates that $\dot{V}O_2$max improves at the same rate as body mass (in boys) or at a slower rate than body mass (in girls). It will be interesting to see how future studies clarify this developmental picture.

The concept of aerobic scope as a means of expressing aerobic reserve independent of body dimensions has already been introduced. The ratio of maximal to resting O_2 uptake doubles between the ages of 6 and 16 years in both boys and girls, matching remarkably well the 50% and 35% decreases, respectively, in 1-mile run times during the same age span. This would suggest that increases in aerobic reserve as the child grows may explain improvements in endurance performance. As reviewed earlier, however, there are questions regarding the conceptual validity of aerobic scope as a marker of aerobic fitness.

Hypothesis #2: **Age-related improvements in endurance performance reflect greater submaximal economy.** The aerobic cost per kg body mass to perform a given weight-bearing activity (economy) progressively diminishes as a child grows. For example, in one study a group of prepubertal boys had a mean $\dot{V}O_2$ per kg of 49.5 ml $\cdot$ kg^{-1} $\cdot$ min^{-1} during flat treadmill running at 6 mph compared to 40.0 ml $\cdot$ kg^{-1} $\cdot$ min^{-1} in young adult men (67). The characterization and explanation for age-related differences in submaximal economy are topics in chapter 11.

Given this improvement in submaximal economy and the relative stability of $\dot{V}O_2$max per kg during growth, it follows that at any given submaximal workload the relative intensity (percentage of $\dot{V}O_2$max) will diminish as the child ages (48). Rowland and Cunningham demonstrated this in their longitudinal evaluation of 20 children tested annually from ages 9 to 13 years (68). Treadmill walking economy, measured at 3.25 mph at an 8% grade, improved from an average of 31.0 to 26.4 ml $\cdot$ kg^{-1} $\cdot$ min^{-1} over the 5 years. These values represented an average of 65.3% of $\dot{V}O_2$max at age 9 and 55.0% of $\dot{V}O_2$max at age 13 (see fig. 6.14).

From this information one would expect older children to perform better in endurance events because they are exercising at a lower relative intensity at a given speed than the younger child. And this should translate into running faster over a given distance or running longer at a certain speed. Body mass scaling exponents for submaximal $\dot{V}O_2$ in children have ranged from .52 to .75 (79)—values similar to those calculated earlier in the context of relating mass to endurance performance. This observation supports improvements in submaximal economy as an important determinant of increases in endurance performance during the childhood years.

Hypothesis #3: **Nonaerobic factors contribute significantly to increases in endurance fitness in children.** There is evidence that factors other than maximal or submaximal O_2 uptake may play a role in the improvements observed in endurance performance of growing children. Cureton et al. evaluated the contributions of height, percent body fat, $\dot{V}O_2$max related to LBM, and 50 yd dash time to 600 yd and mile run time in 196 children ages 7-12 years (23). All these variables were significantly associated

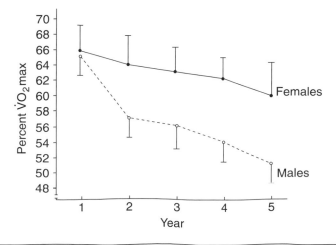

Figure 6.14 Change in relative exercise intensity (percentage $\dot{V}O_2$max) at a given treadmill walking speed in a 5-year longitudinal study of 20 children (from Rowland and Cunningham [68]).

with performance on the two distance runs, but 50 yd dash time and percent body fat were found to be the most important determinants. Similarly, Krahenbuhl and Pangrazi reported that children who placed above the 55th percentile in a 1.6 km run had significantly faster 30 m sprint speed and lower skinfold thicknesses than those who finished below the 45th percentile (46).

Palgi et al. found that anaerobic capacity (by Wingate testing), $\dot{V}O_2$max, percent body fat, and anaerobic threshold all correlated well with 2 km run time in girls and boys 10-14 years old ($r = -.77$, $-.73$, $.55$, and $-.73$, respectively (58). Multiple regression analysis indicated that anaerobic capacity was the most highly related variable.

These findings must be interpreted with caution. They may indicate that anaerobic factors (speed, short-term muscle endurance) are important in the development of endurance fitness in children, an attractive idea given the recognized improvements in anaerobic capacity with age (see chapter 12). Alternatively, however, these findings may signify that anaerobic and aerobic fitness characteristics are closely linked in children, supporting the concept that youngsters are "metabolic non-specialists" (7, p. 16). Furthermore, as Palgi et al. emphasize, "The fact that run time and anaerobic capacity depend on the willingness of the child to give a maximal effort implies that to some extent the common factor of motivation exists in both measurements and may account for some of the relationship" (58, p. 72).

To summarize what we have seen in this section, the physiologic factors responsible for the steady improvements in endurance fitness in growing children have not been well clarified. It is tempting to conclude that a combination of all three of the determinants outlined somehow play a role. The analysis is difficult, considering the natural improvements in strength, speed, maximal O_2 uptake, anaerobic capacity, cognitive abilities, and other factors that parallel endurance performance with increasing age.

GENDER DIFFERENCES

This chapter has referred throughout to sex-related differences that separate aspects of aerobic fitness in boys and girls; in the remainder of this book, attention will focus on how gender influences factors such as muscle strength, submaximal economy, and anaerobic fitness. At this point it is appropriate to reflect on these variations and consider their possible explanations.

Significant average differences in measures of aerobic function are observed in adult men and women (54). Values for $\dot{V}O_2$max per kg in adult men typically are 15-30% greater than those in females, and a similar gender gap is observed in performance in endurance athletic events. From the data presented in this chapter it is apparent that these discrepancies become clearly established at the time of puberty. It is interesting, however, that the same sex-related mean differences in aerobic fitness—although smaller—are observed in prepubertal subjects as early in life as subjects can effectively perform exercise tests.

These prepubertal gender differences are particularly evident in endurance performance. The average 10-year-old boy can run a mile 2 min faster than a girl the same age (1). Mean endurance time for running or walking on a treadmill is typically 10% to 20% longer in prepubertal males than in females (19). However, Åstrand showed only very small differences in the maximal speed a subject could maintain for 5 min of treadmill running in 7-9-year-old boys and girls (13.8 vs. 13.5 km/hr, respectively) (4). Likewise, no gender differences in maximal cycle work were described in 6-15-year-old children by Washington et al. (89).

The sex difference in $\dot{V}O_2$max per kg progressively widens during the course of childhood. According to the cross-sectional data of Krahenbuhl et al., the average 8-year-old boy has a 6% greater maximal O_2 uptake than his female counterpart, but by the age of 12 years the difference is 18% (49).

Average gender differences in aerobic function before the age of puberty are generally not large, however; and to state the obvious, a broad overlap exists between groups of boys and girls. While the practical significance of these differences can therefore be questioned, understanding gender-related influences on aerobic function in children is important from a mechanistic standpoint. Why should girls and boys have different maximal aerobic power and perform differently on aerobic tasks independent of the influences of puberty? Researchers have observed that the magnitude of the performance gap between the sexes appears to exceed that of physiologic differences. This has led to the suggestion that girls are less likely to fulfill their potential for fitness because of social rather than biological constraints (59). In efforts to promote the health-related benefits of exercise in children, then, the gender gap may have significant implications.

Three mechanisms have traditionally been offered to explain gender differences in aerobic fitness in adults: sex-related variations in body composition, hemoglobin concentration, and habitual physical activity. Consequently the potential roles of these influences have been examined in the pediatric age group.

Body Composition

In the young adult, fat-free mass (FFM) per unit stature is 38% greater in males, whereas the percent body fat in women is almost double that of men (9, 52). This means that the body "motor" (i.e., skeletal muscle mass) makes up a significantly smaller proportion of body weight in females. According to Behnke and Wilmore, the percentage of weight accounted for by muscle mass is 45% and 36% for the average young man and woman, respectively (9). Thus in adults, $\dot{V}O_2$max expressed per LBM reduces by one-half the gender differences observed in values related to body weight (80).

These differences are smaller in childhood, but the same patterns are seen. Percent body fat is about 15% in the average 8-year-old boy but 23% in his female counterpart. Differences in FFM per unit stature are less (approximately 6% greater in the boy). This greater relative muscle mass in boys can be expected (a) to improve endurance fitness, since the relative size of their "motor" (skeletal muscle mass) is greater while the "baggage" is lighter, and (b) to account for a greater $\dot{V}O_2$max expressed per kg body mass.

As noted earlier in this chapter, expressing $\dot{V}O_2$max per kg LBM in children will diminish (but generally not eliminate) sex-related differences in maximal aerobic power. Malina and Bouchard suggested that preadolescent and adolescent boys will have, on the average, a 10% greater $\dot{V}O_2$max per kg FFM than girls (52). Cunningham reported that the difference in average $\dot{V}O_2$max in high school male and female runners was reduced from 12% to 5% when values were related to body mass and LBM, respectively (21).

Hemoglobin Concentration

Hemoglobin is responsible for the transport of O_2 in the bloodstream, and even relatively small changes in hemoglobin concentration or total hemoglobin mass can have a profound effect on both maximal O_2 uptake and endurance performance. Since the average adult male has a hemoglobin concentration of 16.0 grams percent compared to 14.0 grams percent in females (24, 31), hemoglobin status has been considered a likely contributor to sex differences in aerobic fitness in adults.

No gender differences in mean hemoglobin concentration are observed before puberty (24). This observation implicates the influence of testosterone on red cell production as the principal factor responsible for gender-related hemoglobin differences in adults. However, even as early as 12-14 years of age, boys may have as much as 0.5 grams percent higher values than girls (24). Aerobic performance in early adolescence may therefore be partially influenced by differences in hemoglobin concentration in boys and girls.

Habitual Activity

Studies quantifying habitual activity in children consistently demonstrate that, on the average, boys are routinely more active than girls (27, 64). The meta-analysis of Eaton and Enns confirmed this observation and suggested that gender differences in activity exist—albeit to a much smaller degree—even in early infancy (27). From the findings of several studies, Rowland created a composite curve of daily energy expenditure for males and females during the course of childhood (64). At all ages beyond 6 years, the boys showed approximately 9% greater activity levels (measured as kcal/kg per day). It is possible, then, that these differences in daily exercise might translate into similar gender discrepancies in both maximal aerobic power and field endurance performance. The role played by variations in usual daily activity levels in influencing $\dot{V}O_2$max, however, does not appear to be large (see chapter 7).

Despite dramatic increases in participation in organized sports by girls, the number of females on athletic teams continues to lag behind that for boys. Data from the National Federation of State High School Associations indicate that throughout the 1980s the participation in high school sports by boys was almost double that of girls (64). These gender differences may also contribute to findings based on comparison of aerobic fitness in male and female children.

Some consider environmental influences an explanation for lower levels of physical activity and sport participation in girls. Opportunities may not be as great for females as for males, and there is a lack of appropriate role models for female athletes (i.e., female coaches and officials). Sexual stereotyping may create psychological barriers for girls, and this can be reinforced by peer conduct (27).

It is difficult to clearly define the extent to which each of the various determinants influences gender differences in aerobic fitness in children. Thomas et al. reviewed fitness testing, anthropometric measurements, and parent questionnaire data to assess sex-related differences in endurance performance in over 12,000 children in the National Children and Youth Fitness Study (85). They concluded that before puberty the major influence on running distance time was body adiposity, whereas hours in outside activity became increasingly influential in the postpubertal years. However, others have emphasized the importance of environmental factors (stereotyped sex role expectations, unequal opportunities for sport involvement) in limiting activity of prepubertal girls (32, 84).

In summary, differences in hemoglobin levels between the sexes are limited to the postpubertal years and probably are of little significance under age 12 years. Body adiposity, on the other hand, clearly influences both performance and $\dot{V}O_2$max variations relative to gender before puberty. Still, considerable sex variance persists in children even when body composition is taken into account (84).

GENETIC INFLUENCES

It is popularly assumed that one's genetic endowment is a major—if not predominant—factor responsible for both laboratory and field measures of aerobic fitness. Certainly the fifth-grade boy who is a "natural" athlete appears to be more born than made. And, as similarly observed in adults, endurance training of the average child will improve $\dot{V}O_2$max, but not to levels even approaching those of prepubertal endurance athletes. As expressed in the traditional adage, to become a star athlete one should choose one's parents carefully.

It might be reasonable to expect genetic factors to exert influence on aerobic power in children by (a) affecting the size and function of O_2 delivery and peripheral extraction systems between individuals, (b) altering the rate of development of O_2 intake in a given child, and (c) governing the degree to which increases (or decreases) in physical activity will improve $\dot{V}O_2$max. From the existing research information one can conclude that (a) is true, but not to the extent commonly believed, (b) has not been studied, and (c) is true in adults but has not been evaluated in children.

The contribution of heredity to interindividual variability in $\dot{V}O_2$max has been traditionally estimated by comparing intrapair differences in maximal aerobic power in monozygous and dizygous twins. This approach is based on the fact that the former share both environmental and genetic influences on $\dot{V}O_2$max whereas the latter should differ only in environmental effects. Using this technique in an early study, Klissouras supported the importance of hereditary factors in determining aerobic fitness in children (44). Exercising 15 pairs of monozygous and 10 pairs of dizygous twins ages 7 to 13 years to exhaustion on a treadmill protocol, he concluded that 93% of the variability in maximal aerobic power is genetically determined.

This study came under criticism, however, because of concerns that other variables influencing aerobic power may not have been adequately controlled (18). Subsequent twin studies have disclosed a wide range of estimates of hereditary influences on $\dot{V}O_2$max, and in general these have indicated a much smaller contribution of the genetic effect on maximal aerobic power than suggested by both common perception and the results of Klissouras (14, 39). Indeed, some have suggested that

heredity is responsible for little, if any, variability in $\dot{V}O_2$max (39). The more recent findings of Bouchard et al. indicate that the true genetic influence may lie between these extremes, with heredity accounting for 40-60% of the phenotypic expression of maximal aerobic power (16).

Lesage et al. concluded that the familial resemblance and heritability estimates for maximal aerobic power are "quite low and generally non-significant" (50, p. 187). In their study of 38 families, the interclass correlation coefficients for $\dot{V}O_2$max per kg and $\dot{V}O_2$max per kg fat-free weight were r = .03 and .10, respectively (p > .05). Malina and Bouchard noted that these results "should not be surprising, because maximal O_2 uptake is a complex phenotype far removed from the action of genes. Maximal O_2 uptake is influenced by the products of hundreds of genes, some pulling the phenotype in one direction and others perhaps affecting it in other directions" (52, p. 325).

Studies in adults indicate that the magnitude of improvement in $\dot{V}O_2$max with endurance training is under genetic control to an extent similar to that for $\dot{V}O_2$max (15). Skilled endurance athletes may thus be blessed with both an inherent high $\dot{V}O_2$max and a greater capacity for improving aerobic power with training. The genetic influence on aerobic trainability in children has not been studied. If the same identification of "high responders" and "low responders" to aerobic training can be assumed in the pediatric age group, the appropriateness of having "untrained controls" in studies addressing aerobic training in children becomes questionable.

Performance on endurance events appears to be more obviously influenced by heredity than is $\dot{V}O_2$max. The contribution of genetic factors to variability of work output during 90 min of cycling in adults has been reported to be 70% (14). The inheritance of psychological factors such as competitiveness, aggression, and motivation may also contribute to familial influences on endurance fitness (18).

SUMMARY

Absolute values of maximal O_2 uptake progressively rise during the course of childhood. Beyond this straightforward observation, there is no clear understanding of (a) the way in which $\dot{V}O_2$max can most appropriately be adjusted for body size, (b) the role of increasing size versus functional changes in the determinants of O_2 uptake, (c) the mechanisms for the distinctive differences between boys and girls, and (d) the means by which changes in $\dot{V}O_2$max might contribute to improvements in endurance performance. These remain the future challenges for developmental exercise physiologists.

There appears to be little question, however, that $\dot{V}O_2max$ per kg, the traditional ratio standard, has serious weaknesses that limit its value as an indicator of "aerobic fitness" in children. $\dot{V}O_2max$ expressed relative to body mass has little use as a marker of field endurance performance except within narrow age groups, since dramatic changes in such performance during the course of childhood are not accompanied by improvements in $\dot{V}O_2max$ per kg. As an indicator of cardiovascular fitness, $\dot{V}O_2max$ per kg is weakened by the influence of body fat, which lowers $\dot{V}O_2max$ per kg without influencing (within limits) cardiac function. In addition, the use of the ratio standard to compare $\dot{V}O_2max$ between groups may produce "spurious" results because $\dot{V}O_2max$ per kg is inversely related to body size. This provides an advantage to smaller subjects while penalizing those who are larger.

But children of the same size, body composition, and biological maturity may differ significantly in $\dot{V}O_2max$ as well, presumably as an expression of inherent aerobic fitness. The amount of physical activity of a child also affects $\dot{V}O_2max$, but, as will be discussed in the next chapter, the variability in usual daily activities cannot be expected to alter aerobic fitness to any great extent. Even with intensive endurance training, improvements in $\dot{V}O_2max$ in children do not typically exceed 10%.

It is critical that any assessment of aerobic fitness in children be performed with an understanding that values for $\dot{V}O_2max$ are significantly influenced by these genetic, developmental, body composition, and activity factors. This holds true for interpreting performance on endurance field events as well as for utilizing $\dot{V}O_2max$ as an expression of maximal aerobic power and cardiovascular fitness.

What We Know

1. Resting metabolic rate (or $\dot{V}O_2$) increases with age during childhood. Expressed relative to either body mass or surface area, however, metabolic expenditure decreases.

2. Maximal O_2 uptake rises as children age. This is largely the result of increases in size of $\dot{V}O_2$-dependent organs during exercise (heart, lungs, blood volume, skeletal muscle).

3. Mean gender differences in $\dot{V}O_2max$ are very small before puberty, but values in males are consistently greater than in females.

4. There has been no evident trend of decreasing aerobic fitness ($\dot{V}O_2max$) in children during the last half decade.

5. Maximal O_2 uptake relative to body mass changes little during childhood in boys and declines in girls. During the same time, dramatic improvements are observed in endurance fitness (in 1-mile run times, for example).

What We Would Like to Know

1. What is the explanation for the decline in mass-relative resting $\dot{V}O_2$ during childhood? In particular, what is the role of tissue-specific metabolic rate?

2. What is the most appropriate denominator for "normalizing" $\dot{V}O_2max$ for increasing body size with growth?

3. How much can prepubertal gender variations in $\dot{V}O_2max$ be explained by differences between boys and girls in body composition, social factors, and habitual physical activity levels?

4. What factors are responsible for the dramatic improvements observed in endurance performance during childhood?

5. How much does improvement in function (as opposed to increased size) of heart, lungs, and skeletal muscle contribute to the rise of $\dot{V}O_2max$ with age?

References

1. American Alliance for Health, Physical Education, Recreation and Dance. Youth fitness testing manual. Washington, DC; 1980.
2. Andersen, K.L.; Seliger, V.; Rutenfranz, J.; Mocellin, R. Physical performance capacity of children in Norway. Eur. J. Appl. Physiol. 33:177-195; 1974.
3. Armstrong, N.; Welsman, J.R. Assessment and interpretation of aerobic fitness in children and adolescents. Exerc. Sport Sci. Rev. 22:435-475; 1994.
4. Åstrand, P.O. Experimental studies of physical working capacity in relationship to sex and age. Copenhagen: Munksgaard; 1952.
5. Åstrand, P.O.; Rodahl, K. Textbook of work physiology. 2nd ed. New York: McGraw-Hill; 1977:p. 155.
6. Bailey, D.A.; Ross, W.D.; Mirwald, R.L.; Weese, D. Size dissociation of maximal aerobic power during growth in boys. Med. Sport 11:140-151; 1987.
7. Bar-Or, O. Pediatric sports medicine for the practitioner. New York: Springer-Verlag; 1983.
8. Bar-Or, O. Pathophysiological factors which limit the exercise capacity of the sick child. Med. Sci. Sports Exerc. 18:276-282; 1986.
9. Behnke, A.R.; Wilmore, J.H. Evaluation and regulation of body build and composition. Englewood Cliffs, NJ: Prentice-Hall; 1974.
10. Bell, R.D.; MacDougall, J.D.; Billeter, R.; Howald, H. Muscle fiber types and morphometric analysis of skeletal muscle in six-year old children. Med. Sci. Sports Exerc. 12:28-31; 1980.
11. Beunen, G.; Malina, R.M. Growth and physical performance relative to the timing of the adolescent spurt. Exerc. Sport Sci. Rev. 16:503-540; 1988.
12. Binkhorst, R.A.; de Jong-van de Ker, M.C.; Vissers, A.C.A. Growth and aerobic power of boys aged 11-19 years. In: Ilmarinen, J.; Valimaki, I., eds. Children and sport. Heidelberg: Springfield; 1984:p. 99-105.
13. Blaxter, K. Energy metabolism in animals and man. Cambridge: Cambridge University Press; 1989:p. 120-179.
14. Bouchard, C. Genetics of aerobic power and capacity. In: Malina, R.N.; Bouchard, C., eds. Sport and human genetics. Champaign, IL: Human Kinetics; 1986:p. 59-88.
15. Bouchard, C. Genetic determinants of endurance performance. In: Shephard, R.J.; Åstrand, P.O., eds. Endurance in sport. Oxford, UK: Blackwell Scientific; 1992:p. 149-162.
16. Bouchard, C.; Lesage, R.; Lortie, G.; Simoneau, J.A.; Hamel, P.; Boulay, M.R.; Perusse, L.; Theriault, G.; Leblanc, C. Aerobic performance in brothers, dizygotic and monozygotic twins. Med. Sci. Sports Exerc. 18:639-646; 1984.
17. Cooper, D.M.; Weiler-Ravell, D.; Whipp, B.J.; Wasserman, K. Aerobic parameters of exercise as a function to body size during growth in children. J. Appl. Physiol. 56:628-634; 1984.
18. Cowart, V.S. How does heredity affect athletic performance? Phys. Sportsmed. 15:134-140; 1987.
19. Cumming, G.R.; Everatt, D.; Hastman, L. Bruce treadmill test in children: normal values in a clinic population. Am. J. Cardiol. 41:69-75; 1978.
20. Cunningham, D.A.; Paterson, D.H.; Blimkie, C.J.R.; Donner, A.P. Development of cardiorespiratory function in circumpubertal boys: a longitudinal study. J. Appl. Physiol. 56:302-307; 1984.
21. Cunningham, L.N. Physiological comparison of adolescent female and male cross country runners. Pediatr. Exerc. Science 2:313-321; 1990.
22. Cureton, K.J. Distance running performance tests in children: what do they mean? JOPERD 53:64-66; 1982.
23. Cureton, K.J.; Boileau, R.A.; Lohman, T.G.; Misner, J.E. Determinants of distance running performance in children: analysis of a path model. Res. Q. 48:270-279; 1977.
24. Dallman, P.R.; Siimes, M.A. Percentile curves for hemoglobin and red cell volume in infancy and childhood. J. Pediatr. 94:26-31; 1979.
25. Davies, C.T.M.; Barnes, C.; Godfrey, S. Body composition and maximal exercise performance in children. Hum. Biol. 44:195-214; 1972.
26. Drabik, J. The general endurance of children aged 8-12 years in the 12 min run test. J. Sports Med. 29:379-383; 1989.
27. Eaton, W.O.; Enns, L.R. Sex differences in human motor activity level. Psych. Bull. 100:19-28; 1986.
28. Eriksson, B.O. Muscle metabolism in children—a review. Acta Paediatr. Scand. Suppl. 283:20-27; 1980.
29. Freedson, P.S.; Goodman, T.L. Measurement of oxygen consumption. In: Rowland, T.W., ed. Pediatric laboratory exercise testing. Champaign IL: Human Kinetics; 1993:p. 91-114.
30. Gardner, G.W.; Edgerton, V.R.; Barnard, R.J. Cardiorespiratory, hematological and physical performance responses of anemic subjects to iron treatment. Am. J. Clin. Nutr. 28:982-986; 1975.
31. Godwin, I.D.; Jencks, J.A. Normal hematological values obtained with a Coulter counter, model S. South. Med. J. 71:47-49; 1978.
32. Hall, E.G.; Lee, A.M. Sex differences in motor performance of young children: fact or fiction? Sex Roles 10:217-229; 1984.
33. Haralambie, G. Skeletal muscle enzyme activities in female subjects of various ages. Bull. Europ. Physiol. Resp. 15:259-267; 1979.
34. Henry, W.L.; Ware, J.; Gardin, J.M.; Hepner, S.I.; McKay, J.; Weiner, M. Echocardiographic measurements in normal subjects. Growth-related changes that occur between infancy and early adulthood. Circulation 57:278-285; 1978.

35. Hermansen, L.; Oseid, S. Direct and indirect estimation of maximal oxygen uptake in pre-pubertal boys. Acta Paediat. Scand. Suppl. 217:18-23; 1971.

36. Heusner, A.A. Energy metabolism and body size. I. Is the 0.75 mass exponent of Kleiber's equation a statistical artifact? Resp. Physiol. 48:1-12; 1982.

37. Holliday, M.A.; Potter, D.; Jarrah, A.; Bearg, S. The relation of metabolic rate to body weight and organ size. Pediat. Res. 1:185-195; 1967.

38. Hollman, W.; Bouchard, C. Untersuchungen uber die Beziehungen zwischen chronologischem und biologischem Alter zu spiroergometrischen Messgrossen, Herzvolumen, anthropometrischen Daten und Skelettmuskelkraft bei 8-18 jahrigen Jungen. (Relations between chronological, skeletal age, and ergometric characteristics, heart volume, anthropometric dimensions, and muscle strength in 8 to 18 year old boys.) Zeitscrift fur Kreislaufforschung 59:160-176; 1970.

39. Howald, H. Ultrastructure and biochemical function of skeletal muscle in twins. Ann. Hum. Biol. 3:455-462; 1976.

40. Jackson, A.S.; Coleman, A.E. Validation of distance run tests for elementary school children. Res. Q. 47:86-94; 1976.

41. Katch, V.L. Use of the oxygen/body weight ratio in correlational analyses: spurious correlations and statistical considerations. Med. Sci. Sports 5:252-257; 1973.

42. Kemper, H.C.G.; Verschuur, R.; de Mey, L. Longitudinal changes of aerobic fitness in youth ages 12 to 23. Pediatr. Exerc. Science 1:257-270; 1989.

43. Kleiber, M. The fire of life. New York: Wiley; 1961:p. 177-225.

44. Klissouras, V. Hertability of adaptive variation. J. Appl. Physiol. 31:338-344; 1971.

45. Knoebel, L.K. Energy metabolism. In: Selkurt, E.E., ed. Physiology. Boston: Little, Brown; 1963:p. 564-579.

46. Krahenbuhl, G.S.; Pangrazi, R.P. Characteristics associated with running performance in young boys. Med. Sci. Sports Exerc. 15:486-490; 1983.

47. Krahenbuhl, G.S.; Pangrazi, R.P.; Burkett, L.N.; Schneider, M.J.; Petersen, G. Field estimation of $\dot{V}O_2$max in children eight years of age. Med. Sci. Sports 9:37-40; 1977.

48. Krahenbuhl, G.S.; Pangrazi, R.P.; Stone, W.J.; Morgan, D.W.; Williams, T. Fractional utilization of maximal aerobic capacity in children 6 to 8 years of age. Pediatr. Exerc. Science 1:271-277; 1989.

49. Krahenbuhl, G.S.; Skinner, J.S.; Kohrt, W.M. Developmental aspects of maximal aerobic power in children. Exerc. Sport Sci. Rev. 13:503-538; 1985.

50. Lesage, R.; Simoneau, J.; Jobin, J.; Leblanc, C.; Bouchard, C. Familial resemblance in maximal heart rate, blood lactate and aerobic power. Hum. Hered. 35:182-189; 1985.

51. Malina, R.M. Growth of muscle tissue and muscle mass. In: Falkner, F.; Tanner, J.M., eds. Human growth. 2. Postnatal growth. New York: Plenum Press; 1978:p. 273-294.

52. Malina, R.M.; Bouchard, C. Growth, maturation, and physical activity. Champaign, IL: Human Kinetics; 1991.

53. Mayers, N.; Gutin, B. Physiological characteristics of elite prepubertal cross country runners. Med. Sci. Sports Exerc. 11:172-176; 1979.

54. McArdle, W.D.; Katch, F.I.; Katch, V.L. Exercise physiology. Energy, nutrition, and human performance. Philadelphia: Lea & Febiger; 1981.

55. Mirwald, R.L.; Bailey, D.A. Maximal aerobic power. A longitudinal analysis. London, ON: Sport Dynamics; 1986.

56. Noakes, T.D. Implications of exercise testing for prediction of athletic performance: a contemporary perspective. Med. Sci. Sports Exerc. 20:319-330; 1988.

57. Orenstein, D.M. Assessment of exercise pulmonary function. In: Rowland, T.W., ed. Pediatric laboratory exercise testing. Champaign, IL: Human Kinetics; 1993:p. 141-164.

58. Palgi, Y.; Gutin, B.; Young, J.; Alejandro, D. Physiologic and anthropometric factors underlying endurance performance in children. Int. J. Sports Med. 5:67-73; 1984.

59. Raithel, K.S. Are girls less fit than boys? Phys. Sportsmed. 15:157-163; 1987.

60. Robinson, S. Experimental studies of physical fitness in relation to age. Arbeitsphysiologie 10:251-323; 1938.

61. Rogers, D.M.; Turley, K.R.; Kujawa, K.I.; Harper, K.M.; Wilmore, J.H. Allometric scaling factors for oxygen uptake during exercise in children. Pediatr. Exerc. Sci. 7: 12-25; 1995.

62. Ross, W.D.; Bailey, D.A.; Weese, C.H. Proportionality and interpretation of longitudinal metabolic function data on boys. In: Lavallee, H.; Shephard, R.J., eds. Frontiers of activity and child health. Ottawa, ON: Pelican; 1977:p. 225-236.

63. Ross Laboratories. Children are different: relation of age to physiologic function. Columbus, OH; 1970.

64. Rowland, T.W. Exercise and children's health. Champaign, IL: Human Kinetics; 1990.

65. Rowland, T.W. Effects of obesity on aerobic fitness in adolescent females. AJDC 145:764-768; 1991.

66. Rowland, T.W. "Normalizing" maximal oxygen uptake, or the search for the holy grail (per kg). Pediatr. Exerc. Sci. 3:95-102; 1991.

67. Rowland, T.W.; Auchinachie, J.A.; Keenan, T.J.; Green, G.M. Physiologic responses to treadmill running in adult and prepubertal males. Int. J. Sports Med. 8:292-297; 1987.

68. Rowland, T.W.; Cunningham, L.N. Walking economy and stride frequency in children: a longitudinal analysis [abstract]. Med. Sci. Sports Exerc. 27 Suppl:S93; 1995.

69. Rubner, M. Ueber den Einfluss der Korpergrosse auf Stoffund Kraftwechsel. Z. Biol. 19:535-562; 1883.

70. Rutenfranz, F.; Andersen, K.L.; Seliger, V.; Klimmer, F.; Berndt, I.; Ruppel, M. Maximum aerobic power and body composition during the pubertal growth period: similarities and differences between children of two European countries. Eur. J. Pediatr. 136:123-133; 1981.

71. Rutenfranz, J.; Mácek, M.; Andersen, K.L.; Bell, R.D.; Vavra, J.; Radvansky, J.; Klimmer, F.; Kylian, H. The relationship between changing body height and growth related changes in maximal aerobic power. Eur. J. Appl. Physiol. 60:282-287; 1990.

72. Sady, S.P.; Katch, V.L. Relative endurance and physiological responses: a study of individual differences in prepubescent boys and adult men. Res. Q. 52:246-255; 1981.

73. Safrit, M.J. The validity and reliability of fitness tests for children: a review. Pediatr. Exerc. Science 2:9-28; 1990.

74. Saltin, B. Physiological adaptation to physical conditioning. Acta Med. Scand. Suppl. 711:11-24; 1986.

75. Sarrus et Rameaux. Memoire adresse a l'Academie Royale. Bull. Acad. Roy. Med. Belg. 3:1094; 1839.

76. Savov, S.G. Physical fitness and skeletal maturity in girls and boys 11 years of age. In: Shephard, R.J.; Lavallee, H., eds. Physical fitness assessment: practice and application. Springfield, IL: Charles C Thomas; 1978:p. 222-228.

77. Schmidt-Nielsen, K. Scaling. Why is animal size so important? Cambridge: Cambridge University Press; 1984:p. 56-98.

78. Shephard, R.J.; Lavallee, H.; Rajic, K.M.; Jequier, J.C.; Brisson, G.; Beaucage, C. Radiographic age in the interpretation of physiological and anthropometric data. Med. Sport 11:124-133; 1978.

79. Sjodin, B.; Svendenhag, J. Oxygen uptake during running as related to body mass in circumpubertal boys: a longitudinal study. Evr. J. Appl. Physiol. 65:150-157; 1992.

80. Sparling, P.B. A meta-analysis of studies comparing maximal oxygen uptake in men and women. Res. Q. 51:542-552; 1980.

81. Sprynarova, S. Longitudinal study of the influence of different physical activity programs on functional capacity of the boys from 11 to 18 years. Acta Paediatr. Belg. Suppl. 28:204-213; 1974.

82. Taylor, C.R.; Weibel, E.R. Design of the mammalian respiratory system. I. Problem and strategy. Resp. Physiol. 44:1-10; 1981.

83. Taylor, G.R.; Maloiy, G.M.C.; Weibel, E.R.; Langman, V.A.; Kaman, J.M.Z.; Seeherman, H.J.; Heglund, N.C. Design of the mammalian respiratory system. III. Scaling maximal aerobic capacity to body mass: wild and domestic animals. Resp. Physiol. 44:25-37; 1981.

84. Thomas, J.R.; French, K.E. Gender differences across age in motor performance: a meta-analysis. Psych. Bull. 98:260-282; 1985.

85. Thomas, J.R.; Nelson, J.K.; Church, G. A developmental analysis of gender differences in health related physical fitness. Pediatr. Exerc. Science 3:28-42; 1991.

86. Unnithan, V.B. Factors affecting submaximal running economy in children [doctoral thesis]. University of Glasgow; 1993.

87. Vanden Eynde, B.; Ghesquiere, J.; van Derven, D.; Vuylsteke-Wauters, M.; Vande Perre, H. Follow-up study of physical fitness in boys aged 10-14 years. In: Ilmarinen, J.; Valimaki, I, eds. Children and sport. Berlin: Springer; 1984:p. 111-118.

88. von Dobeln, W.; Eriksson, B.O. Physical training, maximal oxygen uptake and dimensions of the oxygen transporting and metabolizing organs in boys 11-13 years of age. Acta Paediatr. Scand. 61:653-660; 1972.

89. Washington, R.L.; van Gundy, J.C.; Cohen, C.; Sondheimer, H.; Wolfe, R.R. Normal aerobic and anaerobic exercise data for North American school-age children. J. Pediatr. 112:223-233; 1988.

90. Weibel, E.R. The pathway for oxygen. Cambridge, MA: Harvard University Press; 1984.

91. Welsman, J.; Armstrong, N.; Winter, E.; Kirby, B.J. The influence of various scaling techniques on the interpretation of developmental changes in peak $\dot{V}O_2$ [abstract]. Pediatr. Exerc. Science 5:485; 1993.

92. Zanconato, S.; Buchtal, S.; Barstow, T.J.; Cooper; D.M. ^{31}P-magnetic resonance spectroscopy of leg muscle metabolism during exercise in children and adults. J. Appl. Physiol. 74:2214–2218; 1993.

CHAPTER 7

THE PLASTICITY OF AEROBIC FITNESS

The previous chapters have described the normal growth of $\dot{V}O_2$max in children, with particular attention to the influences of gender, genetic potential, and body composition. We now turn to the question of the plasticity of $\dot{V}O_2$max during childhood—the extent to which normal maturation of maximal aerobic power can be altered by changes in level of physical activity. Of the many determinants of aerobic fitness, physical activity is potentially the most readily altered. If activity significantly influences $\dot{V}O_2$max, then, increasing the level of physical activity would be an appropriate strategy for improving aerobic fitness.

To address this question, we will examine the influence of activity on $\dot{V}O_2$max (1) at the extremes of activity—endurance training and bed rest—as well as (2) within the usual variations in habitual daily activity. There is a general perception that the plasticity of maximal aerobic power in children before the age of puberty may be less than in adults (67). The evidence for this concept will be reviewed and possible explanations explored.

HABITUAL ACTIVITY AND $\dot{V}O_2$MAX

Although the two are often considered almost synonymous, amount of daily physical activity in a child should be clearly distinguished from degree of physical fitness. Activity involves the level of physical movement in the course of a usual day, typically measured in kilocalories of energy expenditure. Physical fitness has been defined in many ways but is generally characterized by how *well* one can perform on a motor task. Thus fitness testing in the school setting measures how fast children can run a mile or how many sit-ups they can do. In this section we will be considering level of daily physical activity as it relates to one particular laboratory index of physical fitness, maximal aerobic power.

First, it is of interest to examine the temporal changes in both physical activity and $\dot{V}O_2$max during the course of childhood. We saw in the previous chapter that absolute levels of $\dot{V}O_2$max rise throughout childhood and adolescence except in girls, who show a plateau at the time of puberty. $\dot{V}O_2$max per kg, on the other hand, remains relatively stable with age in boys but steadily declines in girls. The picture of changes in habitual activity level during childhood is different. Relative to body size or weight, daily energy expenditure progressively falls, both in boys and in girls. As shown in figure 7.1, daily energy utilization in kcal/kg in a 6-year-old is almost twice that of an older adolescent (67).

The explanation for the dramatic decline in daily energy expenditure in growing children is obscure. Many would focus on environmental factors of modern society—television, easy transportation, withdrawal from sports activities—as playing key roles in effecting a more sedentary lifestyle in the childhood years. But it seems likely that the downward curve for activity in children has at least some primary biological basis. One is impressed, for instance, with the similar decline in weight-relative basal metabolic rate with age (see fig. 6.4, page 76) (67). Metabolic energy expended with motor activity during the day may therefore share controlling mechanisms responsible for the energy utilized at rest.

The concept of an "activity-stat" in the central nervous system that influences daily activity levels is supported by experimental data in animals. Anand described studies indicating that animals with lesions in the medial hypothalamus become hypoactive whereas removal or lesions of the rostral hypothalamus, basal ganglia, or ungulate gyrus of the cerebrum cause hyperactive behavior (4). If dopamine metabolism in animals

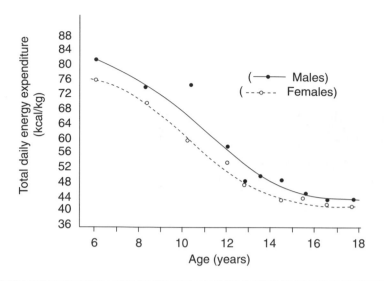

Figure 7.1   Decline in physical activity as indicated by energy expenditure per kg during childhood and adolescence. Reprinted from Rowland 1990.

is selectively inhibited, young animals become increasingly active (87).

If such central neurological control of activity is genetically determined, its influence is not great. When Perusse et al. obtained 3-day activity diaries in 1610 subjects from 375 families, the genetic effect was estimated at 20% of the age- and gender-adjusted variation (61). However, identification of such a central controlling mechanism would have significant importance for exercise scientists. For the bad news, it would suggest that increasing a child's activity (by augmenting physical education classes, for instance) might be counterbalanced by more sedentary activity at other times. For the good news, this knowledge would provide an opportunity to identify factors that could positively influence such an activity-controlling center.

Measurement of Physical Activity

Habitual physical activity is difficult to measure. Whereas maximal aerobic power can be determined relatively easily with exercise testing, an easy, accurate, nonintrusive means of ascertaining a child's daily energy expenditure remains elusive. Indeed, the inability to accurately measure daily activity has served as a major roadblock in efforts to understand not only the natural course of activity throughout life but also the impact of the many potential influences on daily energy expenditure.

More than 30 different techniques have been utilized to assess physical activity, but none has proven sufficiently practical and valid to emerge as a standard method (40). The application of these techniques to children has been the subject of several reviews (7, 28, 80). In general, the easier and more practical a measurement tool is, the less precise it becomes (see fig. 7.2). Diaries and questionnaires, for instance, are easy to administer to large groups of subjects in epidemiologic studies, but children cannot be expected to recall or record activity levels with great accuracy, particularly below the age of 10-12 years (80). At the other end of the scale, caloric expenditure can be accurately recorded in a metabolic chamber or by determining O_2 uptake through indirect calorimetry, but these approaches provide no insight into free-living activity levels of groups of children. New smaller portable devices for measuring O_2 uptake may be useful in determining the caloric requirement of certain forms of activity (59), but this equipment is intrusive and can be expected to alter normal activity levels.

Heart rate is a good indicator of metabolic expenditure and has been commonly employed in studies of activity levels of children (21, 30). Unfortunately, heart rate also accurately reflects such variables as emotional stress, muscle mass involved in exercise, temperature, type of activity, and level of training (80). Lightweight motion sensors have become increasingly popular for measuring activity levels in children, but studies assessing the validity of this approach have shown conflicting results (19).

Direct observation has proven to be an accurate means of measuring activity but has limited practicality except as a way of validating other field techniques (62). The same could be said about the doubly labeled water technique, which appears to be a highly accurate means of evaluating energy expenditure in children

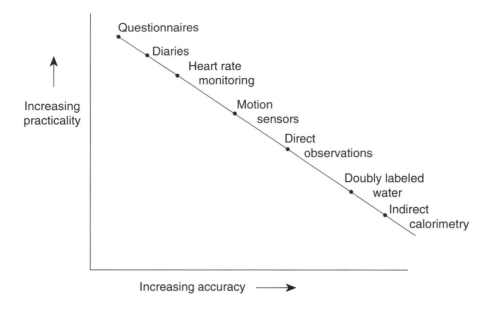

Figure 7.2   Feasibility and accuracy for methods assessing habitual physical activity are inversely related.

(31). But the expense and limited availability of this method will probably restrict its general use in field studies of habitual activity.

Importance of the Fitness-Activity Relationship

Why are we concerned with the effect of activity on $\dot{V}O_2max$? Interest in the relationship between aerobic fitness and habitual activity in children follows from at least two important issues. First, in planning strategies for the evaluation and promotion of exercise for health in children, how do the two interact? And which is the most critical determinant of positive health outcomes? Second, if aerobic trainability is less in children than in adults, how much of the difference is attributable to the greater daily activity level of children?

Children and the Exercise-Health Connection.
The salutary effects of exercise have been recognized since the beginnings of recorded history. Only within the last 30 years, however, has scientific evidence been amassed to validate the positive influence of regular exercise habits on a variety of disease states (see table 7.1). On examination of this list, three features are evident. First, these illnesses constitute the major causes of morbidity and mortality in developed societies. Exercise therefore has the potential for making a significant impact on the health of populations. Second, the diseases listed are essentially all health problems of adults, not children. Even obesity, a common finding in children, does not usually become a health hazard until the adult years. And third, most of these diseases are life-

long problems that begin during the pediatric years but surface clinically only during adulthood. The process of atherosclerosis, for instance, appears to be established during adolescence, but the eventual outcomes of myocardial infarction, stroke, and peripheral vascular disease become manifest in the mid-to-late adult years. This latter observation, of course, is the rationale behind the promotion of not only exercise but also proper diet, limited salt intake, and avoidance of obesity and cigarette smoking in children. Early interventions to ameliorate risk factors as a means of preventing the lifelong progression of atherosclerotic vascular disease appears to be a sound preventive medicine strategy.

Which is more important in influencing these health-related outcomes, physical activity or physical fitness? The answer may relate to the type of health outcome desired. As indicated in table 7.1, physical activity would

Table 7.1   Health benefits of exercise: physical activity or fitness?

	Activity	Fitness
Obesity	x	
Osteoporosis	x	
Coronary artery disease	x	x
Hypertension	x	x
Emotional disorders	x	
Injury prevention		x
Back disease		x

appear to be more important in prevention and/or management of obesity, osteoporosis, and type 2 diabetes mellitus. Physical fitness, particularly in terms of muscle strength, may play a role in prevention of back disease and musculoskeletal injury (especially in sport participation). In some cases (e.g., systemic hypertension), both fitness and activity may play important salutary roles (95). Most studies evaluating outcome measures for coronary artery disease in adults have used indicators of physical activity (weekend leisure activity; daily caloric expenditure of longshoremen) rather than aerobic fitness (64). But there are also some reports in adult subjects of a negative relationship between coronary artery disease morbidity/mortality and fitness measures such as treadmill endurance time and maximal O_2 uptake (48).

Determining the relative importance of activity and fitness to health is important for public health policy makers (71). As noted above, physical fitness is not difficult to measure. Indeed, the batteries of field fitness tests performed routinely in schools are designed to identify children with low health-related fitness. Physical activity, on the other hand, is difficult to assess. If activity and fitness are closely related, measurement of physical fitness by field testing can be assumed to provide information regarding activity as well. If the two are not associated, and if physical activity is deemed highly important for present and future health, the value of the results of field tests of fitness as indicators of health risk is weakened.

A similar analysis can be applied to interventions. Physical fitness is difficult to alter in children, necessitating a training program of certain intensity, duration, and frequency. As will be seen in the sections on training for aerobic fitness and muscular strength in this book, improvements in children are relatively small even after prolonged training regimens. Altering physical activity habits is—at least conceptually—simpler (e.g., the child can walk to the store instead of getting a ride). In reality, of course, the difficulty in encouraging the sedentary 14-year-old to a more active lifestyle is well recognized. It is clear, though, that the strategies used by families, schools, community recreation leaders, and health professionals for improving children's fitness versus their activity levels are very different; improving fitness calls for an exercise training program, whereas changing activity levels calls for efforts at behavior modification. If we can expect activity and fitness to be closely related, we can elect the easiest strategy. If this is not the case, it will be important in planning interventions to pay closer attention to specific health outcomes of improving fitness and activity.

Physical Activity and Aerobic Trainability.
As will be reviewed in the next section, improvements in $\dot{V}O_2max$ after a period of endurance training appear to be less in children than in adults. One of the explana-

tions postulated for this maturity-related difference in aerobic trainability is the inherently higher levels of daily activity levels in children: "The preschool child who characteristically uses his large muscles during many hours of the day is continuing a self-imposed program of physical fitness" (2, p. 88). According to this argument the child is "self-trained" by typical vigorous daily activities, leaving less room for improvement with a formal training regimen. Identifying a relationship between physical activity and aerobic fitness would support this assumption.

That daily activity levels of children significantly influence their $\dot{V}O_2max$ seems immediately unlikely when one examines the nature of these activities. Studies of children's activities confirm what the parent of every 3-year-old child knows: children move from one short-burst activity to another, rarely with any semblance of sustained exercise. In a more scientific context, the intensity of daily activity of children as identified by heart rate monitoring does not satisfy criteria for improving $\dot{V}O_2max$ (at least in adults). These guidelines call for exercise for at least 20 min, three times a week, at a sustained intensity indicated by heart rate 60-90%max (3). Massicotte and MacNab found that improvements in $\dot{V}O_2max$ occurred in boys training at a target heart rate of 170-180 bpm, but that training at rates of 160 bpm and below failed to elicit an aerobic response (46).

Riddoch et al. monitored heart rates in 45 Irish school children over 4 days (63). The boys showed an average total time of 8 min/day during which heart rate was over 70% of $\dot{V}O_2max$, and in the girls the total was only 4 min. In the United States, Gilliam et al. reported that 6-7-year-old boys and girls had heart rates over 160 bpm

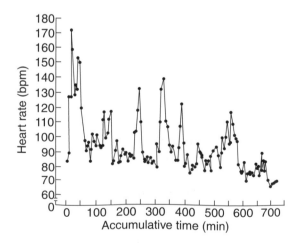

Figure 7.3 A 12 hr heart rate pattern of a 7-year-old girl. Reprinted from Gilliam et al. 1981.

Table 7.2   Is level of habitual activity in children related to maximal aerobic power?

	Study	Activity measure
Yes	Mirwald et al. (50)	Questionnaire
	Atomi et al. (6)	Heart rate
	Fenster et al. (27)	Motion sensor
	Pate et al. (55)	Questionnaire
	Janz et al. (34)	Heart rate
No	Sunnegardh and Brattleby (92)	Questionnaire
	Fenster et al. (27)	Motion sensor
	LaPorte et al. (40)	Motion sensor
	Cunningham et al. (15)	Heart rate
	Armstrong et al. (5)	Heart rate
	Janz et al. (34)	Heart rate
	Al-Hazzaa et al. (1)	Heart rate
	Seliger et al. (85)	Diary

for 21 min/day and 9 min/day, respectively, and that such rates typically appeared in intermittent bursts (30) (see fig. 7.3). The same findings are obtained in older children. Armstrong et al. indicated that only 13% of 13-year-old boys and 6.5% of girls showed a heart rate of over 159 bpm for a 20 min period during 3 days of monitoring (5).

Studies of Activity and Aerobic Fitness.   Given the issues just identified, is there a relationship between habitual physical activity and aerobic fitness in studies in children?

Intuitively, one might expect that the child who is more active throughout the day would exhibit higher levels of $\dot{V}O_2$max. Likewise, it would not be unexpected to find that those with greater maximal aerobic power tended to be more active. By either explanation a close relationship between measures of habitual activity and $\dot{V}O_2$max should be demonstrable.

It is somewhat surprising, then, that the research literature does not support such a strong relationship. Table 7.2 outlines studies that do and do not indicate a significant association between directly measured $\dot{V}O_2$max and level of habitual activity in children. By sheer numbers, the chance of a true activity-fitness relationship would seem to be about 50-50.

AEROBIC RESPONSES TO ENDURANCE TRAINING

An athlete trains to improve performance, recognizing that repetitive stresses of muscular activity (training) trigger adaptive physiologic changes that enhance func-

tional capacity (the fitness effect). This remarkable ability of the human machine to respond to exercise training is observed in all areas of fitness—endurance, speed, strength, and agility—and presumably has its evolutionary roots as a survival mechanism (i.e., a true Darwinian model of survival of the fittest). Our understanding of the means by which repeated muscular stress produces the physiologic characteristics of the fitness effect is scant; moreover, just how such physiologic changes become translated into improved field performance is not altogether clear. Certain features, however, are well recognized. For instance, the fitness effect is highly training-specific (i.e., repeated long-distance runs will not improve muscular strength), and a training effect is not expected unless certain thresholds of exercise frequency and intensity are met.

Improvements in $\dot{V}O_2$max that occur with endurance training reflect integrated enhancement of function throughout the chain of O_2 delivery and peripheral utilization. Increases in maximal aerobic power after training are limited; that is, persistent training in the average individual will never elevate aerobic fitness to the level of a marathon runner. This ceiling of improvement in $\dot{V}O_2$max, as noted previously, is largely genetically determined. The greatest value of $\dot{V}O_2$max following endurance training in a given individual, then, represents the functional limits of that person's aerobic machinery. Studying the responses of $\dot{V}O_2$max to training can therefore provide insight into aerobic metabolic reserve and the way in which it relates to endurance performance.

A formerly sedentary adult who engages in an endurance training program of sufficient duration (over 20 min), intensity (heart rate 60-90%max), and frequency (three times per week) can be expected to demonstrate a predictable set of cardiorespiratory adaptations (3). Maximal cardiac output will rise, a direct result of enhanced maximal stroke volume. The latter occurs because of augmented blood volume and possibly greater cardiac contractility. Improved aerobic capacity of the exercising muscle will be reflected in an increased peripheral O_2 extraction (arteriovenous O_2 difference). Maximal minute ventilation will rise, an effect of increases in both tidal volume and breathing rate. At a given level of submaximal work, heart rate falls while stroke volume is greater (65, 77).

These training-induced alterations in the adult are reflected collectively by an improvement in $\dot{V}O_2$max. The magnitude of increase in maximal aerobic power varies widely. Lortie et al., for instance, reported increases in $\dot{V}O_2$max in previously sedentary adults of 5% to 88% after a 20-week training program (42). It has been stated that overall, adults should improve $\dot{V}O_2$max by 25-30% after appropriate training (32). It is important to recognize, however, that the degree of improvement of

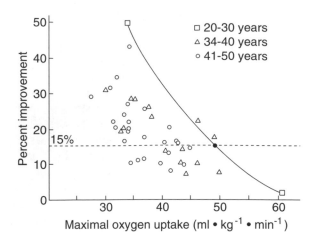

Figure 7.4 Percentage change in $\dot{V}O_2$max with aerobic training relative to initial $\dot{V}O_2$max in adults (from multiple studies). Reprinted from Rowell 1986.

$\dot{V}O_2$max in adult training studies is inversely related to both habitual level of activity and pretraining $\dot{V}O_2$max. This is illustrated in figure 7.4 from Saltin et al. (79), which relates percentage improvement in maximal aerobic power with training to initial $\dot{V}O_2$max in four adult studies.

There is no reason to expect a priori that aerobic trainability should be less in children than in adults. Still, a dampened $\dot{V}O_2$max rise after training in children compared to values in adults was suggested even from the earliest investigations involving pediatric subjects. Bar-Or compiled data on nine such studies in prepubertal children that demonstrated little or no increase in $\dot{V}O_2$max with training (8) (see table 7.3). Two explanations have traditionally been suggested: (1) the aerobic fitness effect might be reliant on hormonal responses (such as testosterone) to training that are absent before puberty, and (2) the high inherent daily activity levels of children may serve to optimize their pretraining $\dot{V}O_2$, diminishing the magnitude of response to training. These issues will be discussed further on in this chapter.

Katch explained the purported blunted aerobic training response in children by the "trigger hypothesis" (36). According to this concept, there is a critical point in a child's life (usually at puberty) before which aerobic trainability will be minimal if $\dot{V}O_2$max changes at all. Katch suggested that "this trigger phenomenon is the result of modulating effects of hormones that initiate puberty and influence functional development and subsequent organic adaptations" (p. 241).

From the training regimens of the studies reviewed in table 7.3, it is apparent that many involved short-burst activities that would not have been expected to improve aerobic fitness (at least by criteria established for adults). Rowland therefore surveyed pediatric training studies with particular attention to identifying those that appeared to conform to such criteria (aerobic activities, three to five sessions per week, at an intensity producing a heart rate of 60-90%max) (66). Of eight such studies, six demonstrated a significant improvement in $\dot{V}O_2$max with training (see table 7.4). The average in-

Table 7.3 Studies in which prepubescents responded to aerobic training with little (< 10%) or no improvement

Reference	Age (years)	Sex	Length	Frequency	Exercise	Increase in $\dot{V}O_2$max (per kg body weight)
				Training regimen		
Ekblom (23)	11	M	6 mo	2/wk	Interval runs, long-distance runs	2.8%
Daniels and Oldridge (18)	10–15	M	22 mo	—	Long-distance runs	None, better running times
Bar-Or and Zwiren (9)	9–10	F,M	9 wk	2–4/wk	All-out interval runs (145 m)	None, better running times
Mocellin and Wasmund (52)	7–10	F,M	7 wk	1–2/wk	All-out runs (800–1000 m)	None, better running times
Stewart and Gutin (89)	10–12	M	8 wk	4/wk	Interval runs at 90% HRmax	None
Lussier and Buskirk (43)	8–12	F,M	12 wk	4/wk	Games, long-distance runs	6.8%, better running times
Yoshida et al. (101)	5	F,M	14 mo	1/wk or 5/wk	Runs (750–1000 m)	None, better running times
Benedict et al. (11)	9–11	F,M	8 wk	4–5/wk	Jumping rope	None

Reprinted from Bar-Or 1989.

crease was 14%, with a range of 7% to 26%. Four other studies that did not conform to aerobic training guidelines failed to show any improvement in $\dot{V}O_2$max.

It was concluded that "these data would appear to indicate that when endurance training programs are of sufficient duration and intensity an improvement in aerobic power in children can be elicited similar to that observed in adults" (66, p. 496). It was pointed out, however, that these studies suffered from serious methodological weaknesses that could have biased results. Many involved only a small number of subjects. Four studies included fewer than 10 children, and none more than 16. Two had no controls. Training intensity was seldom documented, and subject dropouts were reported in only two of the studies. Subjects (e.g., track club members, participants in swimming clubs) were not always representative of the pediatric population, and some reported high pretraining fitness levels.

Pate and Ward performed a similar review of aerobic training studies in prepubertal children (56). They confined their analysis to studies that (a) included a control group, (b) used a "readily interpretable" training protocol (p. 39), (c) used physiological measures, (d) contained a statistical analysis, and (e) had appeared in a peer-reviewed scientific journal. This group comprised 12 training studies in which the age of the children was less than 13 years. In 8 of the 12, $\dot{V}O_2$max rose 1.3-20.5%, with an average rise of 10.4%; mean increase in the control groups was 2.7%. No appreciable change in maximal aerobic power was observed in the other studies.

No clear-cut contributions of mode, pattern, frequency, duration, or intensity of training to magnitude of rise of $\dot{V}O_2$max were noted in this review. Also, no relationship was observed between initial fitness level and amount of improvement in $\dot{V}O_2$max with training. Aerobic fitness failed to improve in two of the four studies involving the youngest subjects but in only one of the eight involving children 10-13 years old. The increase in $\dot{V}O_2$max in the younger subjects was approximately one-half that for the older ones. Even considering the small number of studies involved as well as the problems of testing small children, this information suggests that trainability may be more limited in younger subjects.

Noting that the approximate 10% average increase in $\dot{V}O_2$max seen in these investigations was within the low range typically reported in work with adults, the authors concluded that the analysis provided "convincing evidence that prepubescent boys are physiologically

Table 7.4 Summary of exercise training studies in children which conform to criteria of intensity and duration necessary to improve aerobic fitness in adults

	Brown et al. (13)	Ekblom (23)	Lussier and Buskirk (43)	Eriksson and Koch (25)	Shasby and Hagerman (86)	Daniels and Oldridge (18)	Gilliam and Freedson (29)	Vaccaro and Clarke (96)	Massicotte and MacNab (46)
Subjects									
Number	12	6	16	9	7	14	11	15	9
Sex	F	M	M,F	M	M	M	M,F	M,F	M
Age	8–13	11	8–12	11–13	12–13	10–15	7–9	9–11	11–13
Source	Track club	Elementary school	Volunteers	Volunteers	Physical education class	Volunteers previously running	Volunteers	First year swim training	Volunteers
Controls	Nonendurance track	+	+	0	+	0	+	+	+
Training									
Form	Distance running	Mixed running	Distance running	Distance running	Distance running	Distance running	Aerobic activities	Distance swimming	Bicycle
Duration (wk)	6, 12	24, 128	12	16	12	88	12	28	6
Sessions (min)		45	45	60			25		12
Frequency (per wk)	4–5		4	3	3		4	4	3
Intensity documentation	None	Pulse palpation	Pulse stethoscope	Pulse tape recorder	Pulse palpation	None	Pulse telemetry	None	EKG
Testing	Treadmill	Treadmill	Treadmill	Bicycle	Treadmill	Treadmill	Bicycle	Treadmill	Bicycle
Training effect									
Decreased submax pulse	0	0	+	+	+				+
Increased $\dot{V}O_2$max	+	+	+	+		0	0	+	+
Percent $\dot{V}O_2$ increase	18, 26	10, 3	7	16				10	11

Reprinted from Bar-Or 1989.

adaptive to endurance exercise training" (p. 42). (Only three of the studies included girls, and two of these were among those showing no $\dot{V}O_2$max changes with training.)

Others have critically reviewed the pediatric training literature and reported similar impressions. Shephard contended that if an aerobic training program is conducted according to guidelines recommended for adults, "the maximal oxygen intake of the prepubescent child is increased by about 15%, much as would be anticipated in an older person. There thus seems no good experimental basis for the belief that prepubescent children fail to respond normally to endurance training" (88, p. 209). Similar conclusions were drawn by Sady (76) and Vaccaro and Mahon (97). At the same time, there is general agreement with the observation by Sady that "definitive statements concerning the cardiorespiratory effects of exercise training in children cannot be made [since] few carefully controlled and well-defined exercise training studies including important cardiorespiratory variables have been conducted" (p. 510).

A meta-analysis of 23 studies of aerobic responses to endurance training in children, conducted by Payne and Morrow, provided differing results (58). To be included, studies needed to have involved healthy subjects not over 13 years of age in a controlled design that entailed treadmill or cycle testing. The average pre- and posttest $\dot{V}O_2$max values for the 420 subjects were 46.2 and 48.4 ml $\cdot$ kg^{-1} $\cdot$ min^{-1}, respectively, indicating less than a 5% increase in aerobic fitness from training. No significant difference in the extent of change in $\dot{V}O_2$max was observed between studies that conformed and those that did not conform to accepted criteria for frequency, intensity, and duration of training for increasing aerobic fitness.

Rowland and Boyajian designed a training study in 35 children specifically to avoid the methodological pitfalls of previous investigations (70). Training with endurance activities was conducted for 20-30 min three times a week for 12 weeks in the school setting. Intensity during training, assessed by heart rate monitoring, averaged 166 bpm. Mean increase in treadmill $\dot{V}O_2$max with training was only 6.7%, with no significant differences between boys and girls. The largest individual improvement was 19.7%. One-third of the children demonstrated an increase of less than 3% in $\dot{V}O_2$max with training. Consistent with the observations of Pate and Ward (56), there was no relationship between pretraining $\dot{V}O_2$max and magnitude of improvement with training. This study supports the conclusion from the meta-analysis of Payne and Morrow that aerobic trainability is limited in children compared to adults.

There have been three investigations in which both children and adult subjects underwent training. In each case no significant differences were observed between the two groups. Eisenman and Golding had 12-13-year-old girls and 18-21-year-old women perform running and bench stepping three times a week for 14 weeks (22). Mean improvements in $\dot{V}O_2$max were 17.6% and 16.1%, respectively.

Savage et al. described the effects of a 10-week walk/run training program on $\dot{V}O_2$max. In this study 8 boys (mean age 8 years) and 8 men (mean age 37 years) trained at 40% $\dot{V}O_2$max, and 12 boys and 12 men trained at 75% $\dot{V}O_2$max (82). Significant improvements were limited to the high-intensity training groups (4.6% and 7.9% for the boys and men, respectively). These increases were greater than those for control subjects (p < .05), but the training responses did not differ significantly between the boys and men.

Weber et al. used identical twins as control subjects to examine differences in aerobic fitness of four 10-, 13-, and 16-year-old males after a 10-week run/stepping/cycling training program (100). The 13-year-olds who trained exhibited no significant difference from controls, but the 10- and 16-year-olds showed similar significant increases in $\dot{V}O_2$ compared to the values for their twins.

Maturity-related differences could have been masked in these studies, however, by the small number of subjects (i.e., in the report by Savage et al., improvement in aerobic fitness of the men was actually twice that of the boys—although statistically not different). And it is likely that few of the girls reported by Eisenman and Golding were truly prepubertal.

In summary, then, it appears evident that $\dot{V}O_2$max can be improved with aerobic training in children. In addition, much of the research information suggests that aerobic trainability of children is inferior to that of adults. But the issue is not closed. More than 30 studies addressing this question have been published, representing a wide variety of types of exercise and varied duration and intensity. Many have involved small numbers or inappropriate subjects; others suffer from improper or absent controls and lack of documentation of exercise intensity. And since the magnitude of change of $\dot{V}O_2$max with training has also differed, there is currently no clear-cut answer regarding (1) the extent of aerobic trainability of children or (2) the training criteria necessary for improving aerobic fitness in the prepubertal age group.

Explanations for Possible Maturity-Related Differences in Aerobic Trainability

If it is true that children are quantitatively impaired in comparison to adults in their responses to aerobic training, what mechanisms might be responsible? Suggested explanations have centered around differences in training intensity, inherent activity levels, maturity-related pretraining $\dot{V}O_2$max, and biological influences before and after puberty.

Training Intensity. A sufficient intensity of exercise training has long been recognized as an essential characteristic of programs designed to improve maximal aerobic power. Heart rate has been used commonly as a marker of training intensity, and exercise stimulating a rate of 60-90%max, or 60% of the heart rate reserve (difference between resting and maximal heart rate) has been recommended as a threshold to increasing $\dot{V}O_2$max in adults. There is evidence to suggest, however, that these target heart rate guidelines may not adequately stress O_2 delivery systems in children. If this is the case, diminished aerobic trainability in studies of prepubertal subjects might reflect an inadequate training stimulus.

The concept that children might require a higher target heart rate than adults for improving aerobic fitness comes from an appreciation of maturity-related differences in the anaerobic threshold. Defined as the O_2 uptake coinciding with an abrupt increase in blood lactate during progressive exercise, the anaerobic threshold may act as a more appropriate marker than heart rate of the exercise stress needed to increase $\dot{V}O_2$max. Although the definition is controversial, anaerobic threshold has been considered as the point when O_2 delivery to exercising muscle begins to become inadequate, with a rise in lactate production as anaerobic metabolism ensues (12). A training intensity that approaches, but does not exceed, the anaerobic threshold might be expected to be optimal for stressing and improving O_2 delivery.

Individual values for anaerobic threshold, measured directly by lactate levels or noninvasively by ventilatory parameters (the ventilatory anaerobic threshold, VAT), must be obtained in the exercise laboratory and are impractical for routine clinical or training use. Heart rate at the anaerobic threshold has therefore served as a means of providing target intensity for aerobic training. As will be outlined in chapter 12, anaerobic threshold occurs at a higher relative exercise intensity in children than in adults, and heart rate at anaerobic threshold in prepubertal subjects is greater than the rates indicated by the traditional target levels, noted earlier, for training in adults.

Rowland and Green reported heart rates at VAT in 12 premenarcheal girls during progressive treadmill testing (72). Mean heart rate at VAT was 171 bpm (±12 SD), with a range from 147 to 194 bpm. With use of 60% of heart rate reserve in these girls, the target training rate would have been 159 bpm, and 75% maximal heart rate was 152 bpm. This study therefore indicated that if VAT is a valid target intensity, use of the traditional adult formula would have significantly underestimated the appropriate training stimulus.

Others have reported similar findings. Washington et al. described average heart rate at VAT of 169 bpm and 167 bpm in boys and girls, respectively (99). Tanaka and Shindo found that heart rate at anaerobic threshold (by lactate determinations) averaged 185 bpm in 10-11-year-old boys and 173 bpm in 12-13-year-olds (93). Mahon and Vaccaro reported mean heart rate at VAT of 177 bpm in 29 boys aged 8-13 years (44). These data suggest that heart rate at the anaerobic threshold in children can be expected—on the average—to be approximately 85%max. It is important, however, to recognize the high degree of interindividual variability in all these studies. In the study by Rowland and Green, for instance, 40% of the subjects had a heart rate at VAT that was more than 10 bpm above or below the mean of 171 bpm. For this reason, several authors have emphasized that heart rate at VAT cannot be predicted and as a training target must be individually measured (72, 99).

Nonetheless, this information supports the argument that training studies in children that have shown only minimal changes in $\dot{V}O_2$max may have employed a suboptimal intensity stimulus. The training study of Massicotte and MacNab involving 11-13-year-old boys supports this conclusion (46). Subjects were divided into groups that trained for 6 weeks at a workload producing heart rates of 170-180, 150-160, or 130-140 bpm. Only those who trained at the highest intensity showed significant improvement in $\dot{V}O_2$max.

Similarly, Rowland and Witek studied 15 active children ages 10-11 years who performed walking training for 16 weeks, averaging 4 days/week and 4 miles per session (unpublished data). The average walking speed was 3.5 mph, which produced a mean training heart rate of only 138 bpm (18 SD), equal to 69% of maximal heart rate. Despite the extensive walking program, maximal treadmill testing before and after training indicated no significant changes in $\dot{V}O_2$max (43.7 vs. 42.5 ml · kg^{-1} · min^{-1}) or treadmill endurance time (16.7 vs. 17.5 min).

When a similar walking program was conducted in a group of unfit postpubertal high school subjects, the average training heart rate was 151 bpm, or 79.6%max (74). In this study a small but significant improvement was observed in average maximal O_2 uptake (9.9%), while mean treadmill endurance time increased by 2 min (23% improvement). In these two investigations, then, the same type of exercise training produced different relative intensities in groups of active children and older sedentary adolescents, with different effects on improvement in $\dot{V}O_2$max.

Levels of Habitual Activity. In general, children exhibit a higher level of physical activity during their daily lives than adults. As noted earlier, this observation has led to the suggestion that the greater weight-relative caloric expenditure of children might function as an involuntary "training program," serving to more nearly optimize aerobic fitness than in adults. According to this concept, the degree of improvement in $\dot{V}O_2$max with formal endurance training would consequently be less in children simply because there would be less room for improvement.

The difficulties with this argument have already been outlined. First, analysis of the types of activity in children indicates very little sustained exercise and low overall heart rates. On the basis of critical levels of intensity and duration accepted as necessary for improving $\dot{V}O_2$max during training, then, the daily activities of children would not be expected to optimize aerobic fitness. Second, there appears to be no firm relationship between levels of habitual activity and $\dot{V}O_2$max in children (see table 7.2, page 101). And third, if higher levels of activity minimize improvements in $\dot{V}O_2$max with training, decreased activity or bed rest should cause a greater fall in aerobic fitness in children than in adults. As material at the end of this chapter will suggest, the limited available data do not indicate that this is true.

On the other hand, there is no question that regular daily activities do influence $\dot{V}O_2$max. This is evident from the decline in aerobic fitness that occurs when children as well as adult subjects are placed at bed rest (an issue to be addressed later). Also, there is limited evidence that younger children may have less of a response to aerobic training than older children. If habitual activity levels negatively influence trainability, this would be expected, since physical activity (expressed as weight-relative caloric expenditure) declines progressively during the course of childhood (see fig. 7.1, page 98). In their review, Pate and Ward noted that no improvements in $\dot{V}O_2$max were seen in two of the four studies involving the youngest children (ages 5 to 9 years), while an increase was observed in all but one of the eight training studies conducted with 10-13-year-olds (56). The authors cautioned, however, that these findings might be attributable to difficulties associated with training and exercise testing in younger subjects.

Pretraining $\dot{V}O_2$max.
Depressed aerobic trainability in children has been attributed to the higher level of pretraining $\dot{V}O_2$max in prepubertal subjects compared to adults. It has been consistently observed in adult studies that magnitude of improvement of $\dot{V}O_2$max after a period of endurance training is inversely related to pretraining values of maximal aerobic power (79). Most training studies on postpubertal subjects have been conducted in those with $\dot{V}O_2$max levels of 30-45 ml · kg^{-1} · min^{-1} before the beginning of training. However, the children involved in aerobic training studies have typically had pretraining $\dot{V}O_2$max values of 45-55 ml · kg^{-1} · min^{-1} (97).

The data in figure 7.4 (see p. 102), derived from four studies in adults, suggest that no more than a 10-15% improvement in aerobic fitness might be expected in adult subjects who have pretraining $\dot{V}O_2$max levels commensurate with those usually observed in children. Rowell reviewed adult training studies indicating that a 2-3-month training program in individuals with a mean pretraining $\dot{V}O_2$max of 44 ml · kg^{-1} · min^{-1} resulted in an average increase of 16% (65). He observed that "if $\dot{V}O_2$max is relatively high (e.g., between 50-60 ml · kg^{-1} · min^{-1}), then the increase [in $\dot{V}O_2$max in adults] with 2-3 months of physical conditioning will be only a few percent" (p. 259). These observations raise the intriguing idea that aerobic responses to training might be similar in children and adults if the two groups were matched for pretraining $\dot{V}O_2$max.

Biological Determinants.
It is difficult to assess the possibility that differences in biological mechanisms might be responsible for maturity-related variations in aerobic trainability because (a) the determinants of improvements in $\dot{V}O_2$max with training have not been investigated in children, and (b) the triggers for the "fitness effect" from aerobic training at any age are not well understood.

From the Fick equation, improvements in $\dot{V}O_2$max must reflect increases in maximal stroke volume, heart rate, and/or peripheral O_2 extraction (arteriovenous O_2 difference). Maximal heart rate does not change significantly with training in either adults or children. In adult subjects, training-induced improvements in $\dot{V}O_2$max are reportedly a consequence of both augmented cardiac stroke volume and peripheral O_2 extraction, although the mechanisms by which these are achieved are controversial and the physiological signals that effect these changes remain obscure (65).

Table 7.5 lists the possible determinants that can alter these components of maximal aerobic power and the available data regarding alterations with training in children. It is clear that the pediatric information is sufficiently scant to preclude drawing any conclusions on adult-child differences.

Many of the potential cardiovascular adaptations to endurance training appear to be mediated by alterations in autonomic nervous control, specifically diminished submaximal sympathetic tone, as well as increased plasma volume. The triggers for increasing intracellular aerobic capacity are uncertain.

Clear-cut hormonal changes separate the prepubertal from the postpubertal subject (45), but how these might affect the magnitude of aerobic response to endurance training is unknown. In boys the most obvious hormonal change at puberty is a dramatic rise in serum

Table 7.5 Potential determinants of improvements in $\dot{V}O_2$max following endurance training

Mechanism	Studies in children
Increased stroke volume	Eriksson and Koch (25) 20% increase in SV 12% increase in blood volume

1. Increased preload
    Rise in blood volume
    Resting bradycardia
    Changes in venous capacitance
2. Increased cardiac contractility
3. Decreased afterload	

Increased a-$\overline{v}$ oxygen difference
   Increases in
   1. Hemoglobin mass
   2. Capillary density
   3. Myoglobin concentration
   4. Cellular aerobic enzyme activity
	Koch (38) No change
	
	Eriksson et al. (24)
	30% increase in succinate
	dehydrogenase

testosterone levels. At least in animals, testosterone has a prominent influence on cardiac function. Decreased cardiac output, ejection fraction, and myocardial O_2 uptake are observed when rats are gonadectomized, and these effects are reversed after administration of testosterone (83, 84). In addition, testosterone stimulates skeletal muscle hypertrophy and is an important trigger for red blood cell production.

Levels of growth hormone rise at puberty, and this hormone also serves to provoke increased cardiac function. Studies of growth hormone stimulation for brief periods of time in both animals and humans have indicated significant increases in heart weight, cardiac output, and myocardial contractility (60, 94). As many as two-thirds of patients with acromegaly, or gigantism from excessive growth hormone secretion, exhibit hypertrophic cardiomyopathy (81). In addition, growth hormone has prominent anabolic effects on skeletal muscle and bone tissue.

There may be differences in autonomic activity during exercise that separate children from adults. Maximal levels of circulating norepinephrine, a marker of sympathetic nervous activity, were reported by Lehmann et al. to be 30% lower in a group of 12-year-old boys than in 27-year-old men during treadmill exercise (41). The authors considered this finding indicative of reduced maximum sympathetic activity in the children. Maximal epinephrine levels, reflecting secretory activity of the adrenal medulla, were not different in the two groups.

While these endocrine and neurologic characteristics may (a) separate pre- from postpubertal subjects and (b) affect the O_2 delivery system, it is not at all evident how they might act to influence adaptations of $\dot{V}O_2$ to a training stimulus. Therefore although it is tempting to infer that "it is hormonal regulation that sets the trigger for the organic adaptations and responses to physical conditioning" (36, p. 242), more information will be necessary before we can conclude that endocrinologic changes at puberty are responsible for maturity-related differences in aerobic trainability.

$\dot{V}O_2$ max in Prepubertal Endurance Athletes

Given the extended period of intensive aerobic training that prepubertal endurance athletes undergo, it might be expected that examining their maximal aerobic power would lead to insight into the trainability of children. As outlined in table 7.6, highly trained young athletes do indeed demonstrate higher levels of $\dot{V}O_2$max than the general pediatric population. Unfortunately, however, sport training is not the only factor that separates athletic from nonathletic children. Differences in maximal aerobic power between these two groups might also be apparent (a) if the level of biological maturity of the athletes were more advanced than that of the nonathletes, or (b) if athletes possessed an inherent greater $\dot{V}O_2$max that drew them to participation in sports. The

Table 7.6   Maximal oxygen uptake in child endurance athletes

Author	N	Age	Sex	Sport	$\dot{V}O_2max$ (ml · kg^{-1} · min^{-1})
Van Huss et al. (98)	22	9–15	F	Runners	59.9
	20	9–15	M	Runners	65.9
Daniels and Oldridge (18)	14	10–15	M	Runners	59.5
Nudel et al. (54)	16	8–17	M,F	Runners	61.0
Rowland et al. (74)	10	11–13	M	Runners	61.2
Mayers and Gutin (47)	8	8–11	M	Runners	56.6
Paterson et al. (57)	18	11	M	Multiple	60.8
Baxter-Jones et al. (10)	18	11	M	Swimmers	57.7
	7	11	F	Swimmers	52.2
Sundberg and Elovainio (91)	12	12	M	Runners	59.3
Lehmann et al. (41)	8	12	M	Runners	60.3
Vaccaro and Clarke (96)	15	9–11	M	Swimmers	55.4

cross-sectional studies represented in table 7.6 do not allow one to discriminate between these possibilities.

One observation regarding $\dot{V}O_2max$ in child endurance athletes may have some bearing on the trainability question. These trained competitors typically manifest $\dot{V}O_2max$ values of 60-65 ml · kg^{-1} · min^{-1}, approximately 20-30% higher than values expected from children in the general population (see table 7.5). These observations support the suggestion by Koch that there exists a ceiling of $\dot{V}O_2max$ from training of 60 ml · kg^{-1} · min^{-1} for boys 12-15 years of age (39).

Elite adult male endurance athletes, however, typically have a $\dot{V}O_2max$ of 70-80 ml · kg^{-1} · min^{-1}, which is about 70% greater than that of nontrained men (23). Even by the midteen years, highly trained endurance athletes have significantly higher $\dot{V}O_2max$ values than those who are prepubertal (see table 7.7). This discrepancy has been interpreted as evidence that children before the age of puberty possess a dampened capacity for improvements in maximal aerobic power with training.

It is of course also obvious that adult runners have had the benefit of many additional years of training.

Prepubertal Training Effects in Athletes. Do child endurance athletes improve $\dot{V}O_2max$ with training? The research data are conflicting. Daniels and Oldridge reported physiological responses to 22 months of steady running training in 14 boys 10-15 years of age (18). Absolute values of $\dot{V}O_2max$ increased by 22% during training, but maximal aerobic power expressed relative to body weight remained stable (mean approximately 59.5 ml · kg^{-1} · min^{-1}). Van Huss et al. found no significant changes in $\dot{V}O_2max$ per kg in either male or female elite runners ages 9-15 years during a 3-year training period (mean initial values 65.9 and 54.9 ml · kg^{-1} · min^{-1}, respectively) (98).

However, other studies have indicated that gains in weight-relative aerobic power can be observed in prepubertal children during athletic training. Baxter-Jones et al. measured $\dot{V}O_2max$ serially in 453 athletes in-

Table 7.7   Maximal aerobic power in adolescent endurance athletes

Author	N	Sex	Age	Sport	$\dot{V}O_2max$
Kobayashi et al. (37)	4	M	17	Runners	73.9
Dill and Adams (20)	6	M	17	Runners	72.0
Cunningham (17)	12	M	16	Runners	74.6
Sundberg and Elovainio (91)	12	M	16	Runners	66.4
Faria et al. (26)	15	M	15–19	Cyclists	75.5
Cunningham (17)	12	F	16	Runners	66.1
Cunningham (16)	20	F	15	Runners	62.2

volved in soccer, swimming, gymnastics, and tennis (10). A mixed longitudinal design was employed, with five age cohorts (8, 10, 12, 14, and 16 years) that were each studied for three consecutive years. When age, height, and weight were considered, maximal aerobic power rose in the prepubertal years, indicating an improvement in aerobic fitness beyond that expected as a result of growth and biological maturation. This finding supports the earlier study of Paterson et al., who demonstrated a progressive yearly rise in mean $\dot{V}O_2$max from 62.3 to 67.3 ml · kg^{-1} · min^{-1} in 18 athletic boys during the 3 years preceding the age of peak height velocity (57). Brown et al. trained nine preadolescent girls who were members of track clubs (but who had an average pretraining $\dot{V}O_2$max of only 46.3 ml · kg^{-1} · min^{-1}) (13). $\dot{V}O_2$max per kg increased by 18.5% after 6 weeks of training and by 26.2% after 12 weeks.

Aerobic Trainability in Athletes After Puberty.
The evidence for improvement in weight-relative $\dot{V}O_2$max with athletic training during the teen years is more compelling. Dramatic improvements in $\dot{V}O_2$max per kg have been reported in highly trained Finnish cross-country skiers and cyclists between 14 and 24 years of age (75). In a mixed longitudinal study, values rose from an average of 55 ml · kg^{-1} · min^{-1} in the skiers at age 14 to 80 ml · kg^{-1} · min^{-1} at age 24 years. Values for females were lower, but the rate of improvement was similar. It is difficult to compare these changes with the findings in prepubertal children, however, since the training regimen of the skiers was highly intensive. Weekly training mileage was 20 km at age 14 and increased steadily to almost 150 km/week by age 24.

Murase et al. performed similar serial measurements of $\dot{V}O_2$max in 11 highly trained Japanese males for 5-7 years beginning at age 14 (53). Average maximal aerobic power increased from 65.1 to 72.8 ml · kg^{-1} · min^{-1} (+11.8%) between the ages of 15 and 18 years—a time during which the rise in weight-relative $\dot{V}O_2$max in nontraining controls was only +5.5% (49.1 to 51.8 ml · kg^{-1} · min^{-1}). Of interest is the observation that $\dot{V}O_2$max per kg failed to rise after the age of 18 years in those who continued to train to age 20. Similarly, Miyashita et al. reported that improvements in maximal aerobic power were not seen in highly trained runners between the ages of 19 and 22 years (51).

In the training athletes studied by Baxter-Jones et al., $\dot{V}O_2$max rose progressively in males during each pubertal stage (independent of age, height, and weight), and this phenomenon was most obvious in the swimmers (10). This finding suggests an acceleration of trainability with increasing sexual maturity. No such trend was observed in the females, however.

Zauner and Benson evaluated $\dot{V}O_2$max serially over 3 years by treadmill testing in 15 highly trained swim-

mers (102). Twelve were between 12 and 19 years old (the remainder were younger) and presumably pubertal or postpubertal. Mean $\dot{V}O_2$max per kg rose from mean values of 40.3 to 44.0 to 48.0 ml · kg^{-1} · min^{-1} in the females (n = 7) and from 47.5 to 55.3 to 64.0 ml · kg^{-1} · min^{-1} in the males (n = 8). No control nontraining subjects were studied. Similarly, four elite distance runners reported by Kobayashi et al. improved their mean $\dot{V}O_2$max from 63.8 to 73.9 ml · kg^{-1} · min^{-1} between the ages of 14 and 17 years (37).

Does Puberty Influence Aerobic Trainability?

The information in the preceding section suggests that the pubertal years might offer a particularly advantageous period for improving aerobic fitness in intensely training athletes. Can the same be said for nonathletic adolescents? Should the teen years be a particular focus for improving aerobic fitness? In 1969 Ekblom proposed this very concept—that endurance training during adolescence was critical for establishing a high level of lifelong aerobic fitness (23). Findings of research studies devoted to this issue, however, have been mixed.

Kobayashi et al. described serial measurements of $\dot{V}O_2$max in seven nonathletic boys tested annually from ages 9-10 to 15-16 years (37). Training included activities such as endurance running, soccer, and swimming (1-1.5 hr daily, four to five times per week). Mean age at peak velocity (PHV) was 13.3 years. As shown in figure 7.5, mean $\dot{V}O_2$max per kg rose little until the age of PHV, when values increased from 47.0 to 56.9 ml · kg^{-1} · min^{-1}. Unfortunately, data on control nontraining children during this age span were not obtained.

Mirwald et al. measured $\dot{V}O_2$max yearly in 25 boys between the ages of 7 and 16 years (50). The subjects were grouped by questionnaire as active (n = 14) or inactive (n = 11). $\dot{V}O_2$max was greater in the active boys at all ages, but the difference became greater and reached statistical significance at PHV. The authors concluded that these data "support the contention that the adolescent growth period is a critical period for growth of maximal aerobic power" (p. 411).

There is evidence, too, against puberty as a key time point for maximizing aerobic trainability. In the report by Weber et al. referred to earlier, pre- and postpubertal subjects showed equal improvements in $\dot{V}O_2$max with endurance training (100). In that study, also, the increase in $\dot{V}O_2$max in the circumpubertal 13-year-old twins was the same whether or not the boys participated in a training program.

In summary, several lines of evidence support the importance of the pubertal years as a critical period for optimizing aerobic fitness:

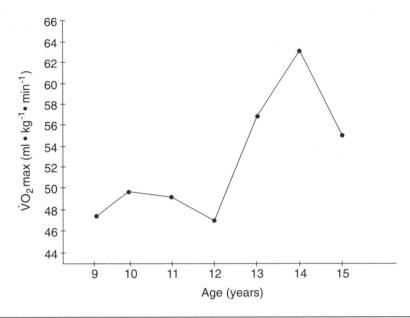

Figure 7.5 $\dot{V}O_2$max changes during training across pubertal years (from Kobayashi et al. [37]).

1. Cross-sectional studies of trained endurance athletes show a significant jump in $\dot{V}O_2$max (about 10 ml $\cdot$ kg^{-1} $\cdot$ min^{-1}) between the prepubertal years and the midteens.
2. That $\dot{V}O_2$max can be appreciably changed with aerobic training in prepubertal athletes appears doubtful. However, major increments in maximal aerobic power are consistently described in older adolescent athletes. But beyond the teen years, continued aerobic training may not significantly alter $\dot{V}O_2$max in endurance athletes.
3. The longitudinal studies of Kobayashi et al. (37) and Mirwald et al. (50) indicate an augmented improvement in $\dot{V}O_2$max from increased physical activity at the time of puberty.

Arguments against this concept can also be mustered:

1. The differences in $\dot{V}O_2$max in cross-sectional and training studies of pre- and postpubertal athletes might be equally well explained by the greater duration, intensity, and regimentation of training in the latter subjects.
2. The cross-sectional data of Weber et al. (100) and others (22, 82) show no differences in aerobic trainability of pre- and postpubertal subjects.

In summary, a considerable body of information argues for a positive effect of puberty in promoting aerobic fitness responses to endurance training. Given the cardiotropic effects of testosterone and growth hormone that become manifest at this time, we are also provided a potential physiological explanation. Further research is necessary to assess how compelling this argument will become.

Comparing Growth and Training Effects

In many cases, the normal physiological changes with exercise that accompany growth mimic those one would expect to result from a period of aerobic training. And, in a similar fashion, the physiological alterations with growth as well as with training are manifest in improvements in endurance athletic performance. These observations have led to the suggestion that an understanding of the relationship between physiological changes and endurance performance in growing children might provide insight into the basic mechanisms for improvement of performance with training at all ages (68).

A comparison of physiological alterations between growth and training is presented in table 7.8. While similarities are clear, there are many obvious differences as well. An increase in maximal aerobic power expressed relative to body weight, for example, is the most salient expression of improvement in aerobic fitness after endurance training, while $\dot{V}O_2$max per kg remains relatively stable throughout childhood and early adolescence in boys and slowly declines during the same period in girls.

Importantly, too, the similarity between the physiological changes with growth and those with training

Table 7.8   Comparison of physiologic changes with growth following endurance training

	Growth	Endurance training
Maximal increase		
$\dot{V}O_2$	x	x
$\dot{V}O_2$ per kg		x
$\dot{V}_E$	x	x
$\dot{V}_E$ per kg		x
Cardiac output	x	x
Stroke volume	x	x
Submaximal decrease		
$\dot{V}O_2$ per kg	x	
Heart rate	x	x
Submaximal increase		
Stroke volume	x	x

does not necessarily imply that the mechanisms inducing these alterations are identical. A decline in heart rate and increase in cardiac stroke volume at a given submaximal work rate are characteristics seen in children while they are growing as well as in people after they train. But these changes could be attributable simply to growth of the cardiac ventricular chambers (a likely explanation in the growing child) or to alterations in autonomic tone with diminished sympathetic neural influences on the heart (more probable as an expression of the training effect).

This illustration of the similarities of changes with growth and training does highlight the critical importance of adequate control subjects in any study evaluating responses to aerobic training in growing children. A 6-year-old boy who does nothing more than sit in front of the television until the age of 12, for instance, will improve his absolute $\dot{V}O_2$max by over 100%! Including nontraining controls in training studies is necessary to separate out the effects of aerobic training from those of normal growth and development.

What constitutes an appropriate control subject in such a study, however, is not altogether clear. After recognizing the need to match subjects for biological age, anthropometric characteristics, and pretraining physical activity, one is still left with accounting for the prominent genetic influence on aerobic trainability. This difficulty can be best solved by utilizing nontraining identical twins as control subjects (100)—a solution not practical for most investigations. Others have used a time series design in which each subject serves as his/her own control through measurement of $\dot{V}O_2$max changes over a period of time immediately before the training program (70, 74).

EFFECTS OF INACTIVITY ON AEROBIC FITNESS

The preceding section addressed the magnitude of improvement in aerobic fitness in children when physical activity is increased by training regimens. These responses provide information on the limits, or ceiling, of function of the O_2 delivery chain in growing children. Little is known, however, about the opposite extreme of $\dot{V}O_2$ plasticity in children—the baseline level of aerobic fitness that accompanies a withdrawal of physical activity.

This information is readily available from studies involving adult subjects who have volunteered for maximal exercise testing before and after a period of complete bed rest. Reported studies have lasted from 7 to 30 days and have demonstrated a decline in $\dot{V}O_2$max ranging from 5% to 28% (14, 33, 35, 49, 78, 90).

This type of investigation has not been performed in prepubertal subjects, presumably because of ethical considerations. But changes in maximal aerobic power that occur after extended inactivity in children would provide useful information surrounding several issues. For instance, if aerobic trainability is inferior in children compared to adults because of their higher levels of habitual physical activity, we would expect children to demonstrate a greater fall in $\dot{V}O_2$max than adults during bed rest. Also, little is known regarding the extent to which daily activity in children contributes to aerobic fitness. Despite concern about the perceived low activity and fitness levels of children, there has been little documentation of the effect of a sedentary lifestyle on maximal aerobic power.

Rowland attempted to provide some information on this issue by measuring $\dot{V}O_2$max serially on five children ages 7 to 11 years who were recovering from an accidental femoral fracture (69). The subjects had been non-weight-bearing for an average of 10.6 weeks (4 weeks in traction, 5 weeks immobilized in a spica cast, 2 weeks on crutches). During the recovery period, average $\dot{V}O_2$max increased from 37.2 to 42.9 ml $\cdot$ kg^{-1} $\cdot$ min^{-1} (13.3%) by the 3rd month, with no significant increase on subsequent monthly maximal tests. At the time of plateau of maximal aerobic power, the children were back to their preaccident level of physical activity by parent report. It was hypothesized that the extent of recovery of $\dot{V}O_2$max reflected that lost during the extended period of bed rest.

From these results it would appear that the effect of prolonged bed rest on aerobic fitness in children is equal to or even less than that in adults, considering that this study involved a period of inactivity three times that reported in most adult studies. This conclusion is tempered by reports that the fall of $\dot{V}O_2$max in adults occurs at a faster rate in the initial stages of bed rest; that is, the relationship between duration of inactivity and fall in aerobic power is not linear, and the degree of decline may be limited beyond 2-3 weeks of bed rest (65). The findings of this limited study do suggest that (1) the contribution of the usual ranges of physical activity to $\dot{V}O_2max$ in children is not large, (2) high levels of habitual physical activity do not explain dampened aerobic training responses in children, and (3) recovery of aerobic function after long periods of immobilization is rapid in this age group.

SUMMARY

While the data are far from convincing, there is reason to suspect that the plasticity of aerobic function in children is depressed before the age of biological maturity. The bulk of evidence from training studies in normal children—although these studies suffer from serious methodological weaknesses—indicates improvements in $\dot{V}O_2max$ that are considerably less than those one would look for in adult subjects.

Both cross-sectional and longitudinal training studies of child endurance athletes suggest that improvements in maximal aerobic power are blunted until after puberty. Intensive training during the teen years, on the other hand, is typically accompanied by a significant rise in $\dot{V}O_2max$, a response that does not appear to persist as the athlete ages. The decline in aerobic fitness that occurs during prolonged inactivity in the child is no more—and may be less—than that in adult subjects.

From the available literature, the plasticity of $\dot{V}O_2max$ surrounding normal daily activities in the typical young adult is estimated as approximately 40-50% (20-25% increase with training, 15-25% decline with bed rest) (78). In prepubertal children the combined aerobic plasticity—

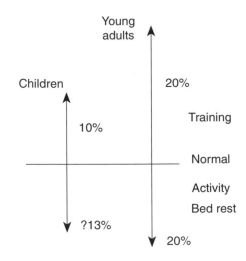

Figure 7.6 Plasticity of $\dot{V}O_2max$ in children and adults. Percentages indicate how $\dot{V}O_2max$ changes from values observed with normal physical activity when subjects are placed at bed rest and when subjects undergo endurance training.

the change in $\dot{V}O_2$ from the value seen with complete bed rest to the value resulting from endurance training—appears to be about 20-25% (see fig. 7.6).

Clearly this is an important issue deserving further investigation. Strategies for interventions for children with low fitness testing scores in the schools may be influenced if little improvement in $\dot{V}O_2max$ can be anticipated with augmented physical activity. Intensive training regimens for prepubertal endurance athletes may be inappropriate if most gains in aerobic fitness cannot be expected until the age of puberty. It will be important, too, to determine whether or not improvements in endurance performance with training are dampened before puberty as is suspected for changes in $\dot{V}O_2max$.

What We Know

1. There is no strong relationship between level of habitual physical activity and aerobic fitness ($\dot{V}O_2max$) in children.
2. Daily activities of children are typically short-burst and nonsustained activities that would not be expected to improve $\dot{V}O_2max$.
3. Improvements in $\dot{V}O_2max$ occur in children after a period of endurance training. These increases are less than those expected in adults.

What We Would Like to Know

1. Why is the $\dot{V}O_2max$ response to endurance training less in children than it is in adults?
2. What thresholds of intensity, duration, and frequency of endurance training in children are important for effecting improvements in $\dot{V}O_2max$?

3. Is puberty a critical time for maximizing responses to aerobic training in both athletes and nonathletes?
4. How much do changes in daily habitual physical activity influence $\dot{V}O_2$max in children?
5. How much can aerobic training in prepubertal children be expected to improve endurance fitness?

References

1. Al-Hazzaa, H.M.; Sulaiman, M.A. Maximal oxygen uptake and daily physical activity in 7- to 12-year old boys. Pediatr. Exerc. Science 5:357-366; 1993.
2. American Academy of Pediatrics. Fitness in the preschool child. Pediatrics 58:88-89; 1976.
3. American College of Sports Medicine. Position statement on the recommended quantity and quality of exercise for developing and maintaining fitness in healthy adults. Med. Sci. Sports Exerc. 10:vii-x; 1978.
4. Anand, B.K. Nervous regulation of food intake. Phys. Rev. 41:677-708; 1961.
5. Armstrong, N.; Williams, J.; Balding, J.; Gentle, P.; Kirby, B. Cardiopulmonary fitness, physical activity patterns, and selected coronary risk factor variables in 11- to 16-year olds. Pediatr. Exerc. Science 3:219-228; 1991.
6. Atomi, Y.; Iwaoka, K.; Hatta, H.; Miyashita, M.; Yamamoto, Y. Daily physical activity levels in preadolescent boys related to $\dot{V}O_2$max and lactate threshold. Eur. J. Appl. Physiol. 55:156-161; 1986.
7. Bar-Or, O. Pediatric sports medicine for the practitioner. New York: Springer-Verlag; 1983.
8. Bar-Or, O. Trainability of the prepubescent child. Phys. Sportsmed. 17:65-81; 1989.
9. Bar-Or, O.; Zwiren, L.D. Physiological effects of frequency and content variation of physical education classes and of endurance conditioning on 9 to 10-year-old girls and boys. In: Bar-Or, O., ed. Pediatric work physiology IV. Natanya, Israel: Wingate Institute; 1973:p. 190-208.
10. Baxter-Jones, A.; Goldstein, H.; Helms, P. The development of aerobic power in young athletes. J. Appl. Physiol. 75:1160-1167; 1993.
11. Benedict, G.; Vaccaro, P.; Hatfield, B.D. Physiological effects of an eight week precision jump program in children. Am. Corr. Ther. J. 5:108-111; 1985.
12. Brooks, G.A. Anaerobic threshold: review of the concept and directions for future research. Med. Sci. Sports Exerc. 17:22-31; 1985.
13. Brown, C.H.; Harrower, J.R.; Deeter, M.F. The effects of cross country running on preadolescent girls. Med. Sci. Sports Exerc. 4:1-5; 1972.
14. Convertino, V.; Hung, J.; Goldwater, D.; DeBusk, R.F. Cardiovascular responses to exercise in middle-aged men after 10 days of bed rest. Circulation 65:134-140; 1982.
15. Cunningham, D.A.; Stapleton, J.J.; MacDonald, I.C.; Paterson, D.H. Daily energy expenditure of young boys as related to maximal aerobic power. Can. J. Appl. Sports Sci. 6:207-211; 1987.
16. Cunningham, L.N. Physiologic characteristics and team performance of female high school runners. Pediatr. Exerc. Science 1:73-79; 1989.
17. Cunningham, L.N. Physiologic comparison of adolescent female and male cross-country runners. Pediatr. Exerc. Science 2.313-321; 1990.
18. Daniels, J.; Oldridge, N. Changes in oxygen consumption of young boys during growth and running training. Med. Sci. Sports 3:161-165; 1971.
19. Danner, F.; Noland, M.; McFadden, M.; DeWalt, K.; Kotchen, J.M. Description of the physical activity of young children using movement sensors and observation methods. Pediatr. Exerc. Science 3:11-20; 1991.
20. Dill, D.B.; Adams, W.C. Maximal oxygen uptake at sea level and 3,090-m altitude in high school champion runners. J. Appl. Physiol. 30:854-859; 1971.
21. DuRant, R.H.; Baranowski, T.; Davis, H.; Rhodes, T.; Thompson, W.O.; Greaves, K.A.; Puhl, J. Reliability and variability of indicators of heart rate monitoring in children. Med. Sci. Sports Exerc. 25:389-395; 1993.
22. Eisenman, P.A.; Golding, L.A. Comparison of effects of training on $\dot{V}O_2$max in girls and young women. Med. Sci. Sports 7:136-138; 1975.
23. Ekblom, B. Effect of physical training on oxygen transport system in man. Acta Physiol. Scand. Suppl. 328:5-45; 1969.
24. Eriksson, B.O.; Gollnick, P.D.; Saltin, B. Muscle metabolism and enzyme activities after training in boys 11-13 years old. Acta Physiol. Scand. 87:485-497; 1973.
25. Eriksson, B.O.; Koch, G. Effect of physical training on hemodynamic response during maximal and submaximal exercise. Acta Physiol. Scand. 87:27-39; 1973.
26. Faria, I.E.; Faria, E.W.; Roberts, S.; Yoshimura, D. Comparison of physical and physiological characteristics in elite young and mature cyclists. Res. Q. Exerc. Sport 60:388-395; 1989.
27. Fenster, J.R.; Freedson, P.S.; Washburn, R.A.; Ellison, R.C. The relationship between peak oxygen uptake and physical activity in 6- to 8-year old children. Pediatr. Exerc. Science 1:127-136; 1989.
28. Freedson, P.S. Field monitoring of physical activity in children. Pediatr. Exerc. Science 1:8-18; 1989.
29. Gilliam, T.B.; Freedson, P.S. Effects of a 12-week school physical fitness program on peak $\dot{V}O_2$, body composition, and blood lipids in 7 to 9 year old children. Int. J. Sports Med. 1:73-78; 1980.

30. Gilliam, T.B.; Freedson, P.S.; Geenan, D.L.; Shahraray, B. Physical activity patterns determined by heart rate monitoring in 6-7 year old children. Med. Sci. Sports Exerc. 13:65-67; 1981.

31. Goran, M.I. Application of the doubly labeled water technique for studying total energy expenditure in young children: a review. Pediatr. Exerc. Science 6:11-30; 1994.

32. Hartley, L.H. Cardiac function and endurance. In: Shephard, R.J.; Åstrand, P.O., eds. Endurance in sport. London: Blackwell Scientific; 1992:p. 72-79.

33. Hung, J.; Goldwater, D.; Convertino, V.A.; McKillop, J.H.; Goris, M.L.; DeBusk, R.F. Mechanisms for decreased exercise capacity after bed rest in normal middle-aged men. Am. J. Cardiol. 51:544-548; 1983.

34. Janz, K.F.; Golden, J.C.; Hansen, J.R.; Mahoney, L.T. Heart rate monitoring of physical activity in children and adolescents: the Muscatine study. Pediatrics 89:256-261; 1992.

35. Kakurin, L.I.; Akhrem-Akhremovich, R.M.; Vanyushina, V. The influence of restricted muscular activity on man's endurance of physical stress, accelerations, and orthostatics. Soviet Conference on Space Biology and Medicine; 1966:p. 110.

36. Katch, V.L. Physical conditioning of children. J. Adol. Health Care 3:241-246; 1983.

37. Kobayashi, K.; Kitamura, K.; Miura, M.; Sodeyama, H.; Murase, Y.; Moyashita, M.; Matsui, H. Aerobic power as related to body growth and training in Japanese boys: a longitudinal study. J. Appl. Physiol. 44:666-672; 1978.

38. Koch, G. Muscle blood flow in prepubertal boys. Effect of growth combined with intensive physical training. In: Borms, J.; Hebbelink, M., eds. Medicine and sport. Basel: Karger; 1978:p. 34-46.

39. Koch, G. Aerobic power, lung dimensions, ventilatory capacity, and muscle blood flow in 12-16 year old boys with high physical activity. In: Berg, K.; Eriksson, B.O., eds. Children and exercise IX. Baltimore: University Park Press; 1980:p. 99-108.

40. LaPorte, R.E.; Cauley, J.A.; Kinsey, C.M. The epidemiology of physical activity in children, college students, middle aged men, menopausal females, and monkeys. J. Chron. Dis. 35:787-795; 1982.

41. Lehmann, M.; Keul, J.; Korsten-Reck, U. The influence of graduated treadmill exercise on plasma catecholamines, aerobic and anaerobic capacity in boys and adults. Eur. J. Appl. Physiol. 47:301-311; 1981.

42. Lortie, G.; Simoneau, J.A.; Hamel, P.; Boulay, M.R.; Landry, F.; Bouchard, C. Responses of maximal aerobic power and capacity to aerobic training. Int. J. Sports Med. 5:232-236; 1984.

43. Lussier, L.; Buskirk, E.R. Effects of an endurance training regimen on assessment of work capacity in prepubertal children. Ann. NY Acad. Sci. 30:734-747; 1977.

44. Mahon, A.D.; Vaccaro, P. Can the point of deflection from linearity of heart rate determine ventilatory threshold in children? Ped Exerc. Science 3:256-262; 1991.

45. Malina, R.M.; Bouchard, C. Growth, maturation, and physical activity. Champaign, IL: Human Kinetics; 1991:p. 329-352.

46. Massicotte, D.R.; MacNab, R.B.J. Cardiorespiratory adaptations to training at specified intensities in children. Med. Sci. Sports 6:242-246; 1974.

47. Mayers, N.; Gutin, B. Physiological characteristics of elite prepubertal cross country runners. Med. Sci. Sports Exerc. 11:172-176; 1979.

48. McBride, P.; Einerson, J.; Hanson, P.; Heindel, K. Exercise and the primary prevention of coronary heart disease. Med. Exerc. Nutr. Health 1:5-15; 1992.

49. McBrine, J.J.; Mazzocca, A.D.; Hayes, J.C.; Roper, M.L.; Barrows, L.H.; Harris, B.A. Adjusting $\dot{V}O_2$max for decrements in strength following 7 days of bed rest [abstract]. Med. Sci. Sports Exerc. 22:S11; 1990.

50. Mirwald, R.L.; Bailey, D.A.; Cameron, N.; Rasmussen, R.L. Longitudinal comparison of aerobic power in active and inactive boys aged 7 to 17 years. Ann. Hum. Biol. 8:404-414; 1981.

51. Miyashita, M.; Miura, M.; Murase, Y.; Yamaji, K. Running performance from the viewpoint of aerobic power. In: Folinsbee, L.J., ed. Environmental stress: individual human adaptations. New York: Academic Press; 1978:p. 183-193.

52. Mocellin, R.; Wasmund, U. Investigations on the influence of a running training programme on the cardiovascular and motor performance capacity in 53 boys and girls of a second and third primary school class. In: Bar-Or, O., ed. Pediatric work physiology IV. Natanya, Israel: Wingate Institute; 1973:p. 279-288.

53. Murase, Y.; Kobayashi, K.; Kamei, S.; Matsui, H. Longitudinal study of aerobic power in superior junior athletes. Med. Sci. Sports Exerc. 13:180-184; 1981.

54. Nudel, D.B.; Hassett, I.; Gurain, A.; Diamant, S.; Weinhouse, E.; Gootman, N. Young long distance runners: physiologic characteristics. Clin. Pediatr. 28:500-505; 1989.

55. Pate, R.R.; Dowda, M.; Ross, J.G. Associations between physical activity and physical fitness in American children. AJDC 144:1123-1129; 1990.

56. Pate, R.R.; Ward, D.S. Endurance exercise trainability in children and youth. In: Grana, W.A.; Lombardo, J.A.; Sharkey, B.J.; Stone, J.A., eds. Advances in sports medicine and fitness. Vol. 3. Chicago: Year Book Medical; 1990:p. 37-55.

57. Paterson, D.H.; McLellan, T.M.; Stella, R.S.; Cunningham, D.A. Longitudinal study of ventilation threshold and maximal O_2 uptake in athletic boys. J. Appl. Physiol. 62:2051-2057; 1987.

58. Payne, V.G.; Morrow, J.R. The effect of physical training on prepubescent $\dot{V}O_2$max: a meta-analysis. Res. Q. Exerc. Sport 64:305-313; 1993.

59. Peel, C.; Utsey, C. Oxygen consumption using the K2 telemetry system and a metabolic cart. Med. Sci. Sports Exerc. 25:396-400; 1993.

60. Penney, D.G.; Dunbar, J.C; Baylerian, M.S. Cardiomegaly and haemodynamics in rats with a transplantable growth hormone secreting tumor. Cardiovasc. Res. 19:270-277; 1985.

61. Perusse, L.; Tremblay, A.; Leblanc, C.; Bouchard, C. Genetic and environmental influences on level of habitual physical activity and exercise participation. Am. J. Epidemiol. 129:1012-1022; 1989.

62. Puhl, J.; Greaves, K.; Hoyt, M.; Baranowski, T. Children's activity rating scale (CARS): description and calibration. Res. Q. Exerc. Sport 61:26-36; 1990.

63. Riddoch, C.; Mahoney, C.; Murphy, N.; Boreham, C.; Cran, G. The physical activity patterns of Northern Irish school children ages 11-16 years. Pediatr. Exerc. Science 3:300-309; 1991.

64. Rigotti, N.A.; Thomas, G.S.; Leaf, A. Exercise and coronary heart disease. Ann. Rev. Med. 34:391-412; 1983.

65. Rowell, L.B. Human circulation. Regulation during physical stress. New York: Oxford University Press; 1986.

66. Rowland, T.W. Aerobic response to endurance training in prepubescent children: a critical analysis. Med. Sci. Sports Exerc. 17:493-497; 1985.

67. Rowland, T.W. Exercise and children's health. Champaign, IL: Human Kinetics; 1990.

68. Rowland, T.W. Trainability of the cardiorespiratory system during childhood. Can. J. Sport Sci. 17:259-263; 1992.

69. Rowland, T.W. Effect of prolonged inactivity on aerobic fitness of children. J. Sports Med. Phys. Fit. 34:147-155; 1994.

70. Rowland, T.W.; Boyajian, A. Aerobic response to endurance training in children: magnitude, variability, and gender comparisons. Pediatrics; 96:654-658; 1995.

71. Rowland, T.W.; Freedson, P.S. Physical activity, fitness, and health in children: a close look. Pediatrics 93:669-672; 1994.

72. Rowland, T.W.; Green, G.M. Anaerobic threshold and the determination of target training heart rates in premenarcheal girls. Pediatr. Cardiol. 10:75-79; 1989.

73. Rowland, T.W.; Unnithan, V.B.; MacFarlane, N.G.; Gibson, N.G.; Paton, J.Y. Clinical manifestations of the "athlete's heart" in prepubertal male runners. Int. J. Sports Med. 15:515-519; 1994.

74. Rowland, T.W.; Varzeas, M.R.; Walsh, C.A. Aerobic responses to walking training in sedentary adolescents. J. Adol. Health 12:30-34; 1991.

75. Rusko, H.K. Development of aerobic power in relation to age and training in cross-country skiers. Med. Sci. Sports Exerc. 24:1040-1047; 1992.

76. Sady, S. Cardiorespiratory exercise training in children. Clin. Sports Med. 5:493-514; 1986.

77. Saltin, B. Cardiovascular and pulmonary adaptation to physical activity. In: Bouchard, C.; Shephard, R.J.; Stephens, T.; Sutton, J.R.; McPherson, B.D., eds. Exercise, fitness and health. A consensus of current knowledge. Champaign, IL: Human Kinetics; 1990:p. 187-203.

78. Saltin, B.; Blomqvist, G; Mitchell, J.H.; Johnson, R.L.; Wildenthal, K.; Chapman, C.B. Response to exercise after bed rest and after training. Circulation 38(Suppl 7):1-78; 1968.

79. Saltin, B.; Hartley, L.H.; Kilbom, A.; Åstrand, I. Physical training in sedentary middle-aged and older men. II. Oxygen uptake, heart rate, and blood lactate concentrations at submaximal and maximal exercise. Scand. J. Clin. Lab. Invest. 24:323-334; 1969.

80. Saris, W.H.M. Habitual physical activity in children: methodology and findings in health and disease. Med. Sci. Sports Exerc. 18:253-263; 1986.

81. Savage, D.D.; Henry, W.L.; Eastman, R.C. Echocardiographic assessment of cardiac anatomy and function in acromegalic patients. Am. J. Med. 67:823-829; 1979.

82. Savage; M.P.; Petratis, M.M.; Thomson, W.H.; Berg, K.; Smith, J.L.; Sady, S.P. Exercise training effects on serum lipids of prepubescent boys and adult men. Med. Sci. Sports Exerc. 18:197-204; 1986.

83. Schaible, T.F.; Malhotra, A.; Ciambrone, G.; Scheuer, J. The effects of gonadectomy on left ventricular function and cardiac contractile proteins in male and female rats. Circ. Res. 54:38-49; 1984.

84. Scheuer, J.; Malhotra, A.; Schaible, T.F.; Capasso, J. Effects of gonadectomy and hormonal replacement on rat hearts. Circulation 6:12-19; 1987.

85. Seliger, V.; Trefny, Z.; Bartunkova, S.; Pauer, M. The habitual activity and physical fitness of 12 year old boys. Acta. Paediatr. Belg. 28 Suppl 1:14-59; 1974.

86. Shasby, G.B.; Hagerman, F.C. The effects of conditioning on cardiorespiratory function in adolescent boys. J. Sports Med. 3:97-107; 1975.

87. Shaywitz, B.A.; Gordon, J.W.; Klopper, J.H.; Zelterman, D.A. The effect of 6-hydroxydopamine on habituation of activity in the developing rat pup. Pharm. Biochem. Behav. 6:391-396; 1977.

88. Shephard, R.J. Effectiveness of training programmes for prepubescent children. Sports Med. 13:194-213; 1992.

89. Stewart, K.J.; Gutin, B. Effects of physical training on cardiorespiratory fitness in children. Res. Q. 47:110-120; 1976.

90. Stremel, R.W.; Convertino, V.A.; Bernauer, E.M.; Greenleaf, J.E. Cardiorespiratory deconditioning with static and dynamic leg exercise during bed rest. J. Appl. Physiol. 41:905-909; 1976.

91. Sundberg, S.; Elovainio, R. Cardiorespiratory function in competitive runners aged 12-16 years compared with normal boys. Acta Paediatr. Scand. 71:987-992; 1982.

92. Sunnegardh, J.; Brattleby, L.E. Maximal oxygen uptake, anthropometry, and physical activity in a randomly selected sample of 8 and 13 year old children in Sweden. Eur. J. Appl. Physiol. 56:266-272; 1987.

93. Tanaka, H.; Shindo, M. Running velocity at blood lactate threshold of boys aged 6-15 years compared with untrained and trained young males. Int. J. Sports Med. 60:90-94; 1985.

94. Thuesen, L.; Christiansen, J.S.; Sorensen, K.E. Increased myocardial contractility following growth hormone administration in normal man. Dan. Med. Bull. 35:193-196; 1988.

95. Tipton, C.M. Exercise and resting blood pressure. In: Eckert, H.M.; Montoye, H.J., eds. Exercise and health. Champaign, IL: Human Kinetics; 1983:p. 32-41.

96. Vaccaro, P.; Clarke, D.H. Cardiorespiratory alterations in 9 to 11 year old children following a season of competitive swimming. Med. Sci. Sports 10:204-207; 1978.

97. Vaccaro, P.; Mahon, A. Cardiorespiratory responses to endurance training in children. Sports Med. 4:352-363; 1987.

98. Van Huss, W.; Evans, S.A.; Kurowski, T.; Anderson, D.J.; Allen, R.; Stephens, K. Physiologic characteristics of male and female age-group runners. In: Brown, E.W.; Branta, C.F., eds. Competitive sports for children and youth. Champaign, IL: Human Kinetics; 1988:p. 143-158.

99. Washington, R.L.; van Gundy, J.C.; Cohen, C.; Sondheimer, H.M.; Wolfe, R.R. Normal aerobic and anaerobic exercise data for North American school-age children. J. Pediatr. 112:223-233; 1988.

100. Weber, G.; Kartodihardjo, W.; Klissouras, V. Growth and physical training with reference to heredity. J. Appl. Physiol. 40:211-215; 1976.

101. Yoshida, T.I.; Ishiko, I.; Muraoka, I. Effect of endurance training on cardiorespiratory function of 5-year-old children. Int. J. Sports Med. 1:91-94; 1980.

102. Zauner, C.W.; Benson, N.Y. Physiological alterations in young swimmers during three years of intensive training. J. Sports Med. 21:179–185; 1981.

CHAPTER 8

RESPONSE TO ENDURANCE EXERCISE: CARDIOVASCULAR SYSTEM

The work assignment of the cardiovascular system during exercise is nothing short of impressive. Consider that the cardiac pump and its peripheral plumbing must (1) provide systemic blood flow for delivering both energy substrate (glucose, fatty acids) and saturated hemoglobin for its oxidation; (2) remove the by-products of exercise metabolism (CO_2, lactic acid); (3) dissipate heat through the cutaneous circulation; (4) transport important regulators of muscle metabolism (such as epinephrine); and (5) maximize flow to exercising muscle through differential regional vasomotor tone.

The means by which the cardiovascular system accomplishes these functions are extraordinarily complex and not well understood. Reduced to simplest terms, cardiac output (Q) can be potentially increased during exercise by a combination of augmented heart rate (HR) and stroke volume (SV); that is, $Q = HR \times SV$. Heart rate is altered through the influences of the autonomic nervous system, while stroke volume is influenced by the interplay of preload (the amount of systemic venous return), myocardial contractility, and afterload (the resistance against which the heart contracts).

This chapter will describe our current understanding of how the cardiac responses to exercise change with exercise during childhood. It will become obvious that this body of knowledge has many gaps, a result largely of the limited technology available for noninvasively measuring cardiovascular function. After a review of this methodology, the characteristics of resting cardiac physiology in children will be presented, followed by a discussion of cardiac functional reserve with exercise as the child grows. We begin, however, with a brief examination of cardiac exercise physiology in mature individuals, for information in children is best assessed in the context of our greater knowledge of the cardiovascular responses of adults to exercise.

THE ADULT MODEL

Cardiac output in the untrained mature human rises to approximately four to five times resting values during a maximal treadmill test. This results mainly from an increase in heart rate, which rises directly with workload to a maximum value that is almost three times the value at rest (approximately 195 bpm in the young adult). Heart rate responses to exercise are mediated by (a) alterations in autonomic nervous input to the sinus node (increases in sympathetic activity and withdrawal of vagal, or parasympathetic, tone) and (b) sympathetic stimulation by increases in plasma epinephrine secreted by the adrenal gland.

During upright exhaustive exercise, stroke volume increases to 1.5-2.0 times resting values, with most of the rise occurring by an intensity equal to 40% of maximal O_2 uptake. This early increase results from augmented ventricular filling (Frank-Starling mechanism), a "replacement" of the diminished ventricular volume that occurs when one assumes the upright position. Increases in stroke volume beyond this level of moderate exercise intensity occur from improved cardiac contractility, a manifestation of the inotropic effects of circulating and neurogenic catecholamines. The stroke volume increases that occur during supine exercise are generally more modest (10-15%).

Maximal heart rate during exercise falls with age during adulthood. At any given age, however, maximal rate is not influenced by cardiovascular fitness, and individual differences in cardiac output reserve are a direct indicator of variations in maximal stroke volume. The ability to generate stroke volume during exercise is thus a key factor in determining one's level of cardiovascular fitness. The factors responsible for these differences are not clear but may involve (1) increased cardiac contractility from augmented sympatho-adrenergic stimulation at maximal exercise, or (2) increased ventricular filling due to a larger end-diastolic dimension (possibly resulting from greater blood volume or more systemic venoconstriction during exercise). From these adult data, certain factors emerge as particularly critical in determining cardiac function during exercise: autonomic nervous and hormonal input, the dimensions of the left ventricle, and blood volume.

This review will attempt to delineate, as far as current research information allows, the extent to which variations in these factors contribute to the changes in cardiovascular function observed with exercise during the childhood years. Several key questions deserve attention:

1. To what extent are growth and size-independent development responsible for the normal evolution of cardiac function during exercise through childhood? Many of the cardiovascular changes during childhood might be expected from growth alone; for example, stroke volume should increase because of normal enlargement of the left ventricle. Others, such as myocardial contractility, could potentially change from alterations in function that are size-independent.
2. Do changes in cardiovascular growth and development occur in a continuum during childhood? Or are these alterations affected principally by the hormonal influences of puberty or achievement of maturity?
3. Which anatomic/physiologic factors are most responsible for increasing cardiac reserve during the growing years?
4. Are there gender differences in the growth and development of cardiac function in childhood?

The discussion in this chapter will be limited to cardiac developmental exercise physiology as it applies to aerobic, or endurance, exercise. The cardiovascular responses to resistance exercise are different and will be reviewed in chapter 13.

MEASUREMENT OF CARDIAC WORK

The lack of a safe, noninvasive, accurate means of measuring cardiac output and function—particularly at high exercise levels—has served as a major roadblock to understanding developmental cardiac exercise physiology.

As a result, the available information is almost entirely descriptive and often contradictory; investigations into mechanisms surrounding cardiovascular changes with growth are particularly lacking. Even with use of a single methodology, intraindividual differences in cardiac output measurements as high as 20% can be observed. It is uncertain whether such findings reflect expected biologic variability or technical imprecision. Particularly vexing is the lack of a "gold standard" technique by which newer methods of estimating cardiac output with exercise can be validated.

Virtually all available techniques require some degree of exercise steady state, making accurate measurements at maximal and near-maximal exercise almost impossible. The artifacts created by respirations and muscular activity cause tests that are useful at rest (echocardiography, systolic time intervals) to be impractical during high-intensity work. Efforts to circumvent some of these problems lead to the study of subjects in positions (i.e., supine) that do not mimic those assumed in normal daily activities or sports events.

Because the means used to examine cardiovascular responses to exercise in children is such a critical issue, it is important to review briefly these techniques and their limitations. As Driscoll et al. have pointed out, "Each requires experience in employing the technique, and the reproducibility of these measurements depends, to a great extent, on the experience and dedication of the investigators" (39, p. 111).

Invasive Methods

Cardiac output is determined from the Fick equation as the O_2 uptake divided by the difference in arterial and mixed venous O_2 content. Each of these components can be measured directly during cardiac catheterization; the systemic and pulmonary circulations are sampled while O_2 uptake is determined by analysis of expired gases. This situation is hardly conducive to the examination of cardiac output responses to exercise in normal children, and data from this approach involve as subjects patients who (1) have known or suspected heart disease, (2) are sedated, and (3) are supine. Moreover, sustained steady state exercise is necessary during blood sampling and $\dot{V}O_2$ measurement. Nonetheless, useful submaximal exercise cardiac output data have been obtained with this technique (71, 113).

One can also estimate cardiac output by measuring the density in the arterial system after injection of dye, of known concentration and volume, in the right side of the heart (dye dilution technique). This method obviates the need for measurement of O_2 uptake, and values can be obtained in approximately 10 s. This technique has been used during cardiac catheterization in studies of cardiac output with exercise in children (27, 66), as well as in the exercise testing laboratory, where an earpiece densitometer is used to measure circulation dye concentration after intravenous injection (62). Similarly, cardiac output can be estimated by changes in temperature recorded by catheter in the right heart after injection of cold infusate (47).

Rudolph pointed out several potential errors in the dye dilution method that he felt limited its accuracy to only 15-20% of actual flow (102): withdrawal of blood for densitometry reading must be absolutely constant, dye must mix fully with circulating blood, and the volume of dye must be measured accurately. He suggested, too, that rapid circulation of blood (as with vigorous exercise) might distort the optical density of the dye, causing error in cardiac output measurement. This may explain why reports in adults indicate that this method overestimates cardiac output during high-intensity exercise (37, 90). It has also been reported that cardiac output estimates by this technique can vary by as much as 30% depending on the sampling site (53).

The validity of the dye dilution technique to assess cardiac output with exercise has not been established in children. Alpert et al. described a correlation coefficient of r = .82 between values of resting cardiac output measured by dye dilution and direct Fick at catheterization in subjects 3-20 years of age (1).

Carbon Dioxide Rebreathing

The Fick equation can also be used to estimate cardiac output (Q) noninvasively through measurement of expired gases by the formula

$$Q = \frac{\dot{V}CO_2}{C_{\dot{v}CO_2} - C_aCO_2}$$

where $\dot{V}CO_2$ is carbon dioxide output (measured from expired gases during steady state collection), $C_{\dot{v}CO_2}$ is venous carbon dioxide content, and C_{aCO_2} is arterial carbon dioxide content. Since the latter requires arterial puncture for direct measurement, estimates of C_{aCO_2} are usually made with conversion equations from the end-tidal CO_2 or from the Bohr equation with measurements of tidal volume, mixed expired PCO_2, volume of respiratory equipment dead space, and assumed value for the subject's physiologic airway dead space.

Mixed venous CO_2 can be estimated by the Collier equilibrium method after the subject rebreathes a gas of known O_2 and CO_2 content (39). In this technique, a plateau of expired PCO_2 is sought when expired alveolar gas CO_2 content reflects mixed venous CO_2 content; a "downstream" correction is often applied for the several mmHg difference between the two. Equations are used to convert both the arterial and mixed venous PCO_2 estimations to CO_2 content for calculation of cardiac output by the Fick equation.

The multiple assumptions and equations involved in this approach confound its accuracy. Marks et al. noted that with nine different means of estimating arterial PCO_2 and four different curves for relating PCO_2 to CO_2 content, it is possible to calculate 36 different values for cardiac output from the same set of data (75). Marks et al. compared these values in six subjects and found differences in cardiac output estimates from 2.0 to 11.1 L/min, with an overall mean and standard deviation of the 36 different estimates of 5.2 (2.3) L/min. They concluded, "This magnitude of error using [CO_2 rebreathing] is dramatic and suggests that extreme caution is advised when interpreting research findings based on these indirect procedures" (pg. 442). In reviewing previous research literature validating the CO_2 rebreathing technique against invasive means of estimating cardiac output, these authors reported an average correlation coefficient of r = 0.82 (range .44 to .96) with exercise.

There has been no systematic evaluation of the validity of the CO_2 rebreathing technique to estimate cardiac output in children. Paterson and Cunningham found that CO_2 rebreathing cardiac output values differed by as much as 15-20% in 12-13-year-old girls during exercise depending on which means of estimating arterial CO_2 content was used (87). In this study, the cardiac output values obtained through use of the downstream correction were 13-16% higher than values obtained without this correction.

Sady et al. reported similar findings in 8-10-year-old children (103). Cardiac output during exercise varied by 9-21% according to the curve used to relate PCO_2 to CO_2 content and up to 19% depending on the physiological dead space prediction equation used.

Reliability studies indicate, however, that the reproducibility of cardiac output values with this technique is reasonably good (75). Considering the high variability of values depending on the calculation method used, there is a need for standardization of the technique and equations employed for making cardiac output estimations in both children and adults.

Estimates of cardiac output during exercise using the CO_2 rebreathing technique are limited to steady state conditions, and measurements at maximal and near-maximal workloads are difficult. This disadvantage is compounded by the disagreeable sensation many children feel in rebreathing increased concentrations of CO_2 at high work intensities. One needs experience in using this technique in order to choose proper bag volumes and CO_2 concentrations. A CO_2 plateau may not be observed if the bag volume is overly large or if CO_2 concentrations are either too great or too small.

Acetylene Rebreathing

The acetylene rebreathing technique also involves estimates of expired gas concentration equilibrium during rebreathing while exercising. With this method, the subject rebreathes from a bag containing a mixture of O_2, helium, acetylene, and nitrogen; pulmonary blood flow (cardiac output) is estimated by the disappearance rate of acetylene concentration in expired air as it is absorbed in the blood. Validation studies in adults indicate a close correlation between acetylene rebreathing values for cardiac output and those derived by direct Fick and dye dilution techniques (23, 120).

Technical issues associated with acetylene rebreathing include (1) the need for instrumentation that can rapidly and accurately measure concentrations of expired gas; (2) the importance of an appropriate volume of gas in the bag, as an overly large or small volume can alter cardiac output estimates; (3) the question of the proper assumed value for the solubility coefficient of acetylene in blood; and (4) avoidance of recirculation of acetylene. This last concern may be particularly pertinent during exercise (39).

Although this technique is well suited for estimation of cardiac output in children (39), its use in the pediatric age group has been limited. Tomassoni et al. have reported cardiac responses using acetylene rebreathing in their rehabilitation program for children with heart disease (118), and Driscoll et al. used this method to assess cardiac function before and after surgery for congenital heart disease (38).

Thoracic Bioimpedance

The ejection of blood from the heart during ventricular systole is associated with changes in electrical resistance in the chest, and these alterations can be mathematically related to cardiac stroke volume. Changes of resistance, or impedance, are measured by spot electrodes applied to the chest and neck, offering a safe, convenient method of estimating cardiac output. Moreover, this technique is unique in providing beat-to-beat stroke volume data without the need for steady state, even at high exercise intensities.

The utility of this method during exercise has been hampered by (1) artifact created by chest wall movement and respiratory efforts, (2) potential errors created by changes in hematocrit and blood resistivity during exercise, (3) unclear influences of differences in body composition and chest wall configuration, and (4) a lack of accuracy suggested by early studies.

Computer technology in newer bioimpedance monitors has minimized artifact effects during exercise, and bioimpedance cardiac output measurements using this equipment have been validated against the thermodilution technique in animals (119), neonates (12), critically ill children (77), and adult surgical patients (4). Correlation coefficients in these studies varied from .82 to .95. Miles and Gotshall reviewed nine studies indicating the validity of impedance cardiography during exercise

(78). Correlation coefficients in these reports ranged from .75 to .95 between cardiac output by impedance and that obtained with CO_2, direct Fick, and dye dilution techniques.

Rowland et al. assessed the validity of this technique during exercise in children and adults, using O_2 uptake as the criterion measure (100). Maximal cardiac values were obtained in 71-94% of subjects. Correlation coefficients between cardiac output and $\dot{V}O_2$ of .65-.80 were somewhat lower than those typically reported with use of other techniques for estimating cardiac output. Test-retest correlation for submaximal cardiac output was r = .97 for 12 subjects tested 1 week apart.

Although this method would be ideal for children because of its safety and convenience, further validity studies are needed to establish its accuracy in determination of cardiac output with exercise.

Doppler Echocardiography

Ultrasound Doppler assessment of aortic flow velocity, coupled with echocardiographic measurement of aortic root diameter, permits a safe noninvasive estimation of cardiac output. Findings in the resting state have been reported to be similar to those obtained by invasive methods (105, 110). Marx et al. assessed the utility of this technique during supine cycle exercise in a group of early-adolescent boys (76). During cycling at 50% $\dot{V}O_2$max, values for Doppler echocardiographic cardiac output correlated reasonably closely to those obtained by CO_2 rebreathing in a separate testing session (r = .86). Adequate Doppler flows could not be obtained in one of five subjects, however, and chest wall motion artifact precluded obtaining maximal values in the majority. The authors suggested that this technique might be valuable for assessing changes in cardiac output relative to O_2 uptake as an indicator of submaximal cardiac function.

THE CHILD'S HEART AT REST

The maintenance of normal resting metabolism is contingent upon adequate body perfusion. The rise in energy requirements associated with growth during childhood must therefore be matched by similar improvements in cardiac output. Since metabolic rate in respect to body mass or surface area is inversely related to body size, one would expect any changes in heart function with growth to be similarly altered. That is, resting cardiac output should reflect basal metabolic rate (BMR), with lower values relative to body size at progressively older ages. (This analysis assumes that peripheral O_2 uptake is independent of age, since $\dot{V}O_2 = Q \times$ a-$\dot{V}$ O_2 uptake. As will be discussed in chapter 10, this is probably a valid conclusion.)

Heart Weight

The mass of the heart relative to body mass is high in newborn babies and declines steadily throughout the pediatric years. The ratio of heart weight to body weight is typically .0073 (males) and .0068 (females) in term newborns (108) but .0043 and .0040, respectively, in adults (112). Heart weights measured by Schulz and Giordano and related to expected body weight norms show an approximate 20% decline from ages 3 to 15 years (96, 108) (see fig. 8.1). Echocardiographic studies have indicated that left ventricular mass during the growing years is more closely related instead to body surface area (BSA) (34, 56).

In the age group old enough for exercise testing, however, the means of normalizing heart mass to body size does not seem critical. When Daniels et al. examined echocardiograms in 6-23-year-old subjects, correlation coefficients were essentially identical between left ventricular mass and both weight and BSA (.83 for males for both; .73 and .74, respectively, for females) (31). Similarly, Scholz et al. reported equally close correlations of body weight and BSA with heart weight in 200 autopsy specimens from birth to age 19 years (107). Only 10 of the hearts in that study were from children with body mass under 10 kg.

Stroke Volume

When echocardiograms are measured over the entire pediatric age span, resting left ventricular end-diastolic dimension is found to relate closely to the cube root of BSA (56). Since left ventricular volume approximates a cube function of end-diastolic diameter, these data suggest that left ventricular size is most closely related to BSA during growth. During the same period, measures of resting left ventricular contractility, such as shortening fraction (diastolic minus systolic dimension, divided by diastolic dimension), are age-independent. This implies that the growth of resting cardiac stroke volume in children is also closely linked to BSA.

Other data indicate that resting stroke volume in children can also be closely related to body weight. Resting cardiac catheterization findings in 29 supine children ages 0-20 years, reported by Krovetz et al., showed correlation coefficients of r = .87 and .90 between stroke volume and body weight and BSA, respectively (66). Average stroke index (stroke volume per BSA) was 44.3 ml/m². The average value calculated for arteriovenous O_2 difference was 44.3 ml/L.

Sproul and Simpson calculated values for supine resting stroke volume from cardiac output (by direct Fick) during cardiac catheterization in 21 normal children ages 6 to 16 years (113). Stroke volume was linearly related to BSA (r = .83) as well as to body weight (r = .81), with a mean stroke index of 42.2 ml/m² over a surface area range of 0.7 to 1.5 m² (see fig. 8.2). Average arteriovenous O_2 difference was 41 ml/L and was not related to age (r = .11). Gutgesell et al. demonstrated similar relationships between echocardiographic left ventricular measurements and weight and BSA (52). Bouchard et al. showed that the ratio of heart volume (by x-ray) and body weight is essentially constant between the ages of 8 and 18 years (17).

The relationship of stroke volume to weight or BSA may be significantly influenced by body composition.

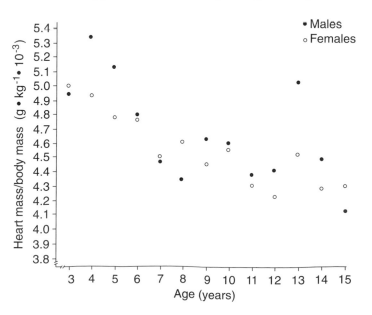

Figure 8.1 Estimated ratio of average heart mass to body mass during the childhood years. Reprinted from Rowland 1991.

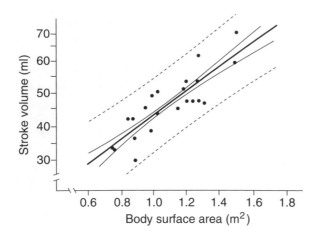

Figure 8.2   Resting stroke volume in children relative to body surface area. Reprinted from Sproul and Simpson 1964.

Several lines of investigation suggest that $\dot{V}O_2$max is closely associated with lean body mass (32, 58, 114); stroke volume and cardiac output may therefore be underestimated in the obese individual when these variables are related to body weight.

In summary, it would appear that increases in resting stroke volume during childhood are associated with increases in left ventricular size, which in turn is directly related to BSA, lean body mass, or total body mass. Current information does not yield insight into which is the proper "normalizing" factor for growth of stroke volume in childhood (20). For children in the age groups typically involved in exercise research (over 8 years), if they are relatively homogenous in body composition, any of the three are probably appropriate. It is unlikely that alterations in afterload, contractility, or preload independent of these anthropometric variables have any significant influence on the growth of resting stroke volume in children.

Heart Rate

Age-related differences in basal heart rates were obtained in the cross-sectional investigations of BMR performed in the early part of the 20th century. These studies were reviewed and their data summarized by Sutliff and Holt in 1925 (115). This information was obtained by palpation of the peripheral pulse in normal healthy subjects in standardized basal conditions (during the postabsorptive state, at least 12 hr after the previous meal, and after lying quietly for at least 30 min).

Basal heart rates decrease progressively throughout the childhood years, falling 10-20 bpm in the age span from 5 to 15 years (see table 8.1). It will be noted that mean values for girls are consistently greater than those

for boys from the age of 9 years on. This influence of gender on basal heart rate persists to the adult years.

These values can be compared to the somewhat higher heart rates reported by Volkmann in 1850 that are presented in the same table (123). These can be best described as resting rather than basal, as subjects were sitting in a chair 2-4 hr after their last meal. It follows that "resting" heart rates taken immediately before exercise testing are neither basal nor resting and are highly (and presumably variably) influenced by anxiety and anticipatory neurohormonal changes.

More recent findings in a mixed longitudinal study from the Child Research Council in Denver were similar to those from the early reports already cited (73) (see fig. 8.3). Basal heart rates were about 15 bpm lower than seated resting rates. Mean heart rate in the basal state was approximately 80 bpm at age 5 and 62 bpm at age 15. After age 10, basal heart rates were about 3-5 bpm faster in girls than in boys.

The fall in basal heart rate during the childhood years tends to parallel the decline in BMR expressed relative to body size (57). Basal metabolic rate (expressed as calories per BSA per hour) drops about 23% in females from age 6 to 16 years, while the basal heart rate falls approximately 20% during the same time span (64).

Investigations in animals consistently show that smaller hearts beat at rest with a great frequency. For example, pulse rates are typically 520-780 bpm in the mouse, but 34-50 bpm in a horse. Measurements of many adult species indicate that resting heartbeat fre-

Table 8.1   Heart rates in different standard states (123, 115)

Years	Resting males and females	Basal males	Females
1	134	116	122
2	111	104	103
3	108	92	86
4	108	100	91
5	103	91	90
6	98	92	88
7	93	89	82
8	94	90	89
9	89	85	92
10	91	75	86
11	87	82	92
12	89	80	85
13	88	81	84
14	87	79	80
15	82	74	80

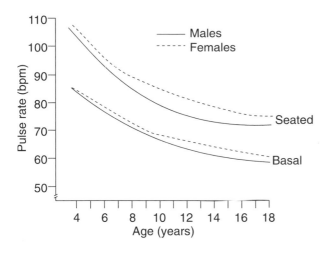

Figure 8.3 Changes with age in basal and seated resting heart rates in boys and girls. Reprinted from Malina and Bouchard 1991.

quency (f_h) relates to body mass (M_b) by the allometric equation

$$f_h = 241 \, M_b^{-0.25}.$$

The exponent –0.25 is identical to that relating weight-relative metabolic rate to body mass in animals (BMR = $70 \, M_b^{-0.25}$) (106). This observation indicates that the decrease in mass-related or BSA-related BMR (or $\dot{V}O_2$) as body size increases is accounted for by a fall in heart rate, while cardiac stroke volume grows in direct proportion to body size. The parallel decline in BMR and basal heart rate during childhood suggests that the same holds true in humans.

What is the mechanism for the slowing of basal and resting heart rate in the childhood years? The resting

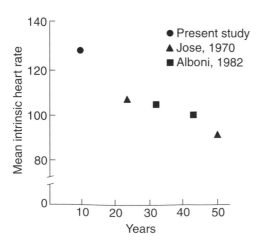

Figure 8.4 Intrinsic heart rate after autonomic blockade in children and adults. Reprinted from Marcus et al. 1990.

heart rate in a child after autonomic blockade (propranolol and atropine) rises approximately 40 bpm, indicating that the intrinsic discharge rate of the sinus node is suppressed by predominantly parasympathetic influence in the nonexercising state (74). Comparison of intrinsic heart rates across age groups using this approach indicates a significantly higher rate in children (130 bpm) compared to young adults (105 bpm) (see fig. 8.4).

These observations suggest that the fall in resting heart rate with age is at least partially independent of autonomic influence, instead principally reflecting intrinsic changes in sinus node depolarization rate. Suggested mechanisms have included changes in sinoatrial nodal membrane ion flux or permeability with age, and alterations in location of the predominant pacemaker cells within the node.

Myocardial Function

There is no evidence that resting myocardial function changes in normal children as they grow. The echocardiographic left ventricular shortening fraction is independent of age, with typical values of about 34-36% (52). The mean velocity of myocardial fiber shortening, a function of systolic myocardial function as well as ventricular preload, tends to decrease with age; but this presumably reflects the progressive fall in heart rate during the same period.

Animal studies have indicated, however, that myocardial contractile properties are diminished in the very young (45). Colan et al. investigated the implications for humans by studying age-related differences in resting contractility in 256 normal children ages 7 days to 19 years (one-third were under 3 years) using echocardiography, phonocardiography, and blood pressure tracings (24) (see fig. 8.5). The left ventricular architecture, as determined by major:minor axis ratio, did not change with growth.

According to LaPlace's law, the normal increase in blood pressure with age should be matched by a proportionately greater ratio of wall thickness to chamber dimension to maintain constant wall stress (21). The study by Colan et al. indicated that the ratio of left ventricular wall thickness to diastolic dimension remained stable with increasing age (24). The resulting increase in wall stress, which was most dramatic in the first few years of life, was offset by the progressive decline in resting heart rate, so no differences in total minute stress were seen with increasing age.

In this study the age-related fall in velocity of fiber shortening was more than could be attributed to increased afterload, suggesting that infants and small children possess greater rather than inferior myocardial contractility compared to older children. Similarly, a

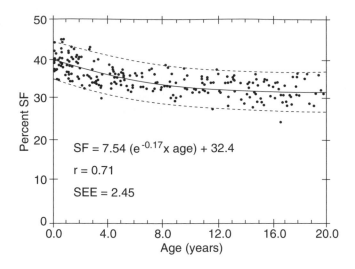

Figure 8.5   Resting left ventricular shortening fraction (SF) during childhood. Reprinted from Colan et al. 1992.

gradual decline in left ventricular shortening fraction was observed from the newborn period (40%) to age 12 years (35%). In summary, then, these authors could present no evidence of impairment of resting cardiac function during the pediatric years.

Other studies using different testing modalities have supported this conclusion. Echocardiographic measures of systolic time intervals by Gutgesell et al. showed that the mean ratio of resting left ventricular pre-ejection period to ejection time (.31), an indicator of cardiac con-

tractility, was independent of age in a group of 145 normal children from birth to 19 years of age (52). Measurements of ventricular ejection fraction by radionuclide angiography in children have demonstrated no differences from values expected in adults (46, 59, 67). Hurwitz et al. studied 90 children and adolescents with normal hearts ranging from 2 months to 20 years of age (59). Average right and left ventricular ejection fractions ranged from 52% to 54% and 62% to 70%, respectively, with no relationship to age (see fig. 8.6).

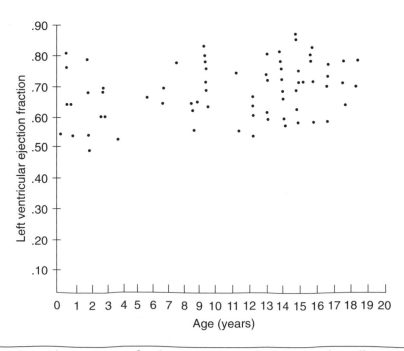

Figure 8.6   Resting left ventricular ejection fraction in children and adolescents by radionuclide angiography. Reprinted from Hurwitz et al. 1984.

Cardiac Output

The pattern of change in resting cardiac output during childhood is a consequence of several trends: ventricular size and stroke volume increase with age in association with body dimensions; heart rate falls in parallel to BMR in relation to body dimensions; and myocardial contractility is independent of age. Since cardiac output is closely related to O_2 uptake (51), resting cardiac output would be expected to progressively decrease relative to body weight or surface area during the pediatric years.

Given the variable influences of emotional state and environment on resting hemodynamic parameters, as well as the imprecision of noninvasive measurements, it is not surprising that studies of resting cardiac output are limited. Longitudinal investigations of resting cardiac output during childhood are nonexistent, and early cross-sectional studies in children typically involved small numbers of sedated subjects evaluated during cardiac catheterization (66, 71).

In 1967, Krovetz et al. described supine cardiac output values obtained by indicator dilution curves in 20 sedated subjects from infancy to age 20 years (66). Cardiac output correlated well with BSA (r = .94), height (r = .94), and weight (r = .91), with a mean cardiac index (output related to BSA) of 4.3 L/min per square meter. In a similar study, Locke et al. found a mean cardiac index of 4.4 L/min per square meter by the direct Fick technique in 23 sedated supine children ages 5 to 16 years (71). The supine cardiac catheterization data in children studied by Sproul and Simpson revealed correlation coefficients of 0.70 and 0.69 with BSA and weight, respectively (113). Mean cardiac index in that study was 4.1 L/min per square meter.

Using impedance cardiography, Barbacki et al. found an almost identical value (4.4 L/min per square meter) in 20 supine boys and girls ages 8-14 years (9). Sholler et al. reported an average cardiac index with Doppler echocardiography of 4.1 L/min per square meter in 41 supine children ages 2-15 years (110). These findings are consistent with the bioimpedance data of Rowland et al. (101), who described a mean cardiac index of 3.0 L/min per square meter in 21 boys (mean age 10.5 years) in the sitting position, since cardiac output can be expected to fall about 25% when one assumes the sitting position (14, 88).

Katori's study of 151 healthy subjects ages 4 to 78, using the earpiece dye dilution method, provided some insight into changes in resting cardiac output during childhood and the relationship of these values to body dimensions (62). In a curve reminiscent of that of absolute O_2 uptake, cardiac output rose from about 4 L/min in the youngest subjects to a peak of 8 L/min in late adolescence, then slowly tapered throughout life. Cardiac output related to mass fell from approximately 240 ml · kg^{-1} · min^{-1} in the younger subjects to 110 ml · kg^{-1} · min^{-1} by adolescence (see fig. 8.7). The decline was less dramatic when cardiac output was expressed relative to BSA, with values of 6 L/min per square meter at age 4 years declining to just above 4 L/min per square meter by adolescence. No differences were seen between boys and girls.

Blood Pressure

Resting systolic, diastolic, and mean systemic blood pressures rise progressively during childhood (73, 116) (see fig. 8.8). The typical blood pressure for a healthy term newborn baby is approximately 70/55 mmHg. At

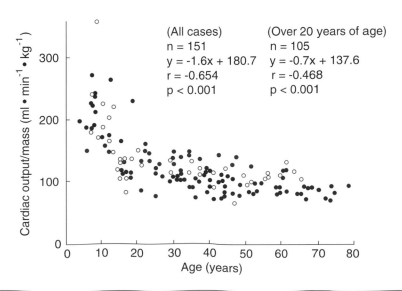

Figure 8.7 Resting cardiac output related to body mass with age. Reprinted from Katori 1979.

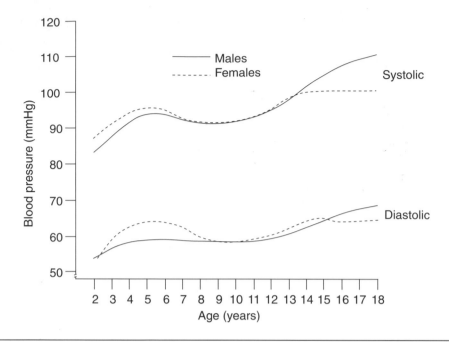

Figure 8.8 Longitudinal changes in resting systolic and diastolic blood pressure during childhood and adolescence. Reprinted from Malina and Bouchard 1991.

age 10 years the average is 100/62, and at age 15 the mean value is 115/65 (73). Since by Ohm's law, blood pressure is the product of flow (stroke volume) and resistance, this increase in blood pressure must reflect changes in these variables. How each contributes to the rise in blood pressure with age is uncertain. Resting stroke volume rises with age as a consequence of increasing left ventricular size. This effect presumably outweighs that of increasing arteriolar radius during growth, although the influence of alterations in the other determinants of peripheral vascular resistance (sympathetic innervation, blood viscosity, local muscle vascular response to metabolites) during childhood is unknown.

Summary

Commensurate with increasing body size, resting cardiac output rises progressively during childhood. Since growth changes in cardiac output can be achieved by increases in stroke volume (a growth-related variable) or heart rate (a size-independent factor), or both, it is helpful to examine which determinant nature "chooses" to augment resting heart function as children grow.

Available research information indicates that increases in cardiac output at rest during childhood are accomplished entirely by a rise in stroke volume; and since myocardial contractility does not change, the increase in stroke volume is a direct expression of increases in heart size. The size of the heart, in turn, is linked to some marker of somatic growth. It is not clear

whether this marker is body weight, surface area, lean body mass, or something else.

Stroke volume, heart size, and the somatic marker are not directly linked to resting metabolic rate, which is disproportionately greater relative to body weight and size in younger subjects. The needs of perfusion to achieve this "excessive" metabolic rate relative to BSA or body weight are met through a higher heart rate in younger children. As children grow, then, resting stroke volume increases, heart rate decreases, and cardiac output rises (but disproportionately to body weight and size).

CARDIOVASCULAR RESPONSES TO EXERCISE

Cardiovascular responses to exercise in children can now be examined in light of the contributions of stroke volume and heart rate to resting cardiac output that have been described. It should again be emphasized that information about maturational changes in these responses is particularly limited. The following data are best regarded as preliminary work, awaiting safer and more accurate technical approaches to measuring cardiac work during exercise.

Heart Rate

Information about heart rate with exercise is the least suspect of the cardiovascular variables, since values can be accurately measured at all intensities of physical activity by electrocardiography or newer electronic methods. It is useful, then, to begin an analysis of cardiovascular responses to exercise with an examination of changes in maximal and submaximal heart rate as the child grows.

Maximal Heart Rate. The peak heart rate demonstrated during an exhaustive, progressive laboratory exercise test is profoundly influenced by subject motivation. This caveat notwithstanding, both cross-sectional and longitudinal studies in healthy children have consistently indicated that maximal heart rates in this setting are stable throughout the growing years (or at least above that age when maximal testing becomes feasible), with values of 195-205 bpm (2, 5, 7, 28, 49, 93, 124). Moreover, these data demonstrate that maximal rates in children are to some extent dependent on the testing modality (cycle vs. treadmill) and type of exercise (walk vs. run) (97). Most studies in children have shown no effects of gender on maximal heart rate.

Bailey et al. tested 51 boys longitudinally over 8 years, beginning at age 8, with a running treadmill protocol (7). Mean maximal heart rate for the entire study was 196 bpm. With the exception of the 1st year, when the average peak rate was 193 bpm, mean maximal rates on serial testing did not vary between years by more than 3 bpm. Rowland and Cunningham tested 9 girls and 10 boys with a maximal treadmill walking protocol annually for 5 years beginning at age 9 (unpublished data). As figure 8.9 shows, no systematic changes in mean values of maximal heart rate were seen with in-

creasing age in either sex; ranges were 2 bpm in the girls and 4 bpm in the boys.

After the late teenage years, maximal heart rate declines throughout life. An average 60-year-old man, for instance, can be expected to reach a rate of 160 bpm during exhaustive exercise (94). While formulas for estimating maximal heart rate for age have been suggested (220 – age in years, or 210 – [0.65 × age]), these are clearly inappropriate for children, whose maximal heart rate is age-independent.

Why children have higher maximal heart rates than at other times in life is unclear. Sympathetic activity appears to be the principal factor responsible for augmenting heart rate above moderate levels of exercise intensity, yet serum norepinephrine levels, a marker of sympathetic activity, have been demonstrated to be 30% *lower* in children than in young adults at peak exercise (68).

Protocols involving treadmill running typically elicit the highest maximal heart rates. Mean peak rate among 327 children tested by Cumming et al. using the Bruce protocol was 200 bpm for both boys and girls (28). The few maximal treadmill running studies in very young subjects (ages 4-6 years) have indicated maximal rates ranging from 199 to 206 bpm, similar to those of older children (29, 111, 127). Maximal rates are typically lower with walking protocols (e.g., Balke), with average values of about 195 bpm (30, 93, 109).

Peak heart rates observed during cycle testing are usually less than those recorded with treadmill exercise. Washington et al. reported average maximal rates with the James protocol of 193 and 196 bpm in 81 boys and

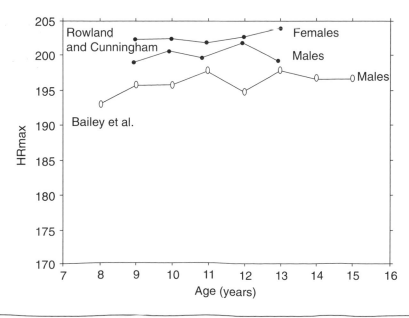

Figure 8.9 Longitudinal changes in maximal treadmill heart rate in two studies. Data from Bailey et al. (7) and Rowland and Cunningham (unpublished data).

70 girls, respectively, who were ages 7-12 years (124). Boileau et al. found that 21 boys ages 11 to 14 years had a mean maximal heart rate of 194 bpm on a walking treadmill test but only 186 bpm during exhaustive cycle exercise (15).

Cumming and Langford determined maximal heart rates in one group of boys using various testing modalities (30). Mean values were 195 and 197 bpm for the Godfrey and James cycle protocols, respectively, 204 bpm for the Bruce treadmill protocol (running), and 198 bpm for the Balke walking protocol.

It is important to recognize that although mean maximal heart rates during childhood are remarkably consistent with age, there is a large variability between individual subjects. The results of Cumming and Langford included a standard deviation for all protocols ranging from 5 to 7 bpm. Sheehan et al. reported a standard deviation of 9 bpm in boys who had a mean maximal rate of 202 bpm during treadmill running (109). This means that two of six subjects could be expected to have a peak rate below 193 or above 211 bpm.

Heart Rate Scope and Reserve.

As the child ages, the resting heart rate falls and maximal rate remains constant. It follows, then, that the difference between the two, termed the *heart rate reserve*, must increase. It has been suggested that the greater reserve in the older child compared to the younger may provide an aerobic advantage for endurance athletic performance (10).

Using the basal data of Malina and Roche (73), and assuming a maximal heart rate of 200 bpm, one can estimate the age-related values for heart reserve. Between the ages of 6 and 12 years, the average boy increases his heart rate reserve from 120 to 133 bpm, a 10% rise. *Heart rate scope,* the quotient of maximal and resting rate, increases from 2.5 to 3.0 during the same time span.

Submaximal Heart Rate.

The heart rate at a given work intensity progressively falls as a child ages. When subjects are cycling at the same submaximal workload, O_2 uptake and cardiac output are not influenced by age. The fall in heart rate might be explained, therefore, simply as secondary to the increase in stroke volume related to normal heart growth. This same change in the relationship of submaximal heart rate and stroke volume is observed after a period of physical training; that is, a rise in stroke volume replaces heart rate in the determination of a given submaximal cardiac output. This training response is considered useful in minimizing myocardial $\dot{V}O_2$ costs during heart work (83). The potential positive effects of this "switchover" on myocardial energy efficiency in the growing child have not been assessed.

The rate of decline in submaximal heart rate has been quantitated on both treadmill and cycle protocols. In a cross-sectional study, Cassels and Morse showed that the mean heart rate in 10-year-olds walking at 3.5 mph on an 8.6% grade was 167 bpm but that in 16-year-old subjects the rate was 147 bpm (22). Bouchard et al. found a mean heart rate of 138 and 100 bpm in 8 and 18-year-old boys, respectively, who were pedaling at a workload of 30 W (17). Godfrey et al. demonstrated that submaximal heart rates were a function of not only body size but also gender (51). Girls exhibited higher rates than the boys, as much as 10-20 bpm at higher work intensities. The reason for gender differences in submaximal heart rates is unclear but may reflect smaller stroke volumes in the girls.

The relationship between heart rate and workload is linear during exercise at moderate intensity in children, but at higher workloads the heart rate tapers as work rate increases. Rowland and Cunningham demonstrated that the mean rate of heart rate deceleration in a group of 12-year-old children was constant above 60% $\dot{V}O_2$max (98). This pattern appears to be similar to that observed in adults, but no direct maturational comparisons have been made. The cause and "rationale" for tapering of heart rate at high work intensities are uncertain. It has been suggested that receptors in the ventricular wall might serve as a "vagal brake" to prevent excessive tachycardia during exercise that would otherwise impair ventricular filling and compromise coronary perfusion (13).

The point at which the heart rate begins to decelerate as work increases (the "*heart rate deflection*") has been shown to correlate closely with ventilatory markers of the anaerobic threshold in both children and adults (19, 48, 72). Whether this implies that the deflection of sinus node activity during high-intensity work is linked to increasing lactic acid concentration and anaerobic metabolism is unknown.

Recovery Heart Rate.

Baraldi et al. demonstrated that heart rate recovery time after maximal exercise increases with work intensity but to a much smaller extent in children than in adults (8). They postulated that the faster recovery of heart rate in children was attributable to their lower catecholamine levels.

The rate of fall in heart rate after exhaustive exercise declines relative to body size and age throughout the course of the pediatric years. One-minute recovery heart rates after maximal cycle testing were 133, 138, and 148 bpm in boys grouped by BSA as < 1.0 m², 1.0-1.19 m², and > 1.2 m², respectively, by Washington et al. (124). The girls showed a similar decline. The younger children tested on the treadmill by Riopel et al. also had a faster fall in heart rate than older subjects despite similar peak rates (93).

Submaximal Heart Rate Kinetics. It has been suggested that children show a more rapid cardiovascular response at the onset of exercise than adult subjects (42). On the basis of observations in his own laboratory, Godfrey concluded, "There is no doubt that children reach a steady state more quickly than adults" (50, p. 30). It has been hypothesized that children might need to rely more on aerobic mechanisms in the early stages of muscular work because of their inferior ability to generate anaerobic energy compared to adults (see chapter 12).

When Sady et al. examined O_2 uptake and heart rate temporal responses to the same relative cycle work intensity in boys and men, however, they observed no differences in rate of rise (104) (see fig. 8.10). Cooper et al. showed that O_2 uptake kinetics were similar at the onset of exercise in 7-9-year-old and 15-18-year-old subjects, but the time to steady state of heart rate was actually slower in the younger children (25).

Stroke Volume

A reasonable hypothesis can now be suggested to describe the changes in components of cardiac reserve with exercise during childhood. First, we know that maximal heart rate during the pediatric years remains constant. Increases in maximal cardiac output as the child grows must therefore solely reflect improvements in maximal stroke volume. Assuming a close link between $\dot{V}O_2max$ and Qmax, it follows that maximal stroke volume per kg body mass should remain relatively constant during childhood in boys and gradually decline in girls (paralleling similar relationships between $\dot{V}O_2max$ and body mass). Heart and left ventricular size is also closely associated with body mass, sug-

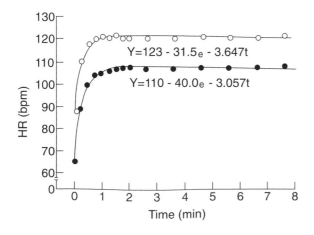

Figure 8.10 Rate of rise in heart rate at submaximal intensity of approximately 40% $\dot{V}O_2max$ shows no difference in children (open circles) and adults. From Sady et al. 1983.

gesting that increases in stroke volume with age are a reflection simply of changes in left ventricular dimensions rather than any alterations in myocardial contractility, afterload, or other factors influencing ventricular preload. The validity of these concepts can be tested by examining studies that have estimated exercise stroke volume in children.

Oxygen Pulse. The crudest but most easily measured indicator of stroke volume during exercise is the O_2 *pulse*, defined as the amount of O_2 consumed by the body for each heartbeat. Consistent with the Fick equation, O_2 pulse is the product of stroke volume and arteriovenous O_2 difference. Investigations in adult subjects have indicated that O_2 pulse during exercise can provide an acceptable estimate of stroke volume. Norris et al., for instance, demonstrated correlation coefficients of 0.73 and 0.97 between O_2 pulse and stroke volume in untrained and trained adult cyclists, respectively, pedaling at 50% $\dot{V}O_2max$ (84). The resting cardiac catheterization data of Sproul and Simpson in children showed a close association between stroke volume and O_2 pulse (r = 0.89) (113).

Studies across a broad range of animal species indicate that the ratio of resting O_2 pulse to body mass is independent of body size (106). Cooper et al. used allometric analysis to show that O_2 pulse at a heart rate of 140 bpm scaled in direct proportion to body weight (26), and Washington et al. demonstrated a linear relationship (r = 0.88) between maximal O_2 pulse and BSA during cycle testing of 151 children 7-12 years old (124). These data support the concept that resting, submaximal, and maximal stroke volume increases directly with body dimensions during childhood.

Maximal Stroke Volume by Carbon Dioxide Rebreathing. Miyamura and Honda provided estimated maximal values of stroke volume with exercise in relation to age and sex (79). These were calculated from cardiac output measurements determined by CO_2 rebreathing within 15 s of exhaustive exercise. Maximal stroke index averaged 65.2 and 56.2 ml/m² in males and females, respectively, who were 9 to 20 years old. These values for maximal stroke index remained stable for both groups over this age range.

Determinants of Stroke Volume With Exercise. Stroke volume can potentially be increased during exercise by either a greater end-diastolic volume (a result of increased filling) or a diminished end-systolic volume (from either augmented myocardial contractility or decreased afterload). Considerable research effort has been expended in adult subjects to determine the relative contributions of these factors to changes in stroke volume with exercise, utilizing echocardiography, radionuclide imaging, and angiography (63). While examples of rather striking contradictory findings can be cited (117, 125), these adult-based data collectively are most consistent with the following pattern.

In the supine position, gravitational effects maximize left ventricular filling even at rest. During progressive exercise in this position, then, no significant changes are observed in left ventricular end-diastolic dimension. Increases in left ventricular shortening fraction during exercise in the supine position are due solely to decreases in left ventricular end-systolic dimension, which in turn result principally from augmented contractility (from increased adrenergic influences on the heart).

Resting stroke volume for someone in the sitting position is generally about 25% less than in the supine position, a result of gravitational reduction in systemic venous return. With the initiation of exercise, the combined effects of systemic venoconstriction and activation of pumping action by contracting leg muscles reverse these hydrostatic effects and "refill" the ventricles. As a result, the initial phase of upright exercise is typified by an increase in end-diastolic dimension; consequently, stroke volume rises by 1.3-1.5 times resting values with an exercise intensity of 40% $\dot{V}O_2$max. Subsequent increases in stroke volume during upright exercise above moderate intensity levels are associated with a decrease in end-systolic dimension and stable end-diastolic dimension. In other words, increases in heart rate maintain pace with augmented systemic venous return to the heart such that there is no enlargement of the left ventricle; increases in stroke volume occur with improvements in myocardial contractility, manifest as a fall in left ventricular end-systolic dimension (61).

Limited data suggest that children respond similarly. Three studies, all involving supine cycle exercise, indicate that end-systolic dimension diminishes and end-diastolic dimension remains stable in young subjects during progressively intense exercise (33, 85, 86).

Oyen et al. measured these dimensions echocardiographically during exercise that produced heart rates of 145-180 bpm in 127 children ages 6-14 years (85). Left ventricular shortening fraction rose during exercise from a mean of 37% to 46%. When the children were separated into three groups by BSA, there was no significant difference in shortening fraction response to exercise; this suggested that the pattern in alterations in cardiac dimensions causing increases in stroke volume are not influenced by biological maturation. Average left ventricular end-diastolic dimension was 3.81 cm at the beginning of exercise in the group with the smallest BSA and 3.72 cm at the highest workload, while the mean end-systolic dimension fell from 2.41 to 2.16 cm. The groups with larger BSA demonstrated a similar pattern (see fig. 8.11).

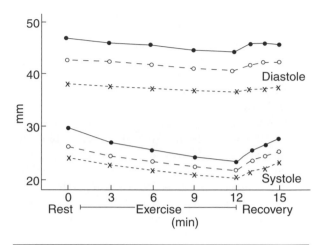

Figure 8.11 Changes in left ventricular systolic and diastolic diameters with exercise and recovery in three different body surface area groups. x------x = BSA < 1.1 m²; O-----O = BSA 1.1-1.4 m²; •———• = BSA > 1.4 m². Reprinted from Oyen 1987.

Dickhuth et al. presented virtually identical findings in an echocardiographic supine exercise study in young adults ages 21-35 years (35). Subjects pedaled up to 150 W with a heart rate of approximately 150 bpm. Mean left ventricular shortening fraction rose from 34% at rest to 42% at 150 W. End-diastolic dimension did not change significantly, while end-systolic dimension steadily declined, from an average of 32 mm at rest to 28.9 mm at 150 W.

At least to a work intensity of 80% maximum, then, there is no echocardiographic evidence that stroke volume determinants are different in children and adults. Two reports of maximal testing in children utilizing gated radionuclide angiography indicate that these systolic and diastolic dimensional changes are also observed at peak exercise. DeSouza et al. exercised 25 asymptomatic children with familial hypercholesterolemia to heart rates of 186 bpm. End-diastolic counts varied little from rest to maximal exercise, while end-systolic counts fell 45% (33). In a radionuclide study of 32 healthy children ages 5-19 years, Parrish et al. found variable responses of left ventricular volume to exercise but a consistent decrease (mean 29%) in left ventricular end-systolic volume (86).

Echocardiograms during recovery from maximal exercise show the same trends. Rowland reported a 10% increase over resting values of left ventricular shortening fraction at 2 min of recovery from exhaustive treadmill exercise in 20 boys (95). Mean end-diastolic dimension was 40.5 mm at rest and 39.0 mm postexercise, while systolic measurements were 25.9 and 21.0, respectively.

Collectively, these echocardiographic and radionuclide angiography data support an increase in myocardial contractility as the primary factor in augmenting stroke volume during exercise in children. There is no apparent change in this pattern as children grow; that is, both qualitative and quantitative alterations in cardiac dimensions with exercise appear to be age-independent.

Cardiac Output. We have seen that increases in maximal stroke volume are entirely responsible for the growth of cardiac reserve during exercise in children, and that improvements in stroke volume are directly proportional to body size, weight, or both. Maximal heart rate, on the other hand, remains constant during the pediatric years, independent of age or body dimensions.

It follows that changes in values for maximal cardiac output during childhood should mirror those of maximal stroke volume. The cross-sectional data of Miyamura and Honda bear this out (79). Mean maximal cardiac output rose from 12.5 to 21.1 L/min in males 9-10 and 19-20 years old, respectively, and from 10.5 to 15.5 L/min in females of similar ages (see fig. 8.12). Average maximal cardiac index was stable in this age span for both genders (mean 12.2 and 10.5 L/min per square meter for males and females, respectively) but was

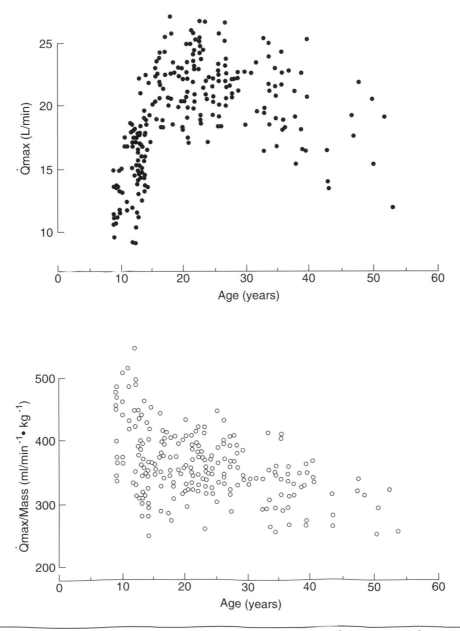

Figure 8.12 Relationship between maximal cardiac output (Q) and age in males. Reprinted from Miyamura and Honda 1973.

consistently higher in the males at every age. In the boys 12 years old and less, the maximal arteriovenous O_2 difference averaged 109 ml/L, while in those 13-20 years old the mean was 135 ml/L.

Gilliam et al. measured maximal cardiac output by the CO_2 rebreathing technique in children during the final 15 s of a progressive cycle exercise protocol (49). Maximal cardiac index fell from 11.8 to 10.5 to 10.0 L/min per square meter in groups ages 6-8, 9-10, and 11-13 years. Maximal stroke index declined from 61.0 to 53.8 to 52.2 ml/m^2 in the same age groups while arteriovenous O_2 difference rose from 122 to 135 to 146 ml/L.

Yamaji and Miyashita studied cardiovascular responses to maximal cycle exercise in 77 healthy but nonathletic boys ages 10-18 years (126). Maximal cardiac output was estimated within 17 s of exhaustion by the CO_2 rebreathing technique. Mean absolute values rose by 100% from age 10 to age 18 (11.0 L/min to 21.4 L/min, respectively). Maximal cardiac index ranged from 10.7 to 13.7 L/min per square meter and showed no clear trend with age. Average values in the presumed prepubertal boys (ages 10-12 years), however, were approximately 1.2 L/min per square meter lower than in the older subjects. Mean maximal arteriovenous O_2 difference averaged 110 ml/L in the prepubertal ages and 125 ml/L in the older boys.

Eriksson and Koch described resting and maximal cardiac output data in nine boys ages 11-13 years (43). Cardiac output was estimated by the dye dilution technique during the final minute of exhaustive upright cycle exercise. Mean stroke index and cardiac index fell from 45 to 36 ml/m^2 (20% decline) and from 3.6 to 2.8 L/min per square meter (22% decrease), respectively, when subjects went from the supine to the sitting position. Average maximal values for cardiac index, stroke index, and arteriovenous O_2 difference were 9.1 L/min per square meter, 48.5 ml/m^2, and 142 ml/L, respectively. The lower values for cardiac output and stroke volume compared to those from other studies may reflect lesser levels of aerobic fitness in these subjects, who had an average $\dot{V}O_2$max of only 38.5 ml · kg^{-1} · min^{-1}.

The authors examined these data from the perspective of previously published results of adult studies at that time (42). They noted that the mean value of stroke volume relative to the cube of body height in this study (19.1 ml/ht^3) was not dissimilar from the values previously reported in nonathletic young men (range 16.7 to 19.1 ml/ht^3). Likewise, the mean maximal arteriovenous O_2 uptake of 142 ml/L was not different from findings obtained in other studies in adults (range 137-147 ml/L).

These data do not indicate any dramatic differences in maximal cardiac output related to body size during growth. Values for maximal cardiac index are reasonably consistent, typically 10-12 L/min per square meter,

with a typical stroke index of 50-60 ml/m^2. There are insufficient data to warrant conclusions regarding gender differences, but the findings of Miyamura and Honda suggest that males can be expected to have 10-20% higher values than females (79).

Myocardial Function

The data just reviewed indicate the expected cardiac response to exercise in children. Other observations, however, have prompted the suggestion that cardiac functional reserve is inferior in prepubertal subjects compared to adults. On the basis of their compilation of findings in the research literature, Bar-Or (10) and Godfrey (50) presented graphic data indicating that children and adolescents have a cardiac output that is at the lower limits of the expected range of adults at any given level of O_2 uptake (see fig. 8.13). These findings have been attributed to a possible "hypokinetic response" of stroke volume to exercise in children that is only partially offset by their higher heart and arteriovenous O_2 difference.

It might be argued that these studies did not involve direct comparisons of adult and child subjects. In fact, in the only cardiac catheterization study that compared children and adults, Krabill et al. found no significant difference in the relationship of changes in cardiac output to O_2 uptake during mild supine exercise between 10 children and 9 adults who had mild pulmonary stenosis (mean right ventricular systolic pressure < 38 mmHg) (65). However, Godfrey noted that in studies using CO_2 rebreathing in his own laboratory, cardiac output rose an average of 20 ml/min for each centimeter increase in body height for children exercising with the

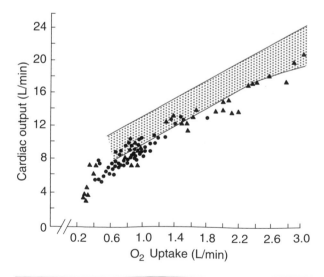

Figure 8.13 Cardiac output versus $\dot{V}O_2$ during exercise in children. Shaded area represents normative data for young adults. Reprinted from Bar-Or 1983.

same O_2 uptake (50). Mocellin et al. showed similar increases in $Q/\dot{V}O_2$ in 12 boys 11.5 to 14 years old compared to 10 subjects 8 to 11.5 years of age (81).

Mocellin felt that these findings could be explained simply by the fact that young children are exercising at a higher relative intensity (percentage $\dot{V}O_2$max) than older children or adults at a given $\dot{V}O_2$ (80). He reasoned that if maximal arteriovenous O_2 difference is independent of age, submaximal values should be related to relative exercise intensity. Thus at a given O_2 uptake during exercise, children should be expected to have a higher arteriovenous O_2 difference and consequently a lower cardiac output.

Further assessment of possible maturity-related changes in myocardial function with exercise can be made by examining exercise factor, radionuclide studies, and measurements of systolic time intervals in children and adults.

Exercise Factor.

Cardiac output is closely linked to O_2 uptake during exercise in both children and adults. The *exercise factor*, the ratio of change in cardiac output to change in O_2 uptake, has been suggested as a marker of myocardial performance during exercise. Normal adult subjects typically show an exercise factor of approximately 6.0 (41, 44, 54); those with congestive heart failure often demonstrate reduced values (55). Among six exercise studies in children, the mean exercise factor was 6.1 (11, 40, 51, 71, 76, 100) (see table 8.2). Therefore, no maturity-related differences in the rate of cardiac response to the metabolic demands of exercise are evident.

Radionuclide Exercise Testing.

Limited information regarding cardiac function with exercise in healthy children is available from studies using radionuclide imaging. DeSouza et al. evaluated 25 subjects ages 8-18 years with familial hypercholesterolemia but no clinical evidence of cardiac disease (33). Gated equilibrium nuclear angiograms were obtained as subjects

Table 8.2 Exercise factor (change in Q relative to $\dot{V}O_2$) in studies of children

Reference	Method	Delta $Q/\dot{V}O_2$
Bar-Or et al. (11)	CO_2 rebreathing	5.7
Marx et al. (76)	Doppler	6.0
Edmunds et al. (40)	CO_2 rebreathing	6.0
Godfrey et al. (51)	CO_2 rebreathing	5.7
Locke et al. (71)	Direct Fick	6.5
Rowland et al. (100)	Bioimpedance	4.4
		8.1

performed supine cycle exercise to exhaustion. Mean left ventricular ejection fraction rose from 63% at rest to 81% (an 18% rise) at maximal exercise. Using a similar protocol, Parrish et al. demonstrated an average rise in left and right ventricular ejection fraction of 9% and 14%, respectively, in 32 children ages 5-19 years without significant heart disease (86).

These results mimic findings obtained in adults. Borer et al. showed increases in left ventricular ejection fraction of 7-30% during maximal supine cycle exercise using the same gated procedure (16). Two studies in adults during maximal upright exercise with first-pass techniques both showed an average increase in ejection fraction of 14% (91, 92).

Systolic Time Intervals.

Measurement of the duration of the components of the cardiac cycle (systolic time intervals, or STIs) provides information regarding the effects of ventricular contractility, preload, and afterload on myocardial performance (69). The time of left ventricular ejection (LVET) is increased with all three of these factors, while the pre-ejection period of systole (between activation and blood ejection, PEP) is shortened as contractility and preload increase. An excellent inverse correlation has been demonstrated between the ratio of PEP to LVET and the ventricular ejection fraction.

Systolic time intervals can be determined by echocardiography, impedance cardiography, or the simultaneous measurement of carotid pulse tracing, electrocardiogram, and phonocardiogram. The artifacts created by body motion have limited the use of STIs during exercise.

Vavra et al. compared STIs using impedance cardiography during submaximal upright cycle exercise between boys ages 11-14 years and 20-30-year-old adults (122). Resting values were age-independent; LVET and PEP both declined with increasing heart rate, and the regression lines were not significantly different between the two groups. These findings suggest that loading conditions and myocardial function are not different during exercise in boys and young men.

Duration of systole and ratio of systole to the total heart cycle length both decrease with exercise. This implies that exercise is accompanied by an increased speed of myocardial fiber shortening (18). Vavra et al. demonstrated that the ratio of systolic duration to cycle length shortens equally in men and boys, suggesting that augmented velocity of myocardial contraction during exercise was equal in the two groups (122).

Cardiac Function During Prolonged Exercise

During extended periods of submaximal exercise at a constant workload, a progressive rise in heart rate and a decline in stroke volume are typically observed (89). Cardiac output remains stable or increases slowly. The most popular explanation for these observations, termed *cardiovascular drift,* is a shift of circulating central blood volume into the cutaneous circulation. Earlier concerns that drift is a reflection of myocardial fatigue appear unwarranted.

Asano and Hirakoba compared cardiovascular changes between 11 boys ages 10-12 years and 12 men ages 20-34 years during a 1 hr period of cycle exercise at 60% $\dot{V}O_2$max (6). Mean values for cardiac output remained constant in both groups, while heart rate rose (152 to 166 bpm and 134 to 154 bpm in the boys and men, respectively). Stroke volume determined by bioimpedance fell (58 to 54 and 98 to 86 ml, respectively). Percentage change in each case was significantly greater in the adults.

In this study, measurement of STIs indicated a progressive fall in PEP/LVET in the adults but not in the children. These findings led the authors to suggest that impairment of myocardial function during prolonged submaximal exercise may be less in children than in adults.

In a similar study, Rowland and Rimany compared cardiac changes using bioimpedance during 40 min of steady-load cycling at 63% $\dot{V}O_2$max in premenarcheal girls and young women (99). The patterns of change were similar in the two groups; heart rate and cardiac output increased, but stroke volume remained stable. The only significant difference between the adults and children was a greater magnitude of rise in heart rate in the women.

Blood Pressure

In adults, the cardiac output response to increasing dynamic exercise workload triggers a progressive rise in systolic blood pressure. At the same time, diastolic pressure typically remains stable or declines slightly, reflecting changes in peripheral vascular resistance. (Blood pressure responses to static, or resistance, exercise are different; these will be addressed in chapter 13.) In general, these patterns have been duplicated in studies of children as well. These findings have been reviewed in detail elsewhere (3, 36).

It is important in assessing this information to recognize the difficulties of accurately measuring blood pressure during exercise, whether by auscultatory methods or use of automatic recording equipment. Artifact from body motion and interference by equipment noise is particularly a problem with treadmill testing. Most problematic is the determination of diastolic pressure. Indeed, after reviewing the research literature, Lightfoot concluded that "in the case of diastolic pressures, the literature seems unanimous that auscultation during exercise does not result in diastolic pressure measurements that bear any relationship to the blood pressures that actually exist in either the central or peripheral areas of the body" (70, p. 299). Also, measurements taken "immediately" at the termination of exhaustive exercise may not accurately reflect true peak levels, since systolic blood pressure falls rapidly at cessation of exercise, as much as 10-20 mmHg/min (82, 93, 121).

Just as resting systolic blood pressure rises with increasing age, so does maximal systolic pressure during

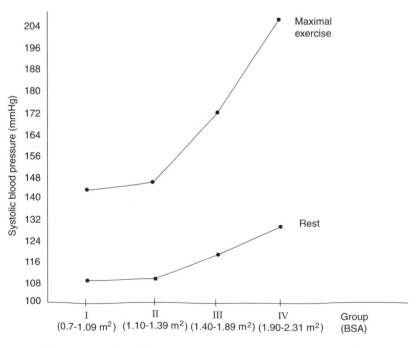

Figure 8.14 Maximal treadmill exercise systolic blood pressure compared to resting values in children of differing body surface area. Drawn from data of Riopel et al. (93).

exercise. This pattern presumably reflects increases in body size rather than chronological age per se. Norms for 279 healthy subjects ages 4-21 years have been reported during maximal treadmill walking (modified Balke protocol) by Riopel et al. (93). Subjects were divided into four categories by BSA. Males with the smallest BSA (0.7-1.09 m²) had mean peak systolic pressures of 142-147 mmHg, while those with the largest (1.90-2.31 m²) showed maximal values of 200-206 mmHg.

As demonstrated in figure 8.14, the rate of increase in peak exercise systolic pressure with increasing size exceeded that of the rise in resting pressures. No significant differences were observed between males and females except in the larger (presumably postpubertal) subjects; in this category, maximal systolic pressures were approximately 15-20 mmHg higher in the males.

Alpert et al. provided similar data for cycle testing (see fig. 8.15), derived from their study of 405 children ages 6 to 15 years (2). Maximal systolic pressure values were directly associated with increasing body size, with an appropriate 30 mmHg increase between children with BSA of 1.0 and 2.0 m². Similar findings have been reported by Washington et al. (124) and James et al. (60). Maximal pressures in these cycle studies were somewhat lower than those reported by Riopel et al. on the treadmill (93). Black children were found to have higher blood pressure responses to exercise than white subjects by both Alpert et al. (2) and Riopel et al. (93).

Reports of changes in diastolic blood pressure with exercise in children have been conflicting, presumably indicative of the technical difficulties of making this measurement. Riopel et al. demonstrated the expected slight decline in maximal diastolic pressures compared to values at rest in their treadmill study (93). However, James et al. reported a 14% rise in diastolic pressure at peak exercise with cycling testing (60), and Washington et al. described similar findings (16% increase in males and 18% rise in females) (124).

Dlin presented data indicating that adolescent athletes show a greater blood pressure response to exercise than do nonathletes (36). This phenomenon may not hold true in younger athletes, however. Van Huss et al. reported that peak systolic blood pressure values were actually lower in 20 male and 21 female elite distance runners ages 9 to 15 years compared to control subjects (166 and 166 mmHg compared to 174 and 173 mmHg, respectively) (121).

SUMMARY

Considering the weaknesses of methodology and study design in the research literature, one is faced with difficulty when attempting to offer dogma regarding developmental cardiac exercise physiology. Still, there is sufficient information to permit the following reasonably feasible construct of the normal cardiac responses to exercise in growing children.

1. Resting heart rate declines during the course of childhood, while stroke volume increases in

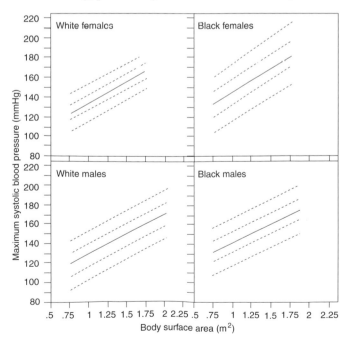

Figure 8.15 Maximal systolic blood pressure during cycle exercise relative to race, gender, and body surface area. Solid line represents 50th percentile of systolic blood pressure. Top line represents 95th percentile confidence band with dashed lines below representing 75th, 25th, and 5th percentile confidence bands. Reprinted from Alpert et al. 1982.

proportion to left ventricular size and body size. The product of the two, cardiac output, parallels increases in O_2 uptake. Both resting Q and $\dot{V}O_2$ relative to body mass or BSA decline as the child grows.

2. Maximal heart rate remains constant throughout childhood. Stroke volume at maximal exercise increases in direct proportion to left ventricular and body size and therefore serves as the determinant of increase in maximal cardiac output in the growing child. The patterns of changes in maximal cardiac output are similar to those of $\dot{V}O_2$, increasing in absolute values but remaining comparatively stable in relation to body weight. Puberty may cause a decline in weight-relative Qmax in females.

3. There is no clear evidence of maturational changes in myocardial performance or cardiac loading conditions. Changes in maximal stroke volume with age appear to be the direct result of increasing left ventricular chamber size.

Clearly, improved insights into normal cardiac changes with growth in children will be contingent upon the development of safer, more accurate, noninvasive means of assessing heart function. Nuclear magnetic resonance imaging and spectroscopy, transesophageal echocardiography, four-dimensional echocardiography, and measurements of heart rate variability are all new techniques that offer promise for increasing our future understanding of cardiac dynamics in the pediatric age group.

What We Know

1. Resting ventricular size and stroke volume increase during the course of childhood in direct relationship to body dimensions. Resting heart rate falls as a consequence of intrinsic sinus node maturation, while myocardial contractility is unchanged.

2. Changes in resting cardiac output parallel those of O_2 uptake, increasing in absolute value but declining relative to body mass.

3. Maximal exercise heart rate is stable in both boys and girls throughout childhood but is dependent on testing protocol.

4. No maturational changes occur in exercise myocardial function during the pediatric years.

What We Would Like to Know

1. How do values of maximal stroke volume and cardiac output change with age? How do these changes relate to increases in body size?

2. What are the characteristics of increases in stroke volume during exercise, particularly at high intensity levels? How much do intrinsic myocardial contractility and increased left ventricular preload contribute to these changes?

3. Is the stroke volume response to exercise in children dampened compared to that of adults?

4. How can gender differences in cardiovascular responses to exercise (particularly heart rate) be explained?

References

1. Alpert, B.S.; Bloom, K.R.; Gilday, D.; Olley, P.M. The comparison between non-invasive and invasive methods of stroke volume determination in children. Am. Heart J. 98:763-766; 1979.

2. Alpert, B.S.; Flood, N.L.; Strong, W.B.; Dover, E.V.; DuRant, R.H.; Martin, A.M.; Booker, D.L. Responses to ergometer exercise in a healthy biracial population of children. J. Pediatr. 101:538-545; 1982.

3. Alpert, B.S.; Fox, M.E. Blood pressure response to dynamic exercise. In: Rowland, T.W., ed. Pediatric laboratory exercise testing. Champaign, IL: Human Kinetics; 1993:p. 67-90.

4. Appel, P.L.; Kram, H.B.; Mackabee, J.; Fleming, A.W.; Shoemaker, W.C. Comparison of measurements of cardiac output by bioimpedance and thermodilution in severely ill surgical patients. Crit. Care Med. 14:933-935; 1986.

5. Armstrong, N.; Williams, J.; Balding, J.; Gentle, P.; Kirby, B. The peak oxygen uptake of British children with reference to age, sex, and sexual maturity. Eur. J. Appl. Physiol. 62:369-375; 1991.

6. Asano, K.; Hirakoba, K. Respiratory and circulatory adaptation during prolonged exercise in 10-12 year-old children and adults. In: Ilmarinen, J.; Valimaki, I., eds. Children and sport. Berlin: Springer-Verlag; 1984:p. 119-128.

7. Bailey, D.A.; Ross, W.D.; Mirwald, R.L.; Weese, C. Size dissociation of maximal aerobic power during growth in boys. Med. Sport 11:140-151; 1978.

8. Baraldi, E.; Cooper, D.M.; Zanconato, S.; Armon, Y. Heart rate recovery from 1 minute of exercise in children and adults. Ped. Res. 29:575-579; 1991.

9. Barbacki, M.; Gluck, A.; Sandhage, K.; Metzner, G. Impedance cardiography in normal children. Cor Vasa 23:190-196; 1981.

10. Bar-Or, O. Pediatric sports medicine for the practitioner. New York: Springer-Verlag; 1983:p. 1-27.

11. Bar-Or, O.; Shephard, R.J.; Allen, C.L. Cardiac output of 10- to 13-year old boys and girls during submaximal exercise. J. Appl. Physiol. 30:219-223; 1971.

12. Belik, J.; Pelech, A. Thoracic bioimpedance measurement of cardiac output in the newborn infant. J. Pediatr. 113:890-895; 1988.

13. Berger, R.A. Applied exercise physiology. Philadelphia: Lea & Febiger; 1982:p. 151.

14. Bevegard, S.; Holmgren, A.; Jonsson, B. The effect of body position on the circulation at rest and during exercise, with special reference to the influence on the stroke volume. Acta Physiol. Scand. 49:279-298; 1960.

15. Boileau, R.A.; Bonen, A.; Heyward, V.H.; Massey, B.H. Maximal aerobic capacity on the treadmill and bicycle ergometer of boys 11-14 years of age. J. Sports Med. 17:153-162; 1977.

16. Borer, J.S.; Kent, K.M.; Bacharach, S.L. Sensitivity, specificity, and predictive accuracy of radionuclide cineangiography during exercise in patients with coronary artery disease. Circulation 60:572-579; 1979.

17. Bouchard, C.; Malina, R.M.; Hollman, W.; Leblanc, C. Submaximal working capacity, heart size, and body size in boys 8-18 years. Eur. J. Appl. Physiol. 36:115-126; 1977.

18. Braunwald, E.; Sarnoff, J.J.; Stainsby, W.N. Determinants of duration and mean rate of ventricular ejection. Circ. Res. 6:319-325; 1958.

19. Bunc, V.; Heller, J.; Leso, J. Kinetics of heart rate responses to exercise. J. Sport Sci. 6:39-48; 1988.

20. Burch, G.E.; Giles, T.D. A critique of the cardiac index. Am. Heart J. 82:424-425; 1971.

21. Burton; A.C. The importance of the size and shape of the heart. Am. Heart J. 54:801-910; 1957.

22. Cassels, D.E.; Morse, M. Cardiopulmonary data for children and young adults. Springfield, IL: Charles C Thomas; 1962.

23. Chapman, C.B.; Taylor, H.L.; Borden, C.; Ebert, R.V.; Keys, A. Simultaneous determinations of the resting arteriovenous oxygen difference by the acetylene and direct Fick methods. J. Clin. Invest. 29:651-659; 1950.

24. Colan, S.D.; Parness, I.A.; Spevak, P.J.; Sanders, S.P. Developmental modulation of myocardial mechanics: age- and growth-related alterations in afterload and contractility. J. Am. Coll. Cardiol. 19:619-629; 1992.

25. Cooper, D.M.; Berry, C.; Lamarra, N.; Wasserman, K. Kinetics of oxygen uptake and heart rate at onset of exercise. J. Appl. Physiol. 59:211-217; 1985.

26. Cooper, D.M.; Weiler-Ravell, D.; Whipp, B.J.; Wasserman, K. Growth-related changes in oxygen uptake and heart rate during progressive exercise in children. Pediatr. Res. 18:845-851; 1984.

27. Cumming, G.R. Hemodynamics of supine bicycle exercise in "normal" children. Am. Heart J. 93:617-622; 1977.

28. Cumming, G.R.; Everatt, D.; Hastman, L. Bruce treadmill test in children: normal values in a clinic population. Am. J. Cardiol. 41:69-75; 1978.

29. Cumming, G.R.; Freisen, W. Bicycle ergometer measurement of maximal oxygen uptake in children. Can. J. Physiol. 45:937-946; 1967.

30. Cumming, G.R.; Langford, S. Comparison of nine exercise tests used in pediatric cardiology. In: Binkhorst, R.A.; Kemper, H.C.G.; Saris, W.H.M., eds. Children and exercise XI. Champaign, IL: Human Kinetics; 1985:p. 58-68.

31. Daniels, S.R.; Meyer, R.A.; Liang, Y.; Bove, K.E. Echocardiographically determined left ventricular mass index in normal children, adolescents and young adults. J. Am. Coll. Cardiol. 12:703-708; 1988.

32. Davies, C.T.M.; Barnes, C.; Godfrey, S. Body composition and maximal performance in children. Hum. Biol. 44:195-214; 1972.

33. DeSouza, M.; Schaffer, M.S.; Gilday, D.L.; Rose, V. Exercise radionuclide angiography in hyperlipidemic children with apparently normal hearts. Nucl. Med. Comm. 5:13-17; 1984.

34. Devereux, R.B. Left ventricular mass in children and adolescents. J. Am. Coll. Cardiol. 12:709-711; 1988.

35. Dickhuth, H.H.; Simon, G.; Heiss, H.W.; Lehmann, M.; Wybitul, K.; Keul, J. Comparative echocardiographic examinations in sitting and supine position at rest and during dynamic exercise. Int. J. Sports Med. 2:178-181; 1981.

36. Dlin, R. Blood pressure response to dynamic exercise in healthy and hypertensive youths. Pediatrician 13:34-43; 1986.

37. Donald, D.E.; Yipintsol, T. Comparison of measured and indocyanine green blood flows in various organs and systems. Mayo Clin. Proc. 48:492-500; 1973.

38. Driscoll, D.J.; Danielson, G.K.; Puga, F.J.; Schaff, H.V.; Heise, C.T.; Staats, B.A. Exercise tolerance and cardiorespiratory response to exercise after the Fontan operation for tricuspid atresia or functional single ventricle. J. Am. Coll. Cardiol. 7:1087-1094; 1986.

39. Driscoll, D.J.; Staats, B.A.; Beck, K.C. Measurement of cardiac output in children during exercise: a review. Pediatr. Exerc. Science 1:102-115; 1989.

40. Edmunds, A.T.; Godfrey, S.; Tooley, M. Cardiac output measured by transthoracic impedance cardiography at rest, during exercise, and at various lung volumes. Clin. Sci. 63:107-113; 1982.

41. Epstein, S.E.; Beiser, G.D.; Stampfer, M.; Robinson, B.F.; Braunwald, E. Characterization of the circulatory response to maximal upright exercise in normal subjects and patients with heart disease. Circulation 35:1049-1062; 1967.

42. Eriksson, B.O. Physical training, oxygen supply and muscle metabolism in 11-13 year old boys. Acta Physiol. Scand. Suppl. 384:1-48; 1972.

43. Eriksson, B.O.; Koch, G. Effect of physical training on hemodynamic response during submaximal and maximal exercise in 11-13 year old boys. Acta Physiol. Scand. 87:27-39; 1973.

44. Ferrer, M.I.; Harvey, R.M.; Cathcart, R.T.; Cournand, A.; Richards, D.W. Hemodynamic studies in rheumatic heart disease. Circulation 6:688-710; 1953.

45. Fisher, D.J.; Towbin, J. Maturation of the heart. Clin. Perinat. 15:421-446; 1988.

46. Fisher, E.A.; Dubrow, I.W.; Hasteiter, A.R. Right ventricular volume in congenital heart disease. Am. J. Cardiol. 36:62-67; 1975.

47. Freed, M.D.; Keane, J.F. Cardiac output measured by thermodilution in infants and children. J. Pediatr. 92:39-42; 1978.

48. Gaisl, G.; Hoffman, P. Heart rate determination of anaerobic threshold in children. Pediatr. Exerc. Science 2:29-36; 1990.

49. Gilliam, T.B.; Sady, S.; Thorland, W.G.; Weltman, A.C. Comparison of peak performance measures in children ages 6 to 8, 9 to 10, and 11 to 13 years. Res. Quart. 48:695-702; 1977.

50. Godfrey, S. Exercise testing in children. London: Saunders; 1974:p. 30.

51. Godfrey, S.; Davies, C.T.M.; Wozniak, E.; Barnes, C.A. Cardiorespiratory response to exercise in normal children. Clin. Sci. 40:419-431; 1971.

52. Gutgesell, H.P.; Paquet, M.; Duff, D.F.; McNamara, D.G. Evaluation of left ventricular size and function by echocardiography. Circulation 56:457-462; 1977.

53. Hanson, J.S.; Tabakin, B.S. Simultaneous and rapidly repeated cardiac output determinations by dye-dilution method. J. Appl. Physiol. 19:275-278; 1964.

54. Harvey, R.M.; Ferrer, M.I.; Samet, P. Mechanical and myocardial factors in rheumatic heart disease with mitral stenosis. Circulation 11:531-551; 1955.

55. Harvey, R.M.; Smith, W.M.; Parker, J.O.; Ferrier, M.I. The response of the abnormal heart to exercise. Circulation 26:341-361; 1962.

56. Henry, W.L.; Ware, J.; Gardin, J.M.; Hepner, S.I.; McKay, J.; Weiner, M. Echocardiographic measurements in normal subjects. Growth-related changes that occur between infancy and early adulthood. Circulation 57:278-285; 1978.

57. Holliday, M.A.; Potter, D.; Jarrah, A.; Bearg, S. The relation of metabolic rate to body weight and organ size. Pediatr. Res. 1:185-195; 1967.

58. Houlsby, W.T. Functional aerobic capacity and body size. Arch. Dis. Child. 61:388-393; 1986.

59. Hurwitz, R.A.; Treves, S.; Kuruc, A. Right ventricular and left ventricular ejection fraction in pediatric patients with normal hearts: first-pass radionuclide angiography. Am. Heart J. 107:726-732; 1984.

60. James, F.W.; Kaplan, S.; Glueck, C.J.; Tsay, J.Y.; Knight, M.J.S.; Sarwar, C.J. Responses of normal children and young adults to controlled bicycle exercise. Circulation 61:902-912; 1980.

61. Karpman, V.L. Cardiovascular system and physical exercise. Boca Raton, FL: CRC Press; 1987:p. 139-140.

62. Katori, R. Normal cardiac output in relation to age and body size. Tokohu J. Exp. Med. 128:377-387; 1979.

63. Keul, J.; Dickhuth, H.H.; Simon, G.; Lehmann, M. Effect of static and dynamic exercise on heart volume, contractility, and left ventricular dimensions. Circ. Res. 48 Suppl 1:163-170; 1981.

64. Knoebel, L.K. Energy metabolism. In: Selkurt, E.E., ed. Physiology. Boston: Little, Brown; 1963:p. 564-579.

65. Krabill, K.A.; Wang, Y.; Einzig, S.; Moller, J.M. Rest and exercise hemodynamics in pulmonary stenosis: comparison of children and adults. Am. J. Cardiol. 56:360-365; 1985.

66. Krovetz, L.J.; McLoughlin, T.G.; Mitchell, M.B.; Schiebler, G.L. Hemodynamic findings in normal children. Pediatr. Res. 1:122-130; 1967.

67. Kurtz, D.; Ahnberg, D.S.; Freed, M.; LaFarge, C.G.; Treves, S. Quantitative radionuclide angiography. Determination of left ventricular ejection fraction in children. Brit. Heart J. 38:966-973; 1976.

68. Lehmann, M.; Keul, J.; Korsten-Reck, U. The influence of graduated treadmill exercise on plasma catecholamines, aerobic, and anaerobic capacity in boys and adults. Eur. J. Appl. Physiol. 47:301-311; 1981.

69. Lewis, R.P. The use of systolic time intervals for evaluation of left ventricular function. Cardiovasc. Clin. 13:335-353; 1983.

70. Lightfoot, J.T. Can blood pressure be measured during exercise? A review. Sports Med. 12:290-301; 1991.

71. Locke, J.E.; Einzig, S.; Moller, J.H. Hemodynamic responses to exercise in normal children. Am. J. Cardiol. 41:1278-1285; 1978.

72. Mahon, A.D.; Vaccaro, P. Can the point of deflection from linearity of heart rate determine ventilatory threshold in children? Pediatr. Exerc. Science 3:256-262; 1991.

73. Malina, R.M.; Roche, A.F. Manual of physical status and performance in childhood. Vol. 2, Physical performance. New York: Plenum Press; 1983.

74. Marcus, B.; Gillette, P.C.; Garson, A. Intrinsic heart rate in children and young adults: an index of sinus node function isolated from autonomic control. Am. Heart J. 112:911-916; 1990.

75. Marks, C.; Katch, V.; Rocchini, A.; Beekman, R.; Rosenthal, A. Validity and reliability of cardiac output by CO_2 rebreathing. Sports Med. 2:432-446; 1985.

76. Marx, G.R.; Hicks, R.W.; Allen, H.D. Measurement of cardiac output and exercise factor by pulsed Doppler echocardiography during supine bicycle ergometry in normal young adolescent boys. J. Am. Coll. Cardiol. 10:430-434; 1987.

77. McKinley, D.F.; Pollack, M.M. A comparison of thoracic bioimpedance to thermodilution cardiac output in critically ill children. Crit. Care Med. 15:358-359; 1987.

78. Miles, D.S.; Gotshall, R.W. Impedance cardiography: non-invasive assessment of human central hemodynamics at rest and during exercise. Exerc. Sport Sci. Rev. 17:231-263; 1989.

79. Miyamura, M.; Honda, Y. Maximum cardiac output related to sex and age. Jap. J. Physiol. 23:645-656; 1973.

80. Mocellin, R. Exercise testing in children with congenital heart disease. Pediatrician 13:18-25; 1986.

81. Mocellin, R.; Sebening, W.; Buhlmeyer, K. Hertzminutenvolumen und Sauerstoffaufnahme in Ruhe and wahrend submximaler Belstungen bei 8-14 jahrigen Jungen. Z. Kinderheilkd 114:323-339; 1973.

82. Nelson, R.R.; Gobel, F.L.; Jorgenson, C.R.; Wang, K.; Wang, Y.; Taylor, H.L. Hemodynamic predictors of myocardial oxygen consumption during static and dynamic exercise. Circulation 50:1179-1189; 1974.

83. Clausen, J.P. Effects of physical training on cardiovascular adjustments to exercise in man. Physiol. Rev. 57:779-815; 1977.

84. Norris, S.R.; Bell, G.J.; Bhambani, Y.N. Oxygen pulse as a predictor of stroke volume during cycle ergometer exercise. Med. Sci. Sports Exerc. 23 Suppl:S158; 1991.

85. Oyen, E.M.; Ignatzy, K.; Ingerfeld, G.; Brode, P. Echocardiographic evaluation of left ventricular reserve in normal children during supine bicycle exercise. Int. J. Cardiol. 14:145-154; 1987.

86. Parrish, M.D.; Boucek, R.J.; Burger, J.; Artman, M.F.; Partain, C.L.; Graham, T.P. Exercise radionuclide ventriculography in children: normal values for exercise variables and right and left ventricular function. Br. Heart J. 54:509-516; 1985.

87. Paterson, D.H.; Cunningham, D.A. Comparison of methods to calculate cardiac output using the CO_2 rebreathing method. Europ. J. Appl. Physiol. 35:223-230; 1976.

88. Poliner, L.R.; Dehmer, G.J.; Lewis, S.E.; Parkey, R.W.; Blomqvist, C.G.; Willerson, J.T. Left ventricular performance in normal subjects. A comparison of the responses to exercise in the upright and supine positions. Circulation 62:528-533; 1980.

89. Raven, P.B.; Stevens, G.H.J. Cardiovascular function and prolonged exercise. In: Lamb, D.R.; Murray, R., eds. Perspectives in exercise science and sports medicine. Vol. 1, Prolonged exercise. Indianapolis: Benchmark Press; 1988:p. 43-74.

90. Reeves, J.T.; Grover, R.T.; Blount, S.G.; Filley, S.G. Cardiac output responses to standing and treadmill walking. J. Appl. Physiol. 16:283-288; 1961.

91. Rerych, S.K.; Scholz, P.; Newman, G.; Sabiston, D.C.; Jones, R.H. Cardiac function at rest and during exercise in normals and patients with coronary heart disease. Ann. Surg. 187:449-464; 1978.

92. Rerych, S.K.; Scholz, P.M.; Sabiston, D.C.; Jones, R.H. Effects of exercise training on left ventricular function in normal subjects: a longitudinal study by radionuclide angiography. Am. J. Cardiol. 45:244-251; 1980.

93. Riopel, D.A.; Taylor, A.B.; Hohn, A.R. Blood pressure, heart rate, pressure-rate product, and electrocardiographic changes in healthy children during treadmill exercise. Am. J. Cardiol. 44:697-704; 1979.

94. Robinson, S. Experimental studies of physical fitness in relation to age. Arbeitsphysiol. 10:251-323; 1938.

95. Rowland, T.W. Post-exercise echocardiography in prepubertal boys. Med. Sci. Sports Exerc. 19:393-397; 1987.

96. Rowland, T.W. "Normalizing" maximal oxygen uptake, or the search for the holy grail (per kg). Pediatr. Exerc. Sci. 3:95-102; 1991.

97. Rowland, T.W. Aerobic exercise testing protocols. In: Rowland, T.W., ed. Pediatric laboratory exercise testing. Champaign, IL: Human Kinetics; 1993:p. 19-42.

98. Rowland, T.W.; Cunningham, L.N. Heart rate deceleration during treadmill exercise in children [abstract]. Pediatr. Exerc. Science 5:463; 1993.

99. Rowland, T.W.; Rimany, T.A. Physiological responses to prolonged exercise in premenarcheal and adult females. Pediatr. Exerc. Science 7:183-191; 1995.

100. Rowland, T.; Staab, J.; Rambusch, J.; Unnithan, V.; Siconolfi, S. Computerized bioimpedance measurement of cardiac output during maximal cycle exercise [abstract]. In: Coudert, J.; Van Praagh, E., eds. Pediatric work physiology. Paris: Masson; 1992:p. 101.

101. Rowland, T.W.; Staab, J.; Unnithan, V.; Siconolfi, S. Maximal cardiac responses in prepubertal and adult males [abstract]. Med. Sci. Sports Exerc. 20 Suppl:S32; 1988.

102. Rudolph, A.M. Congenital diseases of the heart. Chicago: Year Book Medical; 1974:p. 28.

103. Sady, S.P.; Freedson, P.S.; Gilliam, T.B. Calculation of submaximal and maximal cardiac output in children using the CO_2 rebreathing technique. J. Sports Med. 21:245-252; 1981.

104. Sady, S.P.; Katch, V.L.; Villanacci, F.; Gilliam, T.B. Children-adult comparisons of $\dot{V}O_2$ and HR kinetics during submaximal exercise. Res. Q. Exerc. Sport 54:55-59; 1983.

105. Sanders, S.P.; Yeager, S.; Williams, R.G. Measurement of systemic and pulmonary blood flow and QP/QS ratio using Doppler and two-dimensional echocardiography. Am. J. Cardiol. 51:952-956; 1983.

106. Schmidt-Nielsen, K. Scaling. Why is animal size so important? Cambridge: Cambridge University Press; 1984:p. 126-127.

107. Scholz, D.G.; Kitzman, D.W.; Hagen, P.T.; Ilstrup, D.M.; Edwards, W.D. Age-related changes in normal human hearts during the first 10 decades of life. Part I (Growth). A quantitative anatomic study of 200 specimens from subjects from birth to 19 years old. Mayo Clin. Proc. 63:126-136; 1988.

108. Schulz, D.M.; Giordano, D.A. Hearts of infants and children. Arch. Path. 74:464-471; 1962.

109. Sheehan, J.M.; Rowland, T.W.; Burke, E.J. A comparison of four treadmill protocols for determination of maximal oxygen uptake in 10- to 12-year old boys. Int. J. Sports Med. 8:31-34; 1987.

110. Sholler, G.F.; Celermajer, J.M.; Whight, C.M. Doppler echocardiographic assessment of cardiac output in normal children with and without innocent precordial murmurs. Am. J. Cardiol. 59:487-488; 1987.

111. Shuleva, K.M.; Hunter, G.R.; Hester, D.J.; Dunaway, D.L. Exercise oxygen uptake in 3- through 6-year old children. Pediatr. Exerc. Science 2:130-139; 1990.

112. Smith, H.L. The relation of the weight of the heart to the weight of the body with age. Am. Heart J. 4:79-84; 1928.

113. Sproul, A.; Simpson, E. Stroke volume and related hemodynamic data in normal children. Pediatrics 33:912-918; 1964.

114. Sprynarova, S.; Parizkova, J. Changes in the aerobic capacity and body composition in obese boys after reduction. J. Appl. Physiol. 20:934-937; 1965.

115. Sutliff, W.D.; Holt, E. The age curve of pulse rate under basal conditions. Arch. Int. Med. 35:224-241; 1925.

116. Task Force on Blood Pressure Control in Children. Report of the second task force on blood pressure control in children-1987. Pediatrics 79:1-25; 1987.

117. Thompson, W.R.; Shapiro, J.; Thompson, D.L.; Bulawa, W. Comparison of ventricular volumes in normal and post-myocardial infarction subjects. Med. Sci. Sports Exerc. 19:430-435; 1987.

118. Tomassoni, T.L.; Galioto, F.M.; Vaccaro, P.; Vaccaro, J.; Howard, R.P. The pediatric cardiac rehabilitation program at the Children's Hospital National Medical Center, Washington, DC. J. Cardiopulm. Rehab. 7:259-262; 1987.

119. Tremper, K.K.; Hufstedler, S.M.; Burker, S.J.; Zacchari, J.; Harris, D.; Anderson, S.; Roohk, V. Continuous non-invasive estimation of cardiac output by electrical bioimpedance: an experimental study in dogs. Crit. Care Med. 14:231-233; 1986.

120. Triebwasser, J.H.; Johnson, R.L.; Burpo, R.P.; Campbell, J.C.; Reardon, W.C.; Blomqvist, C.G. Noninvasive determination of cardiac output by a modified acetylene rebreathing procedure utilizing mass spectrometer measurements. Aviat. Space Environ. Med. 48:203-209; 1977.

121. Van Huss, W.; Evans, S.A.; Kurowski, T.; Anderson, D.J.; Allen, R.; Stephens, K. Physiological characteristics of male and female age-group runners. In: Brown, E.W.; Branta, C.F., eds. Competitive sports for children and youth. Champaign, IL: Human Kinetics; 1988:p. 143-158.

122. Vavra, J.; Sova, J.; Mácek, M. Effect of age on systolic time intervals at rest and during exercise on a bicycle ergometer. Eur. J. Appl. Physiol. 50:71-78; 1982.

123. Volkmann, A.W. Die Haemodynamik. Leipzig; 1850:p. 407-445.

124. Washington, R.L.; van Gundy, J.C.; Cohen, C.; Soundhemier, H.M.; Wolfe, R.R. Normal aerobic and anaerobic exercise data for North American school-age children. J. Pediatr. 112:223-233; 1988.

125. Weiss, J.L.; Weisfelft, M.L.; Mason, S.J.; Garrison, J.B.; Livengood, S.V.; Fortuin, N.J. Evidence of Frank-Starling effect in man during severe semi-supine exercise. Circulation 59:655-661; 1979.

126. Yamaji, K.; Miyashita, M. Oxygen transport system during exhaustive exercise in Japanese boys. Europ. J. Appl. Physiol. 36:93-99; 1977.

127. Yoshida, T.; Ishiko, I.; Muraoka, I. Effects of endurance training on cardiorespiratory functions of 5-year old children. Int. J. Sports Med. 1:91-94; 1980.

CHAPTER 9

RESPONSE TO ENDURANCE EXERCISE: VENTILATION

Viewed from a cardiopulmonary perspective, exercise can be reduced to a problem simply of gas exchange (59). The metabolic machinery of the exercising muscle cell requires energy from the oxidation of glucose and fatty acids, producing CO_2 as a by-product. Unfortunately, the source of O_2, the ambient air, is far removed from this process of *internal respiration.* The task for the lungs is to appropriately exchange O_2 and CO_2 with the ambient air as (a) the first link of the O_2 delivery chain and (b) the means of "venting" waste CO_2. This process of *external respiration* must be coupled precisely with that of internal respiration; that is, the stability of blood PO_2, PCO_2, and pH must be maintained regardless of the muscle metabolic rate. Sustaining this homeostasis in the face of the dramatic rise in energy cost of exercise draws on the reserves of ventilatory function in the same way it taxes cardiovascular capacity.

These principles hold as true for children as for adults. In examining the ventilatory responses to exercise in growing children, however, it is important to recognize that these changes may reflect not only adaptations to increases in metabolic rate but also (1) the influence of greater body dimensions and/or (2) the development of size-independent organ function.

In many ways, parallels exist between pulmonary and cardiac functions in the gas exchange chain that links skeletal muscle with atmospheric air. During the rise in metabolic rate with exercise, both must respond by augmenting minute volume. This is accomplished by increasing both the rate of function (breaths or heartbeats per minute) and the volume of each function (tidal volume, stroke volume). As the child grows, the heart and

lungs accomplish this by the same basic pattern: stroke volume and tidal volume increase as a result of increasing heart and lung size, respectively. Meanwhile, resting and submaximal heart and breathing rates decline with age, paralleling a decrease in cardiac output and minute ventilation measured relative to body size.

There are also distinct differences between developmental cardiac and pulmonary exercise physiology. For example, cardiac output at all ages is closely linked to metabolic rate both at rest and during exercise. However, younger children, compared to older children and adults, hyperventilate relative to $\dot{V}O_2$. In addition, cardiac output is linearly related to $\dot{V}O_2$ at all exercise intensities. Minute ventilation rises disproportionately to $\dot{V}O_2$ at high levels of work, reflecting not only the high metabolic activity of contracting muscle but also the respiratory drive from excess CO_2 produced by the buffering of lactic acid.

The ease of measuring tidal volume and respiratory rate with exercise has provided more accurate information about the components of ventilation in children than about the components of cardiac output. But insight into the mechanisms surrounding these functions has been hampered by lack of accurate, feasible measurement methodologies during exercise (determinations of dead space, neural drive, CO_2 sensitivity, airway resistance).

This chapter will review our current understanding of changes in ventilatory characteristics at rest and the responses to exercise as children grow. As with the discussion of the cardiovascular system, it is useful to begin with what we know about pulmonary exercise physiology in the adult (9, 58).

THE ADULT MODEL

First, a review of ventilatory definitions is in order. Minute ventilation ($\dot{V}_E$), the air entering or leaving the lungs and airways over the course of a minute, is the product of breathing frequency (f_b) and tidal volume (V_T), the amount of air per breath. Tidal volume can be divided into the air that actually reaches the alveoli and serves for gas exchange (the alveolar ventilation) and the air that simply fills the air passages (dead space). During normal breathing, dead space amounts to approximately 30% of the V_T.

The vital capacity (VC) is the greatest amount of air that can be expelled after a maximal inspiratory effort. This represents the largest volume a person can move in or out of the lungs. The sum of the VC and the air that remains in the lungs afterward (the residual volume) gives the total lung capacity. The maximal voluntary ventilation (MVV) is the greatest minute ventilation that can be achieved in the resting state. $\dot{V}_E$max with exercise in adults is approximately 75% of MVV, indicating that pulmonary capacity is not taxed to its limits with exhaustive activity.

With the onset of exercise, augmented demands for blood oxygenation and CO_2 removal are met by a rise in $\dot{V}_E$. Increases in both V_T and f_b contribute. Tidal volume in adults rises from 15% of VC at rest to 50-60% at maximal exercise, with most of that increase occurring in the lower exercise intensities. The rise in breathing rate, however, is relatively linear, so improvements in $\dot{V}_E$ at near-maximal exercise are principally the product of increasing f_b.

Breathing rate in the typical young adult generally rises from about 12 breaths/min at rest to 40-45 each minute at exhaustion. At the same time, V_T increases from 500 cc to 2500 cc. Consequently, a typical resting $\dot{V}_E$ of 6 L/min can rise to over 100 L/min at exhaustive exercise, about 17 times the resting value.

During the early course of progressively intense exercise, $\dot{V}_E$ rises in close association with both $\dot{V}O_2$ and $\dot{V}CO_2$. At approximately 50-60% $\dot{V}O_2$max, however, the buffering of increasing blood lactic acid by bicarbonate causes excessive CO_2 production beyond that generated by muscle cell metabolism. This additional CO_2 triggers an increase in $\dot{V}_E$, which then rises at a disproportionately greater rate than $\dot{V}O_2$. When blood lactic acid accumulation outstrips buffering capacity at very intense exercise, arterial pH begins to fall, further stimulating $\dot{V}_E$. Therefore, three physiologic factors control the increase in ventilation to $\dot{V}_E$max: (a) CO_2 efflux from contracting muscle cells, (b) CO_2 produced by bicarbonate buffering of lactic acid, and (c) the metabolic acidosis that occurs when buffering of lactic acid is incomplete.

The ventilatory response to exercise just outlined is remarkably effective in maintaining stable P_aO_2, P_aCO_2, and arterial pH levels. Only at high intensity levels does arterial pH fall (usually to about 7.30, although decreases to 7.00 have been observed). The resulting hyperpnea results in a decline in P_aCO_2 from 40 mmHg to 35 mmHg or less. Little change in P_aO_2 is observed with exercise in untrained subjects.

The factors controlling the initiation of the ventilatory responses to exercise appear to be multiple. Acid-base balance and alterations of P_aO_2 and P_aCO_2 are recognized determinants of $\dot{V}_E$. However, since these factors change little, particularly during mild-moderate exercise, the dramatic increase in $\dot{V}_E$ is probably the result mainly of neural factors triggered by musculoskeletal receptors. Other influences such as body temperature and psychological factors also contribute to level of $\dot{V}_E$ attained during exercise.

VENTILATION IN THE RESTING CHILD

From the time a child enters kindergarten until puberty, the weight of the lungs increases nearly threefold, from an average of 211 g to 640 g (46). During this time the resting VC rises from approximately 1000 to 3000 cc, and total lung capacity from 1400 to 4500 cc. (Over this same time span, values for $\dot{V}O_2$max typically increase by a factor of 2.0-2.5.)

Lung structure is not fully developed at the time of birth, and the numbers of both alveoli and airways increase nearly 10 times before a baby reaches adulthood (20). Consequently, the air-tissue interface area in the lung expressed per square meter of body surface area (BSA) rises, from 13.3 in the newborn period to 33.1 at age 4 and 39.5 in adulthood. For the most part, these maturational changes have been completed by 8 years and presumably have little influence on exercise capacity beyond this age. In late childhood and adolescence, increases in air space occur principally through enlargement of existing alveoli and airways.

Resting Lung Volumes

From animal studies we know that smaller mammals have higher resting metabolic rates per body mass than larger mammals. Consistent with this observation, children demonstrate a progressive decline in mass-relative $\dot{V}O_2$ at rest as they grow. Smaller mammals do not, however, have relatively larger lungs; the volume of the lungs relative to body mass remains constant despite animal size (51). In mammals of diverse size, resting V_T relates to mass by the scaling exponent 1.04, breathing frequency by the exponent –0.26, and minute ventilation by the exponent 0.80. The latter, then, nearly matches the scaling factor for resting $\dot{V}O_2$ of 0.76. These size-ventilation relationships in mammals match in many ways those reported in the growing child.

Several authors have described ventilation characteristics in resting healthy children. In general, these data indicate that V_T relative to body size or weight slowly declines and breathing rate falls as the child ages. The net result is a progressive decline in $\dot{V}_E$ expressed relative to body weight (or BSA) through the childhood years. This pattern mirrors that for both resting cardiac output and basal metabolic rate.

Lyons and Tanner reported values for normal total lung volume and its subdivisions in a cross-sectional study of 438 healthy children ages 6 to 14 years (37). Total lung capacity and VC both correlated best with body height, and height cubed produced slightly better correlation coefficients than height alone. Coefficients of .91 and .86 were reported for the cube of height versus VC in males and females, respectively. Values for both VC and total lung volume were slightly but significantly greater in the boys.

These findings supported the earlier work of DeMuth et al., who described allometric relationships of resting VC and height in 147 normal children (4 to 18 years old) (18):

$$\text{Boys VC} = .00216 \times ht^{2.81}$$

$$\text{Girls VC} = .00186 \times ht^{2.82}.$$

The scaling exponents described by DeMuth et al. for VC relative to body weight were .98 and .94 for the boys and girls, respectively. These values approximate those reported for VC relative to mass in animals (1.03) (51). These findings suggest that resting VC increases during childhood approximately in accord with body mass (i.e., VC per kg is independent of age). The observation that the intercept in these equations is smaller in the girls than in the boys (despite similar height exponents) indicates that at the same body size, girls have lower VC values.

In contrast, Åstrand found that VC per kg body mass rose steadily with increasing age during childhood in boys, but not in girls (7). Mean values were 72.3 ml/kg in a group of 7-9-year-old males and 80.8 ml/kg in 14-15-year-olds. Values were 72.3 and 72.1 ml/kg, respectively, in girls of the same ages.

Resting minute ventilation rises during childhood and adolescence, but $\dot{V}_E$ expressed relative to body mass declines. In his study of 93 males ages 6 to 91 years, Robinson reported a fall in resting $\dot{V}_E$ expressed per kg body weight through the pediatric years until age 20 (45). Thereafter, values remained stable throughout the adult years. Jammes et al. found that resting minute ventilation per kg fell dramatically in children before age 10 years but declined only slowly thereafter (32). Mean value was approximately 275 ml $\cdot$ kg^{-1} $\cdot$ min^{-1} at age 10 years and 200 at age 20 years. Minute ventilation per kg reported by Morse et al. in 10-12-year-old subjects was higher than in 13-17-year-olds (average values of 199 vs. 158 ml $\cdot$ kg^{-1} $\cdot$ min^{-1}, respectively) (41).

In Robinson's study, resting V_T declined from 13 to 9 ml/kg over the age span of 6 to 17 years. A similar rate of decline was seen in the children studied by Jammes et al. (32). Gaultier et al. found mean values of 11.3 ml/kg in children 4 to 8 years, 10.1 ml/kg in those between 8 and 12, and 10.0 ml/kg in adults (p < .05 for the first two groups) (25). Cassels and Morse studied girls in age groups 6-8, 8-12, and 12-17 years (11). Tidal volume relative to BSA declined from 321 to 297 to 242 ml/m^2 from the youngest to the oldest age group.

Robinson reported that the proportion of tidal air relative to VC decreased from an average of 23.1% in the youngest boys to 12.6% in the 17-year-olds (45). The authors suggested, however, that the youngest boys may not have produced a true maximal effort during the VC determinations. Morse et al. also described a lower relative utilization of VC for V_T in younger subjects (41). Mean resting V_T/VC was .181 and .153 in groups of subjects ages 10-12 and 13-17 years, respectively.

In Robinson's investigation, mean resting breathing rate decreased from 24 breaths/min at age 6 years to 13 breaths/min at age 17 years (45). A similar decline was described by Gaultier et al. (25). Asmussen reported the relationship between resting breathing rate and body height in 53 children 0-20 years to be

$$f_b = 5969ht^{-1.17}$$

with a correlation coefficient of r = .85 (see fig. 9.1) (6). The scaling exponent for f_b relative to body weight was –.53. It is interesting that this value is almost identical to the factor of –.49 described by Jammes et al. in subjects 6 to 80 years old (32).

Resistance and Compliance

Ventilatory work, duration of inspiration and expiration, and the relation of V_T to f_b are all influenced by the resistance to flow in the airways and the elastance (or stiffness) of the lung (34). It is useful, then, to examine possible alterations of these factors during the growing years.

Resistance (or its inverse, conductance) is created by friction of flow within both the lung and the upper airways. Elastance (or compliance, its inverse) is determined by the elastic properties of the lung, including connective tissue and alveolar surface forces, as well as

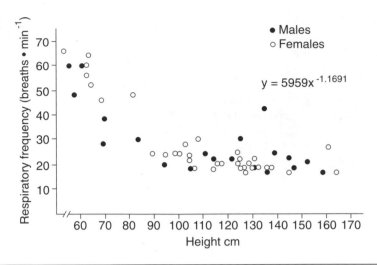

Figure 9.1   Resting breathing frequency relative to body height. Reprinted from Asmussen et al. 1981.

those of the chest wall itself (36, 61). While one might expect that the recognized differences in lung structure as the child grows should affect these properties, the relationships between anatomic development and respiratory function in children remain ill defined (61).

Lung compliance is defined as the change in lung volume for a given pressure, most appropriately expressed relative to a unit lung volume. From the relative stiffness of the lung of the newborn, compliance improves throughout childhood. Most of the improvement, however, occurs in the first 2 years of life, with little change from late childhood to the young adult years (64).

Resistance is expressed by the ratio of pressure and flow within the airways. Values are high in young children, but beyond age 5 years, little change is observed (31).

Lanteri and Sly studied age-related changes in respiratory mechanics in 63 children ages 3 weeks to 15 years during general anesthesia for urological surgery or repair of inguinal hernias (36). All subjects were considered to have normal lungs. An "interrupter technique" was utilized to separately assess the viscoelastic properties of the lung and airway resistance. Airway resistance relative to height declined with the scaling factor of –1.29. At the same time, respiratory system compliance rose relative to height by the exponent 1.76. As indicated by these exponents, the study showed that compliance and resistance do not evolve at the same rate in growing children: the former appears to increase more rapidly than the latter declines.

DeMuth et al. found that scaling factors for height relative to the forced expiratory volume at 50% of VC (an indicator of airway resistance) were 2.28 in boys and 1.87 in girls (19). Exponents were higher for height in respect to peak expiratory flow rates (2.64 and 2.86, respectively). (Interestingly, too, the authors reported a

significant correlation between peak expiratory flow rates and the children's IQ scores. They concluded, "Rather than detecting a mysterious relationship between airway resistance and intelligence, we suggest that the correlations underline the dependency of the peak flow rates on effort and ability to cooperate" [p. 208].)

How these characteristics might become altered in children during exercise is unknown. There is reason to suspect, however, that interactions among exercise-related and growth-related changes in lung mechanics might contribute to age-related differences in respiratory work and dyspnea during physical activity, particularly in younger children.

Diffusion Capacity

The ability of gases to diffuse across the lung-air interface is termed the diffusion capacity, or D_L. The D_L of O_2 is not easily measured, and therefore the D_L for carbon monoxide is usually determined instead. DeMuth and Howatt measured resting D_L for carbon monoxide (D_LCO) in 147 children ages 4-18 years and found that values increased with growth in parallel with lung volumes (17).

Correlation coefficients for D_LCO versus height, weight, and BSA were all approximately 0.90 for both sexes. Scaling exponents for D_LCO relative to height were 2.77 and 2.72, and those for D_LCO relative to weight were .97 and .89, for boys and girls, respectively. These findings indicate a close coupling of D_L and body size during childhood. However, O'Brodovich et al. demonstrated a gradual decrease in values of D_LCO expressed relative to alveolar volume when plotted against body height in subjects 6 to 30 years old (42). This finding suggests growth-related interactions among the components of D_L, pulmonary capillary blood volume, the surface area available for gas exchange, and hemoglobin affinity for O_2.

VENTILATION DURING EXERCISE

Several ventilatory responses to exercise unique to the growing child have intrigued developmental physiologists. The pattern of change in the components of $\dot{V}_E$ during exercise may be different from the pattern in the adult, as children appear to rely more on V_T than on breathing rate at high-intensity work levels. Younger children demonstrate a reduced respiratory efficiency with exercise, manifest as a higher *ventilatory equivalent for O_2*, or $\dot{V}_E$ for a given $\dot{V}O_2$. Children have higher breathing rates during exercise than mature subjects. While this suggests that children breathe more superficially than adults, some research data indicate just the opposite: children have lower values for P_aCO_2 because of higher $\dot{V}_E$ per kg. There is also evidence that neural control mechanisms for ventilation may differ in young children. The explanations for these observations, and the way in which these findings from descriptive studies might be interrelated, are uncertain.

Submaximal Exercise

At a given submaximal work intensity, V_T per kg changes little while breathing rate progressively declines as the child ages. Consequently, $\dot{V}_E$ per kg also falls.

Rowland and Cunningham obtained longitudinal data on 20 children studied yearly from ages 8 to 12 years (unpublished data; see fig. 9.2). At the same submaximal treadmill speed and slope (3.25 mph at 8%), mean breathing rate fell during this period from 45 to 36 bpm. At the same time, V_T per kg remained relatively stable with a value of approximately .021. Average absolute $\dot{V}_E$ rose from 34.2 to 40.8 L/min over the 5 years, while $\dot{V}_E$ per kg declined from .97 to .72 L · min^{-1} · kg^{-1}. In this study, children were exercising at a submaximal intensity (percentage $\dot{V}O_2max$) that declined from 65% to 55% with serial testing.

Rutenfranz et al. presented longitudinal findings in two separate European populations between the ages of 8 and 17 years (50). Submaximal ventilatory responses were described in children exercising at approximately the same relative intensity (65-70% $\dot{V}O_2max$). From ages 12 to 17 years, values for average absolute $\dot{V}_E$ increased in the males from 52.2 to 68.1 L/min but remained stable in the females (47.8 and 47.6 L/min, respectively). Respiratory frequency declined from 39 to 28 bpm in the boys and from 36 to 26 bpm in the girls, while V_T rose from 1.58 to 2.48 L and from 1.52 to 1.87 L in the two groups, respectively.

Cross-sectional data reported by Andersen et al. were similar (1). When 8-16-year-old children were cycling at 50% and 75% of $\dot{V}O_2max$, a steady decline was observed in breathing rate related to age. The fall in rate was more dramatic in the males (about 10 bpm over that age span) than in the females (4-5 bpm). Tidal volume at

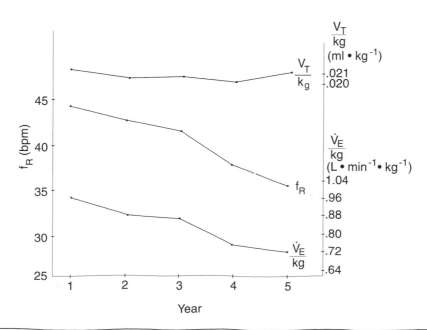

Figure 9.2 Breathing frequency (f_b), minute ventilation per kg ($\dot{V}_E$/kg), and tidal volume per kg (V_T/kg) at the same submaximal treadmill workload in 20 children studied annually for 5 years (Rowland and Cunningham).

a relative workload of 50-60% $\dot{V}O_2$max increased from 530 to 1760 ml in the boys and from 460 to 810 ml in the girls.

Robinson's submaximal findings in boys were obtained at the same absolute workload (treadmill walk at 5.6 km/hr) (45). Breathing rate declined from 49 to 29 bpm between the groups of subjects ages 6 and 17 years, respectively. Absolute $\dot{V}_E$ improved from an average of 21.2 to 48.6 L/min, but $\dot{V}_E$ per kg progressively declined with increasing age; mean values were 1.05 L · kg^{-1} · min^{-1} in the youngest children to 0.67 L · kg^{-1} · min^{-1} in the older adolescents. Average submaximal V_T was 430 ml in the youngest group and 1.73 ml in the older adolescents. When these values are expressed per kg, a small increase with age is seen (.021 at age 6 to .025 at age 17).

Why do children breathe more rapidly than adults at a given submaximal workload? Tidal volume is not relatively smaller in children, and, as will be discussed further on, children actually show a greater $\dot{V}_E$ relative to metabolic requirements during exercise than adults. Presumably the ratio of f_b to V_T is the product of a control system that integrates feedback (pressure/volume) to elicit the breathing pattern that will minimize the work of breathing. The factors determining this optimization of breathing economy remain to be clarified.

Ventilatory Efficiency

There is evidence that children *hyperventilate* during exercise as compared to adults. Robinson reported a progressive increase with age in alveolar PCO_2 during submaximal treadmill walking (45). The average value for 6-year-old boys was 33.0 mmHg and for 17-year-olds 39.6 mmHg. In the 9-15-year-old boys studied by Gadhoke and Jones, mean submaximal end-tidal PCO_2 increased from 36.5 mmHg in subjects with BSA 1.05-

1.19 m^2 to 39.5 mmHg in those with BSA 1.50-1.89 m^2 (24). Similar child-adult differences have been described by Shephard and Bar-Or (53) and by Cooper et al. (12).

Both longitudinal and cross-sectional research data also indicate that children hyperventilate during exercise in relation to metabolic requirements. This ventilatory "inefficiency," indicated by a high $\dot{V}_E/\dot{V}O_2$, is increasingly evident as younger children are tested. When a subject performs a progressive exercise test, $\dot{V}_E/\dot{V}O_2$ initially slowly declines, but at the ventilatory anaerobic threshold, generally about 60-65% $\dot{V}O_2$max, it abruptly rises and continues to increase until exhaustion. At low-to-moderate levels of exercise, then, $\dot{V}_E/\dot{V}O_2$ reflects efficiency of ventilation (in terms of gas exchange), while the ventilatory stimulation from excessive CO_2 resulting from buffering of lactic acid contributes to the ventilatory equivalent for O_2 at intensities above the ventilatory anaerobic threshold.

Mácek and Vavra demonstrated that $\dot{V}_E/\dot{V}O_2$ progressively falls at *all* comparable stages of cycle exercise as larger children are tested (38). Andersen et al. also reported that $\dot{V}_E/\dot{V}O_2$ at the same submaximal relative workload declined with age (see fig. 9.3) (1).

Submaximal $\dot{V}_E$ and $\dot{V}CO_2$ Kinetics

Cooper et al. reported that the rate of rise in $\dot{V}_E$ and $\dot{V}CO_2$ at the onset of submaximal exercise was 30% faster in children ages 7-10 years than in adolescents ages 15-18 years (12). Since CO_2 production relative to a given metabolic work level is expected to be age-independent, it was suggested that this finding may be related to lower storage of CO_2 in prepubertal subjects.

However, Armon et al. found no significant differences in resting whole-body CO_2 stores between adults and children in their study using [^{13}C]-bicarbonate

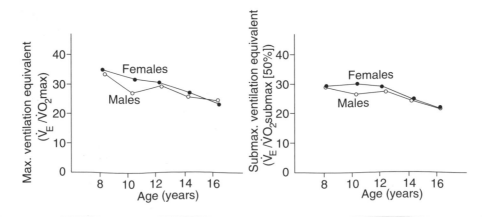

Figure 9.3 Ventilatory equivalent for oxygen ($\dot{V}_E/\dot{V}O_2$) at maximal exercise (left) and at 50% $\dot{V}O_2$max (right) in boys and girls. Reprinted from Andersen et al. 1974.

tracer techniques (4). Zanconato et al. therefore hypothesized that growth-related changes in stored CO_2 might result from mechanisms that are specifically related to exercise (63). Their study of nine healthy 6-10-year-olds and nine healthy adults ages 21-39 years, measuring $^{13}CO_2$ washout after oral ingestion, supported this concept. Resting CO_2 stores did not differ between the two groups. Intermittent exercise did not alter the amount of CO_2 stores in the children but caused an average 31% rise in CO_2 stores in the adults.

The authors suggested three possible explanations for their findings: (1) CO_2 has a greater solubility in fat than in muscle, and children are more lean than adults; (2) children have a lower blood hemoglobin concentration than adults (hemoglobin binds CO_2 and also acts to buffer hydrogen ion when CO_2 is converted to bicarbonate in the blood); and (3) $\dot{V}_E$ and CO_2 production are more closely linked in children than in adults, and this could result in less CO_2 accumulation at the start of exercise. This last concept will be discussed later in this chapter within the context of possible growth-related changes in control of ventilation.

Arterial Blood Gases

Because of ethical constraints against drawing arterial blood samples in children, little direct information is available about alterations in P_aO_2, P_aCO_2, or pH during exercise. Exercise end-tidal PCO_2 (reflecting P_aCO_2) values were about 3 mmHg lower in children compared to adults in the study of Armon et al. (see fig. 9.4) (4).

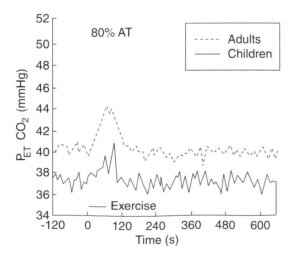

Figure 9.4 End-tidal PCO_2 ($P_{ET}CO_2$) in mmHg in adults and children resting, while exercising at 80% of anaerobic threshold, and during recovery. Reprinted from Armon et al. 1991.

Godfrey et al. obtained arterialized earlobe blood samples on 100 children cycling at approximately one-third and two-thirds of maximal workload (28). Average P_aCO_2 fell from 37.4 to 35.0 mmHg in the boys and from 35.8 to 33.9 mmHg in the girls. Mean arterial pH value for the combined groups declined from 7.38 to 7.37 between the two workloads. These values were considered similar to those previously reported in adult subjects.

Eriksson et al. measured arterial pH, PCO_2, and PO_2 in six boys ages 13-14 years during progressive maximal cycle exercise testing (22). Average pH was 7.39 at rest, 7.35 at 600 kpm submaximal exercise, and 7.27 at exhaustion. Corresponding values for PCO_2 were 39, 36, and 29 mmHg, and those for PO_2 were 98, 95, and 94 mmHg, respectively. In this study, the difference between alveolar and arterial O_2 tension rose from 8 mmHg at rest to 14 mmHg at submaximal exercise to 24 mmHg at maximum. These are values comparable to those seen in exercise testing of adults.

Dead Space Ventilation

The relative stability of P_aCO_2 during mild-to-moderate exercise in children implies that minute alveolar ventilation (V_A) must keep pace with CO_2 production ($\dot{V}CO_2$) as exercise intensity increases. Since minute ventilation is the sum of minute alveolar ventilation plus minute dead space ventilation (V_D),

$$V_A = \dot{V}_E - V_D = f_b(V_T - V_D).$$

As the child grows, f_b progressively falls while V_T increases directly with the child's size. At the same time, $f_b(V_T - V_D)$ remains constant relative to CO_2 production. It would be expected, then, that dead space would increase in approximate proportion to V_T (26). Thus, $\dot{V}_E/\dot{V}O_2$ differences during exercise with increasing age are unlikely to be related to changes in V_D.

Available information from research in children bears this out. The literature review by Radford (43), as well as the investigation of Godfrey and Davies using earlobe blood specimens (27), indicates that the relationship between resting dead space ventilation and body weight remains constant at approximately 1.0 cc/lb throughout the pediatric years. Shephard and Bar-Or calculated dead space from arterialized capillary blood in preadolescent children and adults exercising at 80% $\dot{V}O_2$max (53). No significant differences were observed between the two groups, with V_D/V_T values in the range of 0.20 to 0.25.

Gadhoke and Jones reported no age-related differences in derived values for V_D/V_T in boys 9-15 years old cycling at the same workload (24). Mean values were 0.21, 0.18, and 0.14 at 400, 600, and 800 kpm/min, respectively.

Lung Diffusion Capacity During Exercise

Anderson and Godfrey measured $D_L CO$ at one-third and two-thirds of maximal cycle working capacity in 40 healthy children (2). At the first workload, a significant rise was observed from resting values, but levels increased little between the two submaximal workloads. Highest levels of $D_L CO$ relative to body height are shown in figure 9.5, along with resting values reported by Weng and Levison (60). Diffusing capacity is seen to approximately triple with exercise in children, a rise slightly greater than that reported in adults (23).

Shephard et al. measured lung diffusion capacity relative to O_2 uptake during maximal exercise testing of 10-12-year-old children (52). No tendency for a $D_L CO$ plateau was observed, as values rose in an approximate linear fashion with $\dot{V}O_2$ to subject exhaustion. The authors commented that the slope of the $D_L CO/\dot{V}O_2$ relationship was approximately twice that expected in adults.

Johnson et al. measured membrane diffusing capacity (a measure that eliminates red cell resistance from $D_L CO$) at rest and maximal exercise in four children 8-12 years old and six adults aged 15-28 years (33). No significant differences were observed between the groups, the children and the adults showing a 16.3% and an 18.7% rise, respectively.

As Godfrey emphasized, diffusion of O_2 across the lung surface is not considered critical in O_2 uptake in

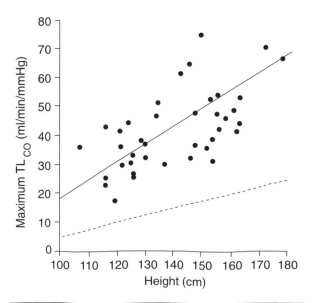

Figure 9.5 Relationship between lung diffusion capacity (TL_{CO}) and height at maximal exercise in children. From data in Anderson and Godfrey (2). Dashed line is resting data of Weng and Levison (60). Reprinted from Godfrey 1974.

humans except under conditions of severely intense exercise (26). This appears to hold as true for children as for adults.

VENTILATION AT MAXIMAL EXERCISE

The highest minute ventilation achieved during exhaustive endurance exercise is driven by (1) CO_2 produced by the maximal aerobic metabolic rate of contracting muscle; (2) CO_2 accumulated by the buffering of lactic acid, a reflection of anaerobic metabolism at high-intensity work levels; and (3) the metabolic acidosis that ensues when this buffering becomes inadequate. $\dot{V}_E max$ increases with lung growth as the child ages. Åstrand reported mean values of 39.8 and 33.9 L/min at age 4-6 years in boys and girls, respectively (7). These numbers increased to 112.9 and 87.9 L/min by age 14-15 years. Similar values have been described by others (45, 50). As with $\dot{V}O_2 max$, these studies show that mean values for $\dot{V}_E max$ are greater for boys at all ages but that these differences are small until the age of puberty.

Several have investigated the relationship of $\dot{V}_E max$ to various anthropometric variables. Mercier et al. studied ventilatory responses to maximal cycle exercise in 76 nonathletic boys ages 10.5 to 15.5 years (40). Lean body mass (LBM, determined by skinfold measurements) was found to explain the greatest percentage of variance in $\dot{V}_E max$, and maximal minute ventilation relative to LBM did not change significantly with age (see fig. 9.6). The allometric scaling factors for $\dot{V}_E max$ relative to height and weight in this study were 2.06 and .68, respectively, indicating that $\dot{V}_E$ per kg decreased with increasing body mass. Although the maximal data of Åstrand show some variability, the same trend is evident in both boys and girls (7). Mean values for $\dot{V}_E max$ per kg at age 4-6 years were 1.94 and 1.85 for the boys and girls, respectively, and at age 14-15 these decreased to 1.59 and 1.49. The boys in Robinson's study, however, showed comparatively stable average values for mass-relative $\dot{V}_E max$ across age groups (45). The 6-year-olds had a mean $\dot{V}_E$ per kg of 1.59; subjects 14-18 years old showed average values of 1.60. The number of subjects for each age group was very small, however (n = 4-9). Morse et al. described no relationship of $\dot{V}_E max$ per kg to age in boys in the age range of 10-17 years (41).

In the longitudinal data of Rutenfranz et al., $\dot{V}_E max$ was linearly related to stature until a height of 160 cm was reached in the girls, whose values then actually decreased (50). In the males, however, the height-$\dot{V}_E max$ relationship continued to be linear to the tallest adolescents studied (170 cm). On the basis of these data, the most practical and accurate measure for normalizing

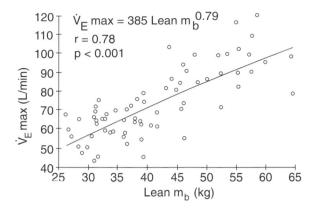

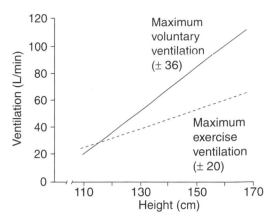

Figure 9.7 Relationship of $\dot{V}_E$max to maximum voluntary ventilation in children of different heights. Reprinted from Godfrey 1974.

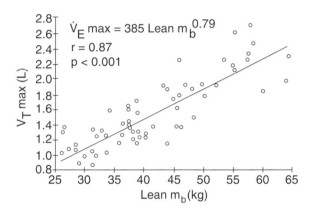

Figure 9.6 Allometric relationship between $\dot{V}_E$max (top) and $V_T$max (bottom) with body mass. Reprinted from Mercier et al. 1991.

$\dot{V}_E$max to increasing body size in children would seem to be body height or body height squared.

The same age-dependent "inefficiency" of ventilation seen at submaximal levels has been observed in most studies at maximal exercise as well. Åstrand reported a steady fall in average maximal $\dot{V}_E/\dot{V}O_2$ values in boys from 40.5 at age 4-6 years to 32.0 at age 14-15 years (7). In girls these values were 37.8 and 33.9, respectively. The findings of Andersen et al. indicated a progressive decline in maximal $\dot{V}_E/\dot{V}O_2$ between the ages of 8 and 16 years, from 33.3 to 24.5 in boys and 34.8 to 23.9 in girls (1) (see fig. 9.3, page 146). The longitudinal study of Rutenfranz et al., however, showed no age trends in maximal ventilatory equivalent for O_2 in either boys or girls (50).

The proportion of MVV attainable by $\dot{V}_E$max during a progressive exercise test to exhaustion appears to be the same in older children as in adults. Godfrey demonstrated that when these two variables were plotted against body height in children, $\dot{V}_E$max generally amounted to 60-70% of MVV (26) (see fig. 9.7). In the smaller children he noted that this number was larger, "partly because they do indeed ventilate relatively more

than older subjects, and partly because they do not cooperate so well with the MVV test" (p. 68-69). Godfrey suggested that the $\dot{V}_E$max/MVV relationship be utilized as a marker of a true exhaustive effort by the exercising subject; that is, if $\dot{V}_E$max is less than 60% of MVV, "the child is probably not trying hard enough" (p. 68-69).

Breathing Frequency

While $\dot{V}_E$max increases during childhood, maximal breathing rate progressively falls (see fig. 9.8). Morse et al. used the equation

$$f_b\text{max} = 60.5 - 0.92(\text{age})$$

to express this relationship in their study of 99 boys ages 10-17 years during treadmill running (41). Mercier et al. found that maximal breathing frequency could be related to body mass (M) in the same age range by the allometric equation

$$f_b\text{max} = 137\, M^{-0.27}.$$

The scaling exponent for LBM was almost identical (−0.28), and that for height (cm) was −0.84 (40).

The decline in maximal breathing frequency during the course of childhood is substantial. In Robinson's study this amounted to a decrease from an average of 62 bpm at age 6 years to 46 bpm at age 18 years (45). Åstrand's treadmill data in the same age range are similar (7). In the boys, $f_b$max fell from an average of 70 bpm to 45 bpm, while the girls showed a decline from 66 to 51 bpm.

Tidal Volume

Tidal volume at maximal exercise steadily rises as children grow (see fig. 9.8). The longitudinal study of

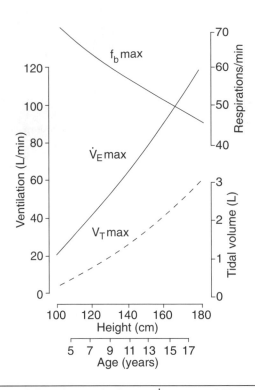

Figure 9.8 Changes in $f_b$max, $\dot{V}_E$max, and $V_T$max with height. Data of Åstrand (7). Reprinted from Godfrey 1974.

Rutenfranz et al. indicated an increase in average $V_T$max from .850 and .740 L in boys and girls, respectively, at age 8 years to 2.08 and 1.78 L by age 15 (50). In accord with the findings of Godfrey just cited, the fraction of VC represented by maximal V_T changed between these ages. There was a significant gender difference, however, with a V_T/VC of .36-.40 in the girls and .40-.48 in the boys. Cross-sectional data in children 8-16 years old from Andersen et al. provided almost identical values (1). Åstrand reported, however, somewhat lower $V_T$max/VC ratios in prepubertal boys compared to adolescents (.48 and .54, respectively) (7).

A child's maximal V_T relative to body weight remains essentially constant during the childhood years. Mercier et al. described scaling factors of wt$^{.96}$ and ht$^{2.90}$ for $V_T$max in children 10.5 to 15.5 years old (40). In that study, however, LBM remained the anthropometric factor that accounted for the greatest percentage of variance (77%) (see fig. 9.6). Åstrand reported stable values of $V_T$max per kg between the ages of 7 and 13 years (approximately 35 and 34 ml/kg for boys and girls, respectively), but the 14-15-year-old boys had higher levels (42 ml/kg) (7).

Much of this work suggests that younger children do not really breathe more "shallowly" during exercise even though their breathing rates are faster. That is, V_T relative to both body dimensions and lung volume re-

mains relatively constant during the years, and breathing rates, while falling progressively, are not disproportionately rapid. By this analysis, and in addition the observation of greater $\dot{V}_E/\dot{V}O_2$ in younger age groups, one would expect maximal minute ventilation expressed relative to body weight to decline as children age. As reviewed in the preceding paragraphs, this conclusion is supported by some—but not all—of the studies examining $\dot{V}_E$max changes during growth.

This pattern is reminiscent of that for cardiac output responses to maximal exercise as the child grows. A volume related directly to organ size (left ventricular dimension for cardiac stroke volume, lung VC for V_T) increases with age. There is currently no convincing evidence that both of these volumes improve functionally with age beyond the improvement that can be attributed to changes in organ size. This volume is multiplied by a size-independent frequency (heart rate, breathing rate) to create a minute volume (cardiac output, ventilation).

But there are differences between lung and heart function at maximal exercise in the growing child as well. Maximal heart rate is independent of age; longitudinal treadmill studies of children in the age range of 8-15 years show stable maximal rates of 195-200 bpm. Peak breathing frequencies at exhaustive exercise, however, decline with increasing age during childhood. Also, cardiac output during exercise in the growing child is closely linked to metabolic rate (O_2 uptake). On the other hand, ventilation relative to $\dot{V}O_2$ at both submaximal and maximal exercise intensities progressively falls with age.

BREATHING PATTERNS WITH EXERCISE

The characteristic rise in $\dot{V}_E$ with increasing exercise intensity is observed in children as in adults: $\dot{V}_E$ is closely related to changes in $\dot{V}O_2$ until approximately 60% $\dot{V}O_2$max, when $\dot{V}_E$ increases disproportionately because of the stimulation of excessive CO_2 produced by the buffering lactic acid. We have some evidence, however, that this break-point at the ventilatory anaerobic threshold may be relatively higher in children than in adults. Chapter 12 will explore this concept in greater detail.

Progressive Exercise

It will be recalled that in the typical adult, increases in ventilation at low-moderate-intensity exercise are accomplished by a rise in both V_T and f_b (39). At higher-intensity work culminating in an exhaustive effort, however, V_T tapers off, and $\dot{V}_E$ is largely the result of a continued linear rise in f_b.

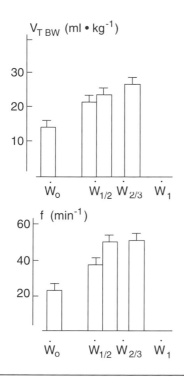

Figure 9.9 Changes in V_T per kg (top) and changes in breathing rate (bottom) at rest, 50% max ($\dot{W}_{1/2}$), 2/3 max ($\dot{W}_{2/3}$), and maximal cycle workload ($\dot{W}_1$) in children. Reprinted from Boule et al. 1989.

Certain data in pediatric exercise studies suggest that this pattern may be different in children. Boule et al. reported ventilatory responses to maximal cycle testing in 18 nonathletic healthy children ages 6 to 15 years (10) (see fig. 9.9). Tidal volume rose linearly with workload

to exhaustion, while breathing rate plateaued at 67% of maximum workload and did not increase further at higher intensities.

Similarly, Rowland and Green demonstrated that the ratio of f_b to V_T rose during a progressive treadmill running protocol in 15 boys 10-14 years old until high intensity levels, when the ratio actually declined (48). This finding contrasted with data for a group of 20 males ages 23-33 years who showed a linear rise of this ratio to maximal exercise. While these findings suggest a blunted breathing rate rise at high workloads in children, Rutenfranz et al. reported a linear response of f_b to increasing exercise intensities up to maximum in 8-, 13-, and 17-year-old subjects (50).

Sustained Submaximal Exercise

During prolonged (40-60 min) periods of steady-load submaximal exercise, the changes in ventilation are very different. Breathing frequency and minute ventilation both slowly rise, while V_T declines (16). This pattern is unusual, since most stimulants of ventilation (chemical or metabolic) cause a rise in V_T. Increases in body temperature may be the most likely explanation for this "ventilatory drift."

The qualitative and quantitative aspects of ventilatory drift do not appear to be different in children and adults. Rowland and Rimany compared ventilatory changes in 11 premenarchal girls ages 9-13 years with those of 13 women aged 20-31 during 40 min of steady-load cycling at an intensity of 63% $\dot{V}O_2max$ (49) (see fig. 9.10). Between 10 and 40 min of exercise, $\dot{V}_E$ rose 7.1% and 11.7% in the girls and women, respectively (p > .05). Meanwhile, breathing rate increased 15% and 14%

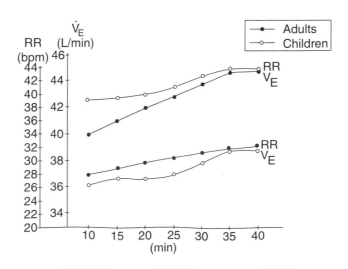

Figure 9.10 Breathing rate (RR) and $\dot{V}_E$ during 40 min of continuous cycling at 60% $\dot{V}O_2$ in girls and women. Reprinted from Rowland and Rimany 1995.

and V_T fell (–6.0 and –2.0%) in the two groups, respectively. There was no significant difference in temperature increase between the girls and women (97.6 to 98.5 °F and 98.2 to 99.4 °F, respectively). Similar findings were described in males by Asano and Hirakoba (5).

WHY IS $\dot{V}_E/\dot{V}O_2$ DURING EXERCISE GREATER IN CHILDREN?

Compared to adults, children ventilate out of proportion to the metabolic demands of exercise. The information in this chapter on age-related differences in ventilatory equivalent for O_2 ($\dot{V}_E/\dot{V}O_2$) as well as P_aCO_2 supports this concept. Moreover, the magnitude of this elevated $\dot{V}_E/\dot{V}O_2$ during exercise is inversely related to the age of the child: there is a continuum of improving ventilation efficiency at both maximal and submaximal work intensities that progresses as the child grows.

The explanation for this inefficiency is uncertain. It is a particularly intriguing question because physiologic processes should not be expected to operate at other than an optimal minimal energy cost. Presumably the exaggerated ventilation response to a given metabolic rate during exercise in children represents the body's need to compromise with yet another "uneconomic" function. While the cause of the child's ventilatory inefficiency is unknown, those attempting to explain the phenomenon have generally viewed it from one of two perspectives—as either (1) a manifestation of increased neural ventilatory drive in children compared to adults, or (2) the effect of size-related differences in ventilation mechanics.

Ventilatory Neural Drive

Several studies support the idea that in comparison to adults, children possess greater ventilatory drive and a lower CO_2 set point (i.e., in the process of homeostasis, ventilation is regulated to maintain a lower P_aCO_2). Why this should be true, however, remains obscure.

Gaultier et al. measured the mouth pressure (P) generated 0.1 s after airways occlusion (a reflection of neural drive to breathe) in 62 children aged 4 to 16 years (25). Values decreased with age (A) as a power function of $P = 8.51A^{-0.62}$. The authors concluded that the higher pressures in young children probably reflect greater neural drive.

Cooper et al. reported the relationship of $\dot{V}_E$ with $\dot{V}CO_2$ during progressive cycle exercise in 128 healthy subjects ages 6 to 18 years (12). The association between the two variables is linear until metabolic acidemia develops at high-intensity exercise and accelerates $\dot{V}_E$. The slope of the line before this respiratory compensation point provides useful information. A lower slope, for instance, can result from an elevated P_aCO_2, while a higher V_D/V_T will increase the slope. Cooper et al. found a small but significant negative relationship between the slope and body weight. Since, as reviewed earlier in this chapter, V_D/V_T appears to be size-independent, the authors suggested that the steeper slope observed in the younger subjects indicated that they possess a lower CO_2 set point.

Armon et al. expanded the findings of Cooper et al. into exercise intensities above the anaerobic threshold (4). They found a closer coupling of $\dot{V}CO_2$ with $\dot{V}_E$ in children compared to adults and obtained lower end-tidal PCO_2 values in the children.

Gratas-Delamarche et al. evaluated ventilation responses to inhaled CO_2 during exercise as a means of assessing maturity-related differences in chemical receptors of respiratory drive centers (30). Subjects were 9 prepubertal boys (mean age 10.3 years) and 10 young adults (mean age 24.9 years). The children demonstrated a lower CO_2 sensitivity threshold (the value of end-tidal PCO_2 when ventilation increased above a steady state level). The younger subjects also exhibited a greater slope of the linear relation between minute ventilation and end-tidal PCO_2, supporting the findings of Cooper et al. (12). These results were considered indicative that children during exercise have a greater sensitivity of respiratory drive centers than adults.

Mechanical Factors

Others have viewed the lower PCO_2, greater $\dot{V}_E$ per kg, and higher $\dot{V}_E/\dot{V}O_2$ values in children as the consequences of size-related differences in ventilatory mechanics. Cotes considered the hyperventilation in children a direct result of their more rapid breathing frequency compared to that of adults (13). "In the case of the ventilation minute volume, the differences in respiratory frequency have the effect that for any level of alveolar ventilation the deadspace ventilation, which is the product of the physiological deadspace and the respiratory frequency, is greater in children than in adults; the ventilation minute volume is increased in consequence" (p. 344).

However, the younger child has a smaller dead space as well as a more rapid breathing rate; thus minute dead space should remain proportional to body size in the same way that V_T does. Indeed, most research data indicate that V_D/V_T remains constant during childhood.

Still, differences in airway dimensions might have some effect on minute ventilation. Gratas-Delamarche et al. suggested that the relative rapid and shallow breathing of children does not permit as efficient washout of alveolar gas as in adults (30). They also proposed that the higher f_b might cause a rise in the total mechanical work of breathing because of an increase in "viscous and turbulent work" (p. 28).

Ventilatory work is strongly influenced by the balance of lung compliance and airway resistance (34). The study by Lanteri and Sly in resting children indicated that these two factors do not necessarily evolve at the same rate during the course of childhood (36). It would not be surprising to find that this is the case also during exercise, and it is interesting to speculate that the change in the relationship of the two factors might influence the "best" economical pattern of exercise ventilation.

Åstrand suggested that the ventilatory "inefficiency" of children might be at least partially related to equipment dead space and therefore be artifactual (7). Because the dead space of the mouthpiece and valve is constant (usually about 50-100 cc), the small child will have a greater relative dead space when using the same equipment as an older child or adolescent. By his calculations, however, Åstrand could not attribute the magnitude of hyperventilation in children to this factor. He concluded that "the difference in ventilation in the different age groups . . . must depend on a dissimilarity in respiratory regulation" (p. 82).

RESPONSES TO ENDURANCE TRAINING

The effects of regular endurance activity in children on ventilatory responses to exercise can be assessed by studying (a) the ventilation profiles of young endurance athletes and (b) changes in ventilatory parameters in nonathletes after a period of aerobic training. The first approach, of course, may be confounded by the influences of genetic predisposition and accelerated biological maturation. It will become apparent from the information in this section that we have no clear-cut picture of the expected ventilatory responses to endurance training, and this is true in both children and adults.

Child Endurance Athletes

Controversy exists about whether there are differences in resting pulmonary volumes and flow rates between child endurance athletes and nonathletes. Vaccaro and Poffenbarger, for instance, could detect no significant differences in resting VC, 1 s forced expiratory volume ($FEV_{1.0}$), or MVV in well-trained 10-14-year-old female runners compared to nonathletic controls (57). However, mean values for all these measures were higher in the athletes. After a season of competitive swim training, the 9-11-year-old children reported by Vaccaro and Clarke showed no differences in changes in VC, $FEV_{1.0}$, or MVV compared to nontraining controls (56).

Bar-Or and Zwiren reported that VC and $FEV_{1.0}$ were similar in 9-10-year-old run-trained boys compared to normally active control subjects (8). Cumming could find no significant correlation between VC or MVV with performance times in an 880 yd run in 13-17-year-old adolescents attending a track camp (14). On the other hand, Andrew et al. described significantly greater values for VC and $FEV_{1.0}$ in both male and female swimmers ages 8-18 years compared to nonathletes, and this difference was evident even in the youngest groups (3).

Vaccaro and Poffenbarger suggested that the discrepancies in these reports might be explained by differences in duration of training (57). Engstrom et al. (21) and Yost et al. (62) observed improved pulmonary function tests in young swimmers after minimum training periods of 32 months. Studies describing no differences in athletic and nonathletic children have generally involved shorter training times. The findings of Sundberg and Elovainio in young competitive endurance runners lend credence to this idea (54). Vital capacity and $FEV_{1.0}$ were not dissimilar between runners and controls at ages 12 and 14 years, but in the 16-year-old group, both variables were significantly greater in the runners. While these findings suggest that adaptive pulmonary changes occur with training (albeit slowly), the authors suggested an alternative explanation: "The 16-year old runners might be a selected group with a hereditary disposition for endurance running. Those lacking this disposition have dropped out before that age when greater demands with respect to training are being placed upon them" (p. 991).

Similar conflicting data regarding differences in VC, $FEV_{1.0}$, and MVV in athletes and nonathletes appear in studies in adults as well (reviewed by Cumming [14]). Cumming concluded that "the controversy over whether [resting pulmonary function] of athletes is actually superior to that of non-athletes, or may improve with training, would suggest that if differences do exist they are slight, and that a high score in these functions is not of great importance in the performance of athletics" (p. 142).

Child endurance athletes tend to have greater $\dot{V}_E max$ than nonathletes, but these differences are often less impressive and more variable than those for $\dot{V}O_2 max$. Unnithan compared exercise findings in 15 run-trained boys (mean age 11.7 years) and 18 control subjects matched for age, height, and weight (55). At a submaximal running speed of 8.0 km/hr, mean values for $\dot{V}_E/\dot{V}O_2$, V_T, f_b, and $\dot{V}_E$ were indistinguishable between the two groups. At maximal exercise there remained no significant differences, although the runners had a $\dot{V}O_2 max$ of 60.5 ml · kg^{-1} · min^{-1} compared to 51.1 ml · kg^{-1} · min^{-1} in the controls. $\dot{V}_E$max values were 71.4 and 64.7 L/min for the two groups, respectively (p > .05).

Similar findings were obtained in the 12-16-year-old runners studied by Sundberg and Elovainio (54). In all age groups, absolute $\dot{V}_E$max was greater in the athletes, but the difference from values for controls (matched for height but not for weight) did not reach statistical significance until age 16. In each age group, however, $\dot{V}O_2$max per kg was approximately 10 ml · kg^{-1} · min^{-1} greater in the runners (p < .05). Clearly, uncertainties regarding the best means of normalizing $\dot{V}O_2$max and $\dot{V}_E$max to body size and composition confound our understanding of these findings.

Gratas et al. described differences in ventilation and occlusion-pressure responses to exercise between athletic and nonathletic boys ages 11-13 years (29). The athletic subjects were training 6 to 15 hr/week in a variety of sports (football, ice skating, table tennis, etc.). At each level of cycle exercise, the trained children exhibited lower values for breathing frequency, ventilatory equivalent for O_2, and $\dot{V}_E$. Mouth occlusion pressures were not significantly different between the two groups at any workload. These findings suggest that young athletes have a more economical breathing pattern than nonathletes but do not show any differences in neural respiratory drive. However, Ramonatxo et al. found greater occlusion pressures in prepubertal than in postpubertal male swimmers, suggesting that ventilatory drive might be higher in the younger subjects (44).

Training Studies

Koch and Eriksson studied ventilatory responses to a 16-week period of exercise training in nine boys aged 11 to 13 years (35). None of the subjects had participated in systematic athletic training before this program. Mean $\dot{V}O_2$max increased from 41.7 to 48.1 ml · kg^{-1} · min^{-1}. The training did not alter resting breathing rate, ventilation, or V_T. At maximal exercise, however, average $\dot{V}_E$ increased from 49.4 to 72.8 L/min, a reflection of a similar rise in V_T, as maximal breathing rate did not change. The mean value for $\dot{V}_E/\dot{V}O_2$max increased with training from 28.9 to 35.1. There were no nontraining control subjects in this study, however.

Children 9 to 11 years old in the study of Vaccaro and Clarke underwent exercise testing before and after a season of competitive swim training (56). $\dot{V}O_2$max improved 17.2% in the swimmers compared to 4.7% in nontraining control children (p < .05). $\dot{V}_E$max increased 19.4% with training and 5.5% in the controls, but this difference was not significant.

Rowland and Boyajian reported a 6.5% increase in $\dot{V}O_2$max in 37 children 10-12 years of age after a 12-week aerobic training program (47). No significant

changes occurred in submaximal breathing rate, V_T, or $\dot{V}_E/\dot{V}O_2$. In comparison to values in a pretraining control period, subjects showed significant increases in $\dot{V}_E$max and $V_T$max with no change in maximal breathing rate or ventilatory equivalent for O_2.

Children who possess high levels of pretraining fitness may not show such changes. Daniels and Oldridge reported no alterations in weight-relative $\dot{V}O_2$max over the course of 22 months of distance running training in 14 boys 10-15 years old (15). Most had some experience with running activities before beginning the program. Similar to O_2 uptake, $\dot{V}_E$max expressed per kg did not change appreciably during the training; however, $\dot{V}_E$max relative to centimeters body height rose from a mean value of .570 at the initial testing to .642 by the end of the 22 months.

SUMMARY

Multiple factors must be taken into account in the attempt to understand the ventilatory responses to exercise in children. Age-related differences in lung size, neural drive, compliance, airway resistance, lung diffusion capacity, CO_2 storage, and blood lactic acid accumulation all may potentially influence the patterns of ventilation that are observed as children grow. In addition, insights into ventilatory changes during maturation are clouded by lack of a clear understanding of the proper anthropometric means of normalizing respiratory measurements to differences in body size. Current research data suggest the following concepts.

1. Resting V_T increases as the lungs grow, while the frequency of breathing progressively declines. Minute ventilation expressed relative to body weight decreases with age. This pattern mimics that for resting metabolic rate.

2. At a given submaximal workload, the same changes are observed; that is, f_b falls with age while V_T and $\dot{V}_E$ increase. Submaximal $\dot{V}_E$ per kg declines as children grow.

3. Maximal values of $\dot{V}_E$max per kg also decrease with age, but $\dot{V}_E$max appears to be closely associated with the square of body height. Maximal f_b decreases progressively throughout childhood.

4. These ventilatory patterns are similar in boys and girls, but mean values for volume measures are typically slightly greater for the males at all age levels.

5. Compared to adults, children demonstrate greater $\dot{V}_E$ relative to the metabolic requirements of exercise. This is evidenced by higher values for $\dot{V}_E/\dot{V}O_2$ and $\dot{V}_E$ per kg and lower P_aCO_2 at all levels of exercise. These characteristics become less

obvious as children age. Maturity-related differences in ventilation responses to exercise may reflect variations in neural respiratory drive, lung mechanics, or both.

6. Athletic training does not appear to consistently alter resting lung volumes and dynamics, but $\dot{V}_E$ improves similarly to $\dot{V}O_2$. Increases in minute ventilation with endurance training are entirely a manifestation of improved V_T, as f_b remains unchanged.

What We Know

1. Resting lung V_T increases with age in childhood but declines slowly relative to body size. Breathing rate at rest also progressively falls. Therefore, resting ventilation per kg body mass falls as children age.

2. During submaximal work, children breathe more rapidly than adults. A progressive decline in maximal breathing rate is also observed during the pediatric years.

3. Children hyperventilate during exercise in comparison to adults, showing lower alveolar PCO_2 and higher $\dot{V}_E/\dot{V}O_2$.

4. Maximal exercise ventilation rises with age in close proportion to body height. Maximal V_T per kg is stable throughout childhood.

What We Would Like to Know

1. How do changes in airway resistance and lung compliance influence ventilatory responses to exercise during childhood?

2. Why do young children have a lower ventilatory efficiency (i.e., higher $\dot{V}_E/\dot{V}O_2$) during exercise?

3. What mechanisms explain the more rapid breathing rates in children at a given submaximal workload compared to adults?

4. How can maximal ventilatory responses to exercise be best related to increased body size?

5. How does pulmonary function differ in athletes and nonathletes, and how do these factors change with endurance training?

References

1. Andersen, K.L.; Seliger, V.; Rutenfranz, J.; Messel, S. Physical performance capacity of children in Norway. Part III. Respiratory responses to graded exercise loadings—population parameters in a rural community. Eur. J. Appl. Physiol. 33:265-274; 1974.

2. Anderson, S.D.; Godfrey, S. Transfer factor for CO_2 during exercise in children. Thorax 26:51-54; 1971.

3. Andrew, G.M.; Becklake, M.R.; Guleria, J.S.; Bates, D.V. Heart and lung functions in swimmers and non-athletes during growth. J. Appl. Physiol. 32:245-251; 1972.

4. Armon, Y.; Cooper, D.M.; Zanconato, S. Maturation of ventilatory responses to 1-minute exercise. Pediatr. Res. 29:362-368; 1991.

5. Asano, K.; Hirakoba, K. Respiratory and circulatory adaptation during prolonged exercise in 10-12 year old children and in adults. In: Ilmarinen, J.; Valimaki, I., eds. Children and sport. Berlin: Springer-Verlag; 1984:p. 119-128.

6. Asmussen, E.; Secher, N.H.; Andersen, E.A. Heart rate and ventilatory frequency as dimension-dependent variables. Eur. J. Appl. Physiol. 46:379-386; 1981.

7. Åstrand, P.O. Experimental studies of physical working capacity in relation to sex and age. Copenhagen: Munksgaard; 1952.

8. Bar-Or, O.; Zwiren, L. Physiological effects of increased frequency of physical education classes and of endurance conditioning on 9-10 year old girls and boys. In: Pediatric work physiology: proceedings of the Fourth International Symposium. Wingate, Israel: Wingate Institute for Physical Education; 1973:p. 183-198.

9. Berger, R.A. Applied exercise physiology. Philadelphia: Lea & Febiger; 1982:p. 205-237.

10. Boule, M.; Gaultier, C.; Girard, F. Breathing pattern during exercise in untrained children. Respir. Phys. 75:225-234; 1989.

11. Cassels, D.E.; Morse, M. Cardiopulmonary data for children and young adults. Springfield, IL: Charles C Thomas; 1962:p. 52-77.

12. Cooper, D.M.; Kaplan, M.R.; Baumgarten, L.; Weiler-Ravell, D.; Whipp, B.J.; Wasserman, K. Coupling of ventilation and CO_2 production during exercise in children. Pediatr. Res. 21:568-572; 1987.

13. Cotes, J.E. Lung function. Assessment and application in medicine. 4th ed. Oxford, UK: Blackwell Scientific; 1979:p.344.

14. Cumming, G.R. Correlation of athletic performance with pulmonary function in 13 to 17 year old boys and girls. Med. Sci. Sports 1:140-143; 1969.

15. Daniels, J.; Oldridge, N. Changes in oxygen consumption of young boys during growth and running training. Med. Sci. Sports 3:161-165; 1971.

16. Dempsey, J.A.; Aaron, E.; Martin, B.J. Pulmonary function and prolonged exercise. In: Perspectives in exercise science and sports medicine. Vol. 1, Lamb, D.R.; Murray, R., eds. Prolonged exercise. Indianapolis: Benchmark Press; 1988:p. 75-124.

17. DeMuth, G.R.; Howatt, W.F. III. Pulmonary diffusion. Pediatrics 35 Suppl:185-193; 1965.

18. DeMuth, G.R.; Howatt, W.F.; Hill, B.M. I. Lung volumes. Pediatrics 35 Suppl:162-175; 1965.

19. DeMuth, G.R.; Howatt, W.F.; Hill, B.M. V. Forced flow rates. Pediatrics 35 Suppl:200-210; 1965.

20. Dunnill, M.S. Postnatal growth of the lung. Thorax 17:329-334; 1962.

21. Engstrom, I.; Eriksson, B.O.; Karlberg, P.; Saltin, B.; Thoren, C. Preliminary report on the development of lung volumes in young girl swimmers. Acta Paediatr. Scand. Suppl. 217:73-76; 1971.

22. Eriksson, B.O.; Grimby, G.; Saltin, B. Cardiac output and arterial blood gases during exercise in pubertal boys. J. Appl. Physiol. 31:348-352; 1971.

23. Filley, G.; MacIntosh, D.J.; Wright, G.W. Carbon monoxide uptake and pulmonary diffusing capacity in normal subjects at rest and during exercise. J. Clin. Invest. 33:530-539; 1954.

24. Gadhoke, S.; Jones, N.L. The responses to exercise in boys aged 9-15 years. Clin. Sci. 37:789-801; 1969.

25. Gaultier, C.; Perret, L.; Boule, M.; Buvry, A.; Girard, F. Occlusion pressure and breathing pattern in healthy children. Respir. Physiol. 46:71-80; 1981.

26. Godfrey, S. Exercise testing in children. London: Saunders; 1974.

27. Godfrey, S.; Davies, C.T.M. Estimates of arterial PCO_2 and their effect on the calculated values of cardiac output and dead space on exercise. Clin. Sci. 39:529-537; 1970.

28. Godfrey, S.; Davies, C.T.M.; Wozniak, E.; Barnes, C.A. Cardiorespiratory response to exercise in normal children. Clin. Sci. 40:419-431; 1971.

29. Gratas, A.; Dassonville, J.; Beillot, J.; Rochcongar, P. Ventilatory and occlusion-pressure responses to exercise in trained and untrained children. Eur. J. Appl. Physiol. 57:591-596; 1988.

30. Gratas-Delamarche, A.; Mercier, J.; Ramonatxo, M.; Dassonville, J.; Prefaut, C. Ventilatory response of prepubertal boys and adults to carbon dioxide at rest and during exercise. Eur. J. Appl. Physiol. 66:25-30; 1993.

31. Hogg, J.C.; Williams, J.; Richardson, J.B. Age as a factor in the distribution of lower-airway conductance and in the pathologic anatomy of obstructive lung disease. N. Engl. J. Med. 282:1283-1287; 1970.

32. Jammes, Y.; Auran, Y.; Gouvernet, J.; Delpierre, S.; Grimaud, C. The ventilatory pattern of conscious man according to age and morphology. Bull. Europ. Physiopath. Resp. 15:527-540; 1979.

33. Johnson, R.L.; Taylor, H.F.; Lawson, W.H. Maximal diffusing capacity of the lung for carbon monoxide. J. Clin. Invest. 44:349-355; 1965.

34. Jones, N.L. Dyspnea in exercise. Med. Sci. Sports Exerc. 16:14-19; 1984.

35. Koch, G.; Eriksson, B.O. Effect of physical training on pulmonary ventilation and gas exchange during submaximal and maximal work in boys aged 11 to 13 years. Scan. J. Clin. Lab. Invest. 31:87-94; 1973.

36. Lanteri, C.J.; Sly, P.D. Changes in respiratory mechanics with age. J. Appl. Physiol. 74:369-378; 1993.

37. Lyons, H.A.; Tanner, R.W. Total lung volume and its subdivisions in children: normal standards. J. Appl. Physiol. 17:601-604; 1962.

38. Mácek, M.; Vavra, J. Anaerobic threshold in children. In: Binkhorst, R.A.; Kemper, H.C.G.; Saris, W.H.M., eds. Children and exercise XI. Champaign, IL: Human Kinetics; 1985:p. 110-113.

39. McArdle, W.D.; Katch, F.I.; Katch, V.L. Exercise physiology. Energy, nutrition, and human performance. Philadelphia: Lea & Febiger; 1981:p. 154-196.

40. Mercier, J.; Varray, A.; Ramonatxo, M.; Mercier, B.; Prefaut, C. Influence of anthropometric characteristics on changes in maximal exercise ventilation and breathing pattern during growth in boys. Eur. J. Appl. Physiol. 63:235-241; 1991.

41. Morse, M.; Schultz, F.W.; Cassels, D.E. Relation of age to physiological responses of the older boy (10-17 years) to exercise. J. Appl. Physiol. 1:683-709; 1949.

42. O'Brodovich, H.M.; Mellins, R.B.; Mansell, A.L. Effects of growth on the diffusion constant for carbon monoxide. Am. Rev. Respir. Dis. 125:670-673; 1982.

43. Radford, E.P. Ventilation standards for use in artificial respiration. J. Appl. Physiol. 5:451-460; 1954.

44. Ramonatxo, M.; Mercier, J.; Abdallah El-Fassi-Ben, R.; Vago, P.; Prefaut, C. Breathing pattern and occlusion pressure during exercise in pre and peripubertal swimmers. Respir. Physiol. 65:351-364; 1986.

45. Robinson, S. Experimental studies of physical fitness in relation to age. Arbeitsphysiologie 10:318-323; 1938.

46. Ross Laboratories. Children are different: relation of age to physiologic function. Columbus, OH; 1970.

47. Rowland, T.W.; Boyajian, A. Aerobic response to endurance training in children. Pediatrics; 96:654-658; 1995.
48. Rowland, T.W.; Green, G.M. The influence of biological maturation and aerobic fitness on ventilatory responses to treadmill exercise. In: Dotson, C.O.; Humphrey, J.H., eds. Exercise physiology. Current selected research. New York: AMS Press; 1990:p. 51-59.
49. Rowland, T.W.; Rimany, T.A. Physiological responses to prolonged exercise in premenarcheal and adult females. Pediatr. Exerc. Science 7:183-191; 1995.
50. Rutenfranz, J.; Andersen, K.L.; Seliger, V.; Klimmer, F.; Ilmarinen, J.; Ruppel, M.; Kylian, H. Exercise ventilation during the growth spurt period: comparison between two European countries. Eur. J. Pediatr. 136:135-142; 1981.
51. Schmidt-Nielsen, K. Scaling. Why is animal size so important? Cambridge: Cambridge University Press; 1984:p. 99-103.
52. Shephard, R.J.; Allen, C.; Bar-Or, O.; Davies, C.T.M.; Degre, S.; Hedman, R.; Ishi, K. The working capacity of Toronto schoolchildren. Part II. Canad. Med. Ass. J. 100:705-714; 1969.
53. Shephard, R.J.; Bar-Or, O. Alveolar ventilation in near maximum exercise. Data on pre-adolescent children and young adults. Med. Sci. Sports 2:83-92; 1970.
54. Sundberg, S.; Elovainio, R. Cardiorespiratory function in competitive endurance runners aged 12-16 years compared with ordinary boys. Acta Paediatr. Scand. 71:987-992; 1982.
55. Unnithan, V. Factors affecting submaximal running economy in children [doctoral thesis]. Glasgow: University of Glasgow; 1993.
56. Vaccaro, P.; Clarke, D.H. Cardiorespiratory alterations in 9 to 11 year old children following a season of competitive swimming. Med. Sci. Sports 10:204-207; 1978.
57. Vaccaro, P.; Poffenbarger, A. Resting and exercise respiratory function in young female child runners. J. Sports Med. 22:102-107; 1982.
58. Wasserman, K. Breathing during exercise. N. Eng. J. Med. 298:780-785; 1978.
59. Wasserman, K. Coupling of external to internal respiration. Am. Rev. Respir. Dis. 129 Suppl:S21-S24; 1984.
60. Weng, T.; Levison, H. Standards of pulmonary function in children. Am. Rev. Respir. Dis. 99:879-894; 1969.
61. Wohl, M.E.B.; Mead, J. Age as a factor in respiratory disease. In: Chernick, V., ed. Disorders of the respiratory tract in children. 5th ed. Philadelphia: Saunders; 1990:p. 175-181.
62. Yost, L.J.; Zauner, C.W.; Jaeger, M.L. Pulmonary diffusing capacity and physical working capacity in young competitive swimmers and untrained youths. Physiologist 20:103-108; 1977.
63. Zanconato, S.; Cooper, D.M.; Barstow, T.J.; Landaw, E. $^{13}CO_2$ washout dynamics during intermittent exercise in children and adults. J. Appl. Physiol. 73:2476-2482; 1992.
64. Zapletal, A.; Paul, T.; Samanek, M. Pulmonary elasticity in children and adolescents. J. Appl. Physiol. 40:953–958; 1976.

CHAPTER 10

RESPONSE TO ENDURANCE EXERCISE: PERIPHERAL FACTORS

Compared to the cardiovascular and ventilation responses to exercise, the following peripheral factors contributing to aerobic fitness in children lie largely shrouded in mystery:

- Hemoglobin concentration
- Total hemoglobin mass
- Blood volume
- Oxygen-hemoglobin dissociation curve
- Muscle capillarization
- Mitochondrial density
- Myoglobin concentration
- Aerobic enzyme activity

These variables are collectively manifest as the *peripheral arteriovenous oxygen (a-$\bar{v}$ O_2) difference,* an indicator of the total amount of O_2 extracted by the tissues. According to the Fick equation, a-$\bar{v}$ O_2 difference multiplied by cardiac output determines O_2 uptake.

Some quick arithmetic illustrates the key role of these peripheral factors in establishing one's level of aerobic fitness. Oxygen uptake at maximal exercise may reach 10 to 20 times resting values, depending on age and fitness. Achieving this magnitude of O_2 uptake clearly exceeds the capability of the heart to generate cardiac output. In fact, without the contribution of increases in peripheral O_2 extraction with exercise, maximal cardiac output in an adult would have to reach 100 L/min to achieve expected levels of $\dot{V}O_2$max (35). The negative impact on aerobic fitness created by chronic illnesses that affect a-$\bar{v}$ O_2 difference (anemia, muscle disease) is further witness to the critical importance of these factors in determining exercise performance (2).

The paucity of research information on peripheral aerobic factors in children reflects problems of both limited methodology and ethical constraints. There have, for instance, been few direct measurements of a-$\bar{v}$ O_2 difference in children, the limited data having been obtained in the resting state at the time of cardiac catheterization. Values of a-$\bar{v}$ O_2 difference during exercise in young subjects have been derived from measurements of O_2 uptake and estimates of cardiac output. The questionable accuracy of the latter (see chapter 8) compounds the uncertainty of calculated values for peripheral O_2 extraction. Equally problematic, the ethical issues surrounding muscle biopsies in children have restricted our knowledge of metabolic changes within the exercising muscle during the growing years.

This chapter will summarize current information regarding the changes in peripheral factors that contribute to aerobic fitness during childhood. It is tempting to speculate that these alterations might significantly influence the development of endurance performance with increasing age. There are, however, no data available to directly support or refute this idea.

THE ADULT MODEL

At rest, the O_2 content (product of hemoglobin concentration and its O_2-binding capacity) of arterial blood in the adult is approximately 19 ml O_2/100 cc blood. Mixed venous O_2 content (i.e., that measured on the right side of the heart) is typically 14 ml/100 cc. Consequently, the a-$\bar{v}$ O_2 difference of an adult in the resting state can be expected to be about 5 ml/100 cc. During progressively intense exercise, arterial O_2 content changes little, while increased O_2 extraction by the contracting muscles causes the mixed venous value to fall. At maximal exercise the mixed venous O_2 content may be as low as 2-3 ml/100 cc, resulting in a maximal a-$\bar{v}$ O_2 difference of 16 ml/100 cc. In the early stages of lower extremity exercise (running, cycling), femoral venous O_2 content is significantly lower than that in mixed venous samples. However, progressive vasoconstriction in nonexercising tissues causes femoral and mixed venous values to be similar at maximal exercise, when over 85% of available O_2 is extracted from the bloodstream by contracting muscles (1, 35, 39, 44).

In a nonathletic young adult, O_2 uptake usually increases from rest to maximal exercise by a factor of about 14. Cardiac output rises to four times resting values, while the increase in a-$\bar{v}$ O_2 difference is slightly more than threefold. While a trained endurance athlete can improve $\dot{V}O_2$max to 20 times resting levels, maximal a-$\bar{v}$ O_2 difference may be no greater than in the nonathlete (39).

A redistribution of blood flow away from nonexercising tissue by arteriolar vasoconstriction of splanchnic and renal vascular beds also improves O_2 delivery to exercising muscle. Blood flow through the splanchnic vessels declines from 1100 ml/min at light exercise to 300 ml/min at maximal exercise, and a similar decline is observed in blood supply to the kidneys. At the same time, muscle blood flow increases by a factor of 5 (35).

During a progressive exercise test, a-$\bar{v}$ O_2 difference steadily rises, but some data suggest that most of the increase occurs in the early stages. Saltin described values reaching half of maximum by 30-40% $\dot{V}O_2$max (42). This tapering of a-$\bar{v}$ O_2 difference at high-intensity exercise mimics a similar pattern observed in heart rate (see chapter 8).

Sufficient blood hemoglobin concentration is important for aerobic fitness, and values correlate with maximal O_2 uptake. Athletes tend to exhibit a slightly lower hemoglobin concentration than nonathletes, resulting from dilution of hemoglobin from an increased plasma volume effect of training.

Capillary density of muscle, mitochondrial volume, and activity of cellular aerobic enzymes all influence the ability of muscle to utilize aerobic metabolism during exercise. A period of physical training enhances each of these factors. Improvements in the content of oxidative enzymes may correlate more closely with aerobic work capacity (the ability to sustain endurance activities) than with $\dot{V}O_2$max, however. This may reflect a greater utilization of lipids for oxidation during sustained exercise in subjects who have a higher content of cellular aerobic enzymes.

The aerobic function of skeletal muscle is also influenced by distribution of fiber types. Fibers may be *slow-twitch* (type 1), rich in mitochondria and high in aerobic enzyme content for endurance exercise, or *fast-twitch* (type 2), possessing the ability to generate energy rapidly for short-burst activities. The distribution of these two fiber types varies from muscle to muscle in a given person as well as between individuals. All research evidence is not consistent, but most data indicate that the distribution of these fibers is genetically fixed, although the metabolic activities of both types can be enhanced with training.

ARTERIOVENOUS OXYGEN DIFFERENCE

Limited information suggests that the a-$\bar{v}$ O_2 difference both at rest and during exercise is age-independent and that values for children and adults are similar. Resting values are available from two studies of children involving direct measurement during supine cardiac catheterization. Sproul and Simpson reported a mean value for a-$\bar{v}$ O_2 difference of 4.1 ml/100 ml in a group of normal, healthy children between the ages of 6 and 16 years (48). No relationship was observed between a-$\bar{v}$ O_2 difference and age (r = .11). Similarly, Krovetz et al. found an average a-$\bar{v}$ O_2 difference of 4.4 ml/100 ml in 29 children who were 0-20 years of age (26).

Maximal Exercise

Yamaji and Miyashita estimated a-$\bar{v}$ O_2 difference at maximal exercise from CO_2 rebreathing measurements of cardiac output determined within 17 s of the end of the test (51). The subjects were 77 Japanese boys ages 10-18 years. Considerable variability in mean maximal aerobic power was observed in the different age groups (38.6 ml $\cdot$ kg^{-1} $\cdot$ min^{-1} for the 10-year-olds, for instance, and 50.5 ml $\cdot$ kg^{-1} $\cdot$ min^{-1} for the 14-year-olds). Maximal a-$\bar{v}$ O_2 difference ranged from 10.3 ml/100 ml to 13.3 ml/100 ml with no clear-cut age trend.

Johnson et al. measured maximal O_2 uptake and estimated maximal cardiac output by acetylene rebreathing in subjects 8-28 years old (17). Average calculated a-$\bar{v}$ O_2 differences in children ages 8-12 years and adults ages 15-28 years were 15.2 and 15.9 ml/100 ml, respectively.

Eriksson reported resting and maximal values for a-$\bar{v}$ O_2 difference in nine boys ages 11-13 years (11). The results were obtained by calculation from cardiac output estimated by the dye dilution technique during cycle exercise. The average resting value of 4.5 ml/100 ml is consistent with values from the studies done during cardiac catheterization. During the final minute of exhaustive exercise, a-$\bar{v}$ O_2 difference rose to a mean of 14.2 ml/100 ml. This compares with maximal a-$\bar{v}$ O_2 difference findings in four studies in adults, which averaged 14.0 ml/100 ml (11).

On the other hand, Miyamura and Honda reported that the average calculated maximal a-$\bar{v}$ O_2 difference in 9-12-year-old boys was 10.9 ml/100 ml while the value in subjects 13-20 years of age was 13.5 ml/100 ml (36). In that study, maximal cardiac output was determined by CO_2 rebreathing. Using the same technique, Gilliam et al. also showed an age-related increase in maximal a-$\bar{v}$ O_2 difference (13). Values were 12.2, 13.5, and 14.6 ml/100 ml in children 6-8, 9-10, and 11-13 years old, respectively.

Training Effects

Results of studies examining the influence of aerobic training on peripheral O_2 extraction in adults have been conflicting. Saltin et al. (43) and others (6, 15, 38, 42) have reported that approximately half of improvements in $\dot{V}O_2$max after training of adult subjects can be accounted for by an increase in maximal a-$\bar{v}$ O_2 uptake. These results are consistent with reports of improved muscle capillarization, increased mitochondrial density, and greater myoglobin and cellular aerobic enzyme content triggered by regular endurance exercise. However, other investigators describe no significant changes in peripheral O_2 extraction after training, reporting that increases in $\dot{V}O_2$max are entirely the result of improvements in maximal cardiac output. For example, adult athletes with an average maximal O_2 uptake of 5.2 l min[-1] have been observed to have no significantly greater a-$\bar{v}$ O_2 difference at maximal exercise than nonathletes with a $\dot{V}O_2$max of 3.2 l min[-1] (39).

Eriksson studied the influence of a 16-week aerobic training program on peripheral O_2 extraction in nine boys 11-13 years old (11). Average maximal O_2 uptake rose from 39 to 45 ml · kg[-1] · min[-1]. No significant change in a-$\bar{v}$ O_2 difference was observed either at rest or at maximal exercise following training. Improvements in maximal cardiac output in these boys were therefore entirely responsible for augmented aerobic fitness from the training program.

Pattern of Increased Arteriovenous Oxygen Difference With Exercise

As noted previously, studies in adults suggest a curvilinear rise in peripheral O_2 extraction during progressive exercise, with the greatest increase occurring at low intensity levels. In adult athletes, a-$\bar{v}$ O_2 difference has been reported to actually plateau at near-maximal exercise (39). Rowland et al. described the same pattern in calculating exercise a-$\bar{v}$ O_2 from $\dot{V}O_2$ and cardiac output (by thoracic bioimpedance) in 10-12-year-old boys (see fig. 10.1) (40). In the study of Eriksson, however, the

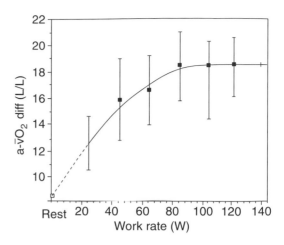

Figure 10.1 Pattern of arteriovenous O_2 difference with progressive exercise in children.

rise in a-$\bar{v}$ O_2 difference with increasing exercise intensity was strictly linear (11).

HEMATOLOGICAL FACTORS

The transport of O_2 by blood constitutes a critical link in the chain of O_2 delivery to exercising muscle. Maturational changes in hemoglobin concentration, total hemoglobin mass, blood volume, and characteristics of the hemoglobin-O_2 dissociation curve might therefore be expected to influence the development of aerobic fitness in children.

Hemoglobin

The concentration of hemoglobin in the blood rises slowly during the course of childhood. Values in the prepubertal years are similar in boys and girls, but at the onset of puberty the increase in hemoglobin concentration accelerates in males and plateaus in females.

Dallman and Siimes produced percentile curves for hemoglobin levels in children derived from 9946 subjects ages 0.5 to 16 years (see fig. 10.2) (8). From these data one can predict that the average 2-year-old boy or girl with a hemoglobin concentration of 12.6 g/dl will show a rise to 13.7 g/dl by age 12. During the early teenage years, we see a major escalation of values for males, presumably the effect of testosterone on red cell production. The average value for a 16-year-old boy (15.2 g/dl) is 10.9% greater than that of a girl the same age (13.7 g/dl). Changes in hemoglobin concentration with age are presumably not a reflection of changes in body dimensions. Studies in mature animals have shown that hemoglobin concentration is similar in all species and is independent of animal size (45).

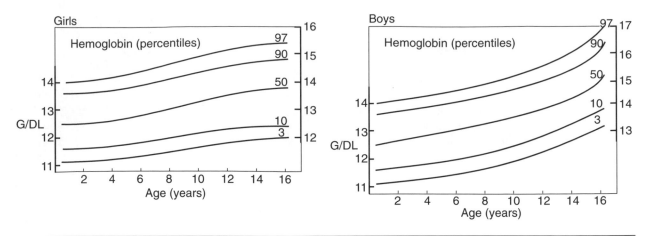

Figure 10.2   Changes in hemoglobin concentration with growth during childhood. Reprinted from Dallman et al. 1979.

A gram of fully saturated hemoglobin will hold 1.34 ml of O_2. It follows that the O_2-carrying capacity of hemoglobin improves for boys from 16.8 ml/100 cc at age 2 years to 20.3 ml/100 cc at age 16. The increase is less dramatic in females (16.8 rising to 18.4 ml/100 cc). As values of mixed venous O_2 content with maximal exercise are not available in children, the effect of their lower arterial O_2 content on O_2 delivery is uncertain. If adults can lower venous content to 2-3 ml/100 ml at exhaustive exercise, children would appear to have less a-$\bar{v}$ O_2 reserve than adults (see fig. 10.3). The data on this question, presented earlier in this chapter, are mixed: it is not clear whether differences in peripheral

O_2 extraction with maximal exercise exist between prepubertal and postpubertal subjects.

In this regard, it is of interest to note that the 11-13-year-old boys studied by Eriksson had maximal a-$\bar{v}$ O_2 differences almost identical to those previously described in adult subjects but utilized 86% of their O_2-carrying capacity versus 73-77% in the adult studies (11). This suggests that the lower hemoglobin concentration in normal children compared to adults does not adversely influence a-$\bar{v}$ O_2 difference during exercise. It is not difficult to hypothesize, however, that the capacity for *increasing* peripheral O_2 extraction with aerobic training might consequently be limited in prepubertal

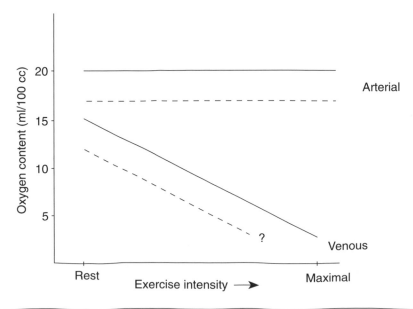

Figure 10.3   Arteriovenous O_2 difference with exercise in children (- - -) and adults (—). Lower values of arterial and venous O_2 content in children suggest possible limitation of O_2 uptake at maximal exercise.

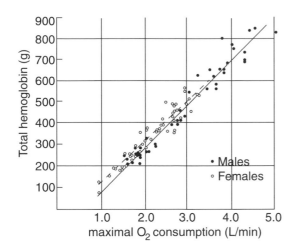

Figure 10.4 Relationship of total body hemoglobin with O_2 uptake in children. Reprinted from Åstrand 1952.

subjects. This restriction, based on a lower blood hemoglobin concentration, could contribute to the smaller improvements in $\dot{V}O_2$max seen with endurance training programs in children (see chapter 7).

Age-related changes in hemoglobin concentration are reflected in alterations in the red blood cell mass. Mean hematocrit values (volume of red cells packed by centrifugation) are 35.5% at age 2 years and 39.0% at age 12 (46). The average hematocrits in the mature male and female are 47% and 42%, respectively.

Åstrand demonstrated a close linear relationship between total body hemoglobin content and maximal O_2 uptake across all age levels and in both sexes (1) (see fig. 10.4). He found that total hemoglobin per body mass was essentially stable and gender-independent in

the prepubertal years, with values of approximately 7.7 g/kg. At puberty there was no change in the girls, but values rose to 10.0 g/kg in the boys.

Training Effects. There is no evidence that blood hemoglobin levels are influenced by either aerobic fitness or endurance training in children. The nine boys ages 11-13 years in Eriksson's study had a mean concentration of 14.7 g/100 ml after 16 weeks of aerobic training compared to a pretraining value of 14.2 g/100 ml (11). As will be noted later, however, total hemoglobin values improved with training. Sundberg and Elovainio could find no significant differences in hemoglobin concentrations between endurance runners and nonathletes 12-16 years old (50). Rowland et al. assessed the hematological status of female high school cross-country runners (n = 20), swimmers (n = 15), and nonathletes (n = 30). Mean hemoglobin concentrations for the three groups were 13.3, 13.3, and 13.4 g/dl, respectively (41).

Oxygen-Hemoglobin Dissociation Curve. The O_2-hemoglobin dissociation curve describes the influence of changes in blood PO_2 on percentage of hemoglobin that is bound with O_2. A shift of this curve to the right facilitates O_2 release at the tissue level and should be expected to improve the amount of O_2 available for aerobic metabolism during exercise. Factors that can influence such a shift include increases in acidity, temperature, CO_2 content, and concentration of 2,3-diphosphoglycerate (2,3-DPG), a substance produced by anaerobic metabolism within the red blood cells (35).

Cassels and Morse studied the influence of age on the shape of the O_2-hemoglobin dissociation curve at rest (5). As illustrated in figure 10.5, a slight shift to the right in the steep portion of the curve was observed in

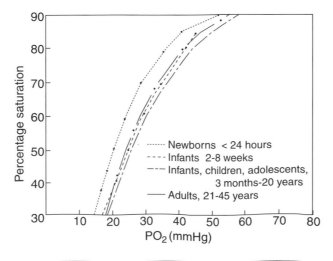

Figure 10.5 Oxygen-hemoglobin dissociation curve in humans relative to age. Reprinted from Cassels and Morse 1962.

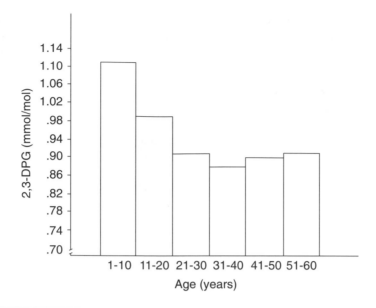

Figure 10.6   Changes in red blood cell 2,3-DPG concentration with age. Data from Kalofoutis et al. (18).

children and adolescents compared to adults. A similar shift has been found in adults after physical training (6), but this has not been studied in children. Claussen suggested that the small enhancement of O_2 release to the muscle created by this rightward shift is unlikely to contribute significantly to improvements in a-$\bar{v}$ O_2 difference (6).

It is not clear which of the several factors that influence the position of the O_2-hemoglobin dissociation curve are responsible for this age difference. An inverse relationship between hemoglobin and 2,3-DPG concentrations has been described (9). Kalofoutis et al. reported changes in red blood cell 2,3-DPG with age (see fig. 10.6) (18). Subjects ages 1 to 10 years old exhibited 11% higher values than those 11 to 20 years. A similar decline was observed in the third decade of life; values stabilized thereafter. These findings suggest that increased 2,3-DPG levels in children might serve to help compensate for lower arterial O_2 content resulting from decreased hemoglobin concentrations.

An examination of O_2-dissociation curves of animals (see fig. 10.7) reveals a consistent rightward shift in smaller animals: the smaller the animal, the greater is the facility for O_2 unloading at the tissues (45). This finding has been considered consistent with the need of smaller animals to sustain relatively higher metabolic rates. The pattern cannot be ascribed to difference in hemoglobin concentration, which is size-independent.

Blood Volume

Total blood volume increases with growth of the child. Koch described mean values in boys of 2.4 L at age 10 years, increasing to 4.0 L at age 16 (21). Resting blood

volumes per kg body mass reported by Cassels and Morse did not change appreciably between the ages of 7 and 17 years (mean of .089 L/kg) (5). When blood volume is expressed relative to body surface area, however, a progressive increase is observed as children grow.

Animal studies also show that relative blood volume is independent of mass, with a usual value of 60-70 cc/kg. Stahl presented an equation for relating blood

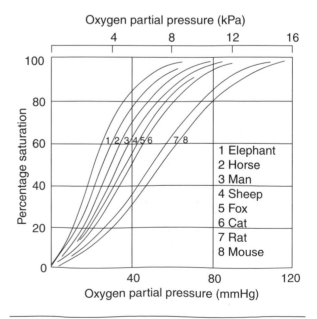

Figure 10.7   The O_2-hemoglobin dissociation curve in animals relative to body size. Reprinted from Schmidt-Nielsen 1984.

volume (V_b in ml) in animals relative to body mass (M, in kg): $V_b = 65.6 M^{1.02}$ (49).

Responses to Acute Exercise. Cassels and Morse exercised boys 12-17 years old to exhaustion on a treadmill in order to examine changes in blood volume (5). Values declined between 4.8% and 6.9%, with the smaller decrease in the younger age groups. It is difficult to tell whether these results truly indicated age-related differences in blood volume responses to acute exercise. In a separate test, subjects exercised at steady state moderate intensity for 15 min. Blood volume changes ranged from −4.8% to −7.1%, with no discernible age trend.

Mácek et al. evaluated changes in plasma volume from hematocrit values during prolonged exercise in children (32). Ten prepubertal boys exercised on a cycle and treadmill at 40% and 60% $\dot{V}O_2$max for 60 min. No changes were observed at 60%max, but at 40%max a 1% fall in hematocrit was observed, limited to the first 10 min. This was interpreted as a mild hemodilution at onset of endurance exercise. In adults, however, slight hemoconcentration has been observed in similar studies.

Responses to Training. Two studies, one longitudinal and the other cross-sectional, have indicated a relationship of aerobic fitness with blood volume and total hemoglobin in children. Eriksson reported an increase in blood volume from 2.92 to 3.28 L (12.3%) in 12 boys 11-13 years old after 16 weeks of endurance training (p < .01) (11). Total hemoglobin rose from 389 g to 428 g (10%), while blood hemoglobin concentration did not change. These alterations occurred while $\dot{V}O_2$max improved from 1.86 L/min to 2.21 L/min (an 18.8% increase). These responses are similar to those observed in adults (11).

Koch and Rocker described plasma volume and hemoglobin values in eight athletic 13-15-year-old boys (22). The subjects, who had a mean $\dot{V}O_2$max of 59.6 ml · kg^{-1} · min^{-1}, were participating regularly in a number of sports activities, including soccer, running, badminton, and ice hockey. Average plasma volume was 59.1 ml/kg, considerably greater than the expected mean of 44 ml/kg for 13-16-year-old nonathletes reported by Krasilnikoff and Weeks (23). However, no significant difference was found in weight-relative plasma volume between these athletic young adolescents and two groups of trained adult distance runners 17-20 and 24-30 years of age (mean $\dot{V}O_2$max 62.6 ml · kg^{-1} · min^{-1}).

MUSCLE AEROBIC CAPACITY

Little information is available about age-related differences in the aerobic machinery of the peripheral muscle cell, and these data are limited to studies of children in the resting state. Consequently, descriptions of the characteristics of muscle enzyme content and mitochondrial density in growing children can be expected to reflect principally maturational changes in the resting metabolic rate. How these alterations affect metabolism during exercise, as well as how these changes might be manifest in the normal evolution of endurance performance with age, is uncertain.

Animal Studies

An examination of studies evaluating muscle aerobic capacity in animals is important, because these reports indicate that tissue concentrations of aerobic enzymes and mitochondria in mature animals of various species are inversely related to body size. This is not altogether surprising, since mass-related O_2 uptake also diminishes as animals become larger. The findings suggest, then, that muscle aerobic capacity in children should decrease as they age in direct relationship with the normal decline in basal metabolic rate (relative to mass), both trends reflecting an increase in body size.

In his classic 1950 study, Krebs examined the metabolic rates of tissue slices in vivo of nine species ranging from mice to horses (24). Weight-relative rates of tissue O_2 uptake declined with increasing body size. Metabolic rates in liver slices, for instance, were almost three times greater in the mouse than in the horse. Martin and Fuhrman showed similar differences in the rates of muscle respiration in the mouse and dog (33). In these studies, the changes in tissue metabolism were not of sufficient magnitude, however, to entirely explain whole-body-weight-specific metabolic rates in the intact organism.

The components of muscle aerobic capacity of animals also scale inversely to body size. Kunkel et al. reported that muscle content of cytochrome oxidase was related to body mass by the scaling exponent −0.24 (27). In his study of rats, rabbits, sheep, and cattle, Smith found that the total number of mitochondria in the liver was proportional to body mass to the power 0.72 (47). Mathieu et al. reported that the density of mitochondria in 13 animal species was inversely related to body weight (34). In 10 animal species varying in size by a factor of 10^5, Emmett and Hochachka showed that the catalytic activities of muscle aerobic enzymes scaled inversely to body mass (10). (They also found that, in contrast, enzymes important for cellular anaerobic metabolism increased in their activity in larger animals. This will be discussed in chapter 12.) In summary, these studies all indicate that aerobic activity per gram of muscle decreases with increasing animal size.

In reviewing this literature, Hochachka concluded that the allometric scaling pattern of aerobic enzyme activity was a quantitative rather than a qualitative phenomenon (16). That is, "the large differences in enzyme activity per gram muscle is due to the amount of enzyme rather than to its catalytic efficiency" (p. 2). The same appears to hold true for mitochondrial differences. Over the broad range of animals, the O_2 consumption of a given volume of mitochondria is similar. "This means that muscles in small homeotherms have very high metabolic capacities compared to large animals because they amplify the number of copies of mitochondria, not because their mitochondria are catalytically more efficient" (p. 2).

Muscle Enzyme Content

The scope of size difference between children and adults is far less than that for the animals in the reports cited, but the same size-related trends in muscle oxidative capacity appear to be evident. Eriksson described findings of quadriceps femoris muscle biopsies in three groups of normal boys ages 11-15 years (11). Activities of succinate dehydrogenase (SDH) and phosphofructokinase (PFK) were determined as markers of aerobic and anaerobic enzyme function, respectively. Average SDH activity was 5.3 compared to 4.0 µmol/(g × min) observed in a group of 26 untrained men 24-52 years old. Respective values for PFK were 8.4 and 25.3 µmol/(g × min). These findings are consistent with the relationships observed between size and metabolic function in animals: anaerobic capacity increases with animal size, while the aerobic potential decreases (16).

Berg et al. reported similar findings in a study of resting quadriceps muscle enzyme activities in children 4-8, 12-14, and 16-18 years old (4). Activities of PFK, aldolase, and lactic dehydrogenase, all reflecting anaerobic metabolism, rose progressively with increasing age. Over the same age span the activities of the aerobic enzymes citrate synthetase and fumarase declined (see fig. 10.8). The authors examined the ratio of muscle fumarase to PFK activity in the three groups to assess the influence of age on the relationship of aerobic to anaerobic capacity. The ratio was .52 in the youngest children, .27 in the 12-14-year-olds, and .24 in the oldest subjects (see fig. 10.9).

Haralambie compared aerobic and anaerobic enzyme activities of vastus lateralis biopsies of 13-15-year-old adolescents with those of 22-42-year-old adults (14). There were no significant differences in glycolytic enzyme activities, including PFK, between the two groups. However, 5 of 6 aerobic enzymes of the tricarboxylic acid cycle had higher activities in the adolescent subjects. No significant gender differences were observed in either age group for 21 of the 22 enzymes studied.

There are few data on the changes in muscle aerobic capacity with endurance training in the childhood years. Five of the boys reported by Eriksson underwent 6 weeks of aerobic training (11). Maximal O_2 uptake expressed relative to the square of body height improved by 5.6%. Training resulted in a 30% increase in SDH activity (5.4 to 7.0 µmol/[g × min]), while PFK activity almost doubled (8.4 to 15.4 µmol/[g × min]). However,

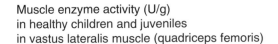

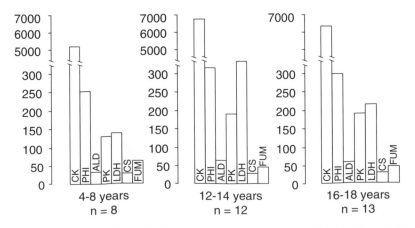

Figure 10.8 Muscle enzyme activity in healthy children. CK = creatine kinase; PHI = hexose phosphate isomerase; ALD = aldolase; PK = pyruvate kinase; LDH = lactic dehydrogenase; CS = citrate synthetase; FUM = fumarase. Reprinted from Berg, Kim, and Keul 1986.

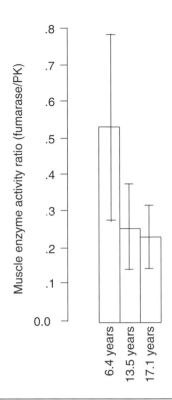

Figure 10.9 Ratio of muscle fumarase to pyruvate kinase in boys and girls of different ages, reflecting the ratio of aerobic to anaerobic activity (1 = 6.4 years; 2 = 13.5 years; 3 = 17.1 years). Reprinted from Bell et al. 1980.

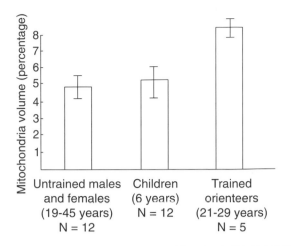

Figure 10.10 Mitochondrial volume density in muscle biopsies of children versus trained and untrained adults. From Bell et al. 1980.

even with training the PFK values were only 60% of those reported in untrained adults.

Fournier et al. examined the effects of running training and detraining on vastus lateralis enzyme activities in 12 boys in the postpubertal age group (16-17 years) (12). Half of the subjects were involved in sprint training, four times a week for 3 months, while the remainder participated in endurance training. Those training by endurance running increased $\dot{V}O_2$max from 58.4 to 64.3 ml · kg⁻¹ · min⁻¹; SDH activity, indicative of muscle aerobic capacity, rose 42%, while PFK did not change significantly. The sprint-trained boys demonstrated a similar rise in maximal aerobic power (59.5 to 63.2 ml · kg⁻¹ · min⁻¹), but no significant increase in SDH. However, activity of PFK rose 21%. Both groups were studied again after 6 months of detraining, when the training-induced gains in $\dot{V}O_2$max, SDH, and PFK were found to have been abolished.

From the limited research data, then, one can suggest that muscle aerobic capacity (as indicated by resting enzyme activities) declines during the childhood years. This pattern is consistent with the fall in metabolic rate related to body dimensions over the same period. It is important to note that this decline in aerobic enzyme ac-

tivity is occurring at the same time that endurance performance (i.e., 1-mile run time) progressively improves.

Endurance training appears to cause dramatic improvements in muscle aerobic capacity in the circumpubertal years. These changes are far greater than training-induced increases in $\dot{V}O_2$max or endurance performance.

Mitochondrial Density

The information just reviewed would lead one to expect children to exhibit a greater density of mitochondria in skeletal muscle. But the only study to address this question failed to demonstrate any important differences between young children and adults. Bell et al. obtained needle biopsy specimens from the vastus lateralis muscle in seven girls and six boys (mean age 6.4 years) (3). Mean maximal O_2 uptake for the group was 45.2 ml · kg⁻¹ · min⁻¹. On the average, mitochondria made up 5.54% of the total volume of the muscle fiber. This value is "slightly greater" than that reported for untrained adult men and women (4.9%) (p. 31; see figure 10.10).

The mitochondrial density of the children was found to be significantly correlated with the percentage of slow-twitch fibers (r = 0.69). However, no association was detected between $\dot{V}O_2$max and mitochondrial density (r = 0.39).

MUSCLE FIBER TYPES

The relative composition of slow- and fast-twitch fibers in the muscles of children has been reported by several investigators. Lexell et al. studied sections of vastus lateralis muscle from the autopsies of previously healthy males ages 5 to 37 years (29). These cross-sectional data showed that the proportion of type 2 fibers rose significantly from the ages of 5 years (about 35%) to 20 years (about 50%). The authors considered these findings as indicative of a transformation of type 1 to type 2 fibers during this time period.

In a similar study, Oertel examined fiber types in postmortem material from 113 subjects ages 1 week to 20 years who had died from accidents (37). The proportion of type 1 fibers increased from 40% at birth to about 60% by age 2 years. After that time the relative percentages of type 1 and type 2 fibers remained constant.

The muscle biopsy study in 6-year-olds by Bell et al. showed that 59% of fibers were slow-twitch, 20% were fast-twitch, and 21% were classified as fast-twitch oxidative, an intermediate fiber type (3). A significant correlation was observed between mitochondrial density and distribution of slow-twitch fibers (r = .69). Lundberg et al. reported 59% type 1 fibers in vastus lateralis muscle biopsies of 25 healthy children ages 2 months to 11 years (30). A similar slow-twitch fraction was described by Eriksson in 16 boys ages 12-15 years (60%) (11).

Although limited in number, these studies indicate a remarkably consistent finding of about 60% slow-twitch fibers in vastus lateralis muscle of children. This value is higher than that typical of sedentary adult subjects (usually about 35-45%) but is typical of percentages reported in trained adult endurance athletes (52-61%) (11). (Costill et al. have reported frequency of slow-twitch fibers as high as 90-98% among the world's best distance runners [7].)

It is tempting to conclude that the higher percentage of slow-twitch fibers in nonathletic children as compared to adults reflects greater muscle aerobic capacity in prepubertal subjects. Indeed, this finding complements both the animal and human data indicating greater aerobic enzyme activity in smaller individuals. However, distribution of fiber types has been considered genetically fixed, as most studies have failed to indicate changes with training. The high percentage of slow-twitch fiber types of the elite adult athlete appears, therefore, to be based on hereditary endowment rather than training adaptations.

Data on the response of muscle fiber composition to physical training in children is scant but is consistent with the studies in adults. Fournier et al. could find no change in percentage of slow- and fast-twitch fibers after 3 months of either sprint or endurance training in 16-17-year-old boys (12). Five 11-year-old boys reported by Eriksson had 54.8% slow-twitch fibers after 2 weeks of endurance training and 48.9% at 6 weeks (11). These values were considered within the normal variability of the biopsy method.

MUSCLE BLOOD FLOW

Koch investigated muscle blood flow during exercise in two studies of nine boys 1 year apart using the 133-xenon clearance method (20). Subjects were actively training in a number of sports and had an average maximal O_2 uptake of 59.5 ml $\cdot$ kg^{-1} $\cdot$ min^{-1}. The boys were initially studied at age 12 years; blood flow was determined (1) in the tibialis anterior muscle immediately after maximal ischemic resistance work and (2) in the vastus lateralis muscle during submaximal and maximal cycle exercise. The former is presumed to represent maximal blood flow capacity. Maximal blood flow (MBF) was significantly higher after the ischemic test than at maximal cycle exercise, and both values were greater than those observed in young adults. Also, in contrast to the pattern seen in adults, MBF rose continuously to maximal exercise levels. The percentage of MBF during maximal cycle exercise relative to ischemic work was lower in boys than in adults. The author noted, "If one considers this ratio as a measure of the MBF actually used in relation to the total flow reserve capacity, this implies that these boys used a smaller proportion of their total reserve capacity during maximal work" (p. 44).

The boys were studied again at 13 years of age, with changes indicating a trend toward the adult pattern (21). Peak MBF was reached at submaximal cycle exercise, and the percentage of MBF on this test relative to ischemic MBF increased. The absolute MBF on both tests declined from the values on the first evaluation but were still somewhat higher than in adult subjects.

This single investigation, then, suggests that muscle blood flow may be greater in children than in adults. This idea is consistent with animal studies dating back to the 1920s showing that smaller animals have greater capillary densities than larger ones (25). More recent reports suggest, however, that factors such as habitual use of the muscle may be more important than scaling considerations in determining capillary density. A very high capillary density is observed in the chewing jaw muscles of the sheep, for example (45).

The redistribution of blood flow that occurs during exercise prominently affects O_2 delivery to exercising muscle. Vasoconstriction of nonexercising vascular beds (e.g., renal, splanchnic) in the adult permits over 80% of cardiac output to be diverted to the working muscle.

Changes in organ blood flow with exercise have not been evaluated in children. As noted by Mácek, however, there is reason to suspect that the quantitative aspects of redistribution might be different in prepubertal subjects (31). Diminished norepinephrine levels at maximal exercise compared to those in adults suggest that children have less sympathetic activity (28); one should expect this to result in a lower capacity for peripheral vasoconstriction during high-intensity exercise. Besides causing less shunting of blood to exercising muscle, diminished vasoconstriction could result in relatively greater liver blood flow and enhanced hepatic clearance of metabolites (e.g., lactate) during exercise in children. This hypothesis awaits future research investigation.

SUMMARY

Much needs to be learned about the peripheral factors that affect aerobic fitness in children. The little information gained in research to date, however, suggests several intriguing concepts surrounding the development of these factors in the growing child. These changes may profoundly influence both O_2 metabolism and endurance performance.

Several independent lines of investigation indicate that the aerobic "fire" of the muscle cells burns less intensely as the child ages (19). This is, of course, in ac-

cord with the observation that total O_2 uptake relative to body size declines throughout the course of childhood. The activity of aerobic enzymes appears to be greater in children than in adults, and this is consistent with animal data indicating that oxidative enzyme activity scales inversely with body mass. Muscle blood flow may be greater during exercise in children. Limited biopsy and autopsy information also suggests that the percentage of slow-twitch oxidative muscle fibers is larger in children than in adults.

On the other hand, the increase in blood hemoglobin concentration, particularly in males at puberty, should be expected to improve O_2 delivery with age. Most data suggest that the younger child is not hampered by a smaller arterial O_2 content, as a-$\bar{v}$ O_2 difference both at rest and during exercise appears to be age-independent. It is possible, however, that the smaller improvements in $\dot{V}O_2$max with endurance training in children could reflect a limited reserve in ability to improve peripheral O_2 extraction.

What We Know

1. The a-$\bar{v}$ O_2 difference at rest and maximal exercise appears to be independent of age.

2. Blood hemoglobin concentration rises slowly during childhood, without gender differences. At puberty, significant increases are observed in males secondary to bone marrow stimulation by testosterone.

3. Athletic training does not influence hemoglobin concentration in children.

4. Blood volume relative to body mass does not change during childhood.

What We Would Like to Know

1. How do peripheral factors such as a-$\bar{v}$ O_2 difference, muscle aerobic capacity, and plasma volume respond to exercise training in children?

2. What is the normal pattern of change in peripheral O_2 extraction during progressive exercise?

3. Are muscle aerobic capacity, muscle fiber types, and capillary density of muscle different in children compared to adults?

4. Does the lower hemoglobin concentration and resulting decreased O_2-carrying capacity in children compared to adults limit aerobic fitness or response to aerobic training in children?

References

1. Åstrand, P.O. Experimental studies of physical working capacity in relationship to sex and age. Copenhagen: Munksgaard; 1952.

2. Bar-Or, O. Pathophysiological factors which limit the exercise capacity of the sick child. Med. Sci. Sports Exerc. 18:276-282; 1986.

3. Bell, R.D.; MacDougall, J.D.; Billeter, R.; Howald, H. Muscle fiber types and morphometric analysis of skeletal muscle in six-year-old children. Med. Sci. Sports Exerc. 12:28-31; 1980.

4. Berg, A.; Kim, S.S.; Keul, J. Skeletal muscle enzyme activities in healthy young subjects. Int. J. Sports Med. 7:236-239; 1986.

5. Cassels, D.E.; Morse, M. Cardiopulmonary data for children and young adults. Springfield, IL: Charles C Thomas; 1962:p. 23-34.

6. Claussen, J.P. Effect of physical training on cardiovascular adjustments to exercise in man. Physiol. Rev. 57:779-815; 1977.

7. Costill, D.L.; Fink, W.J.; Pollock, M.L. Muscle fiber composition and enzyme activities of elite distance runners. Med. Sci. Sports 8:96-100; 1976.

8. Dallman, P.R.; Siimes, M.A. Percentile curves for hemoglobin and red cell volume in infancy and childhood. J. Pediatr. 94:26-31; 1979.

9. Eaten, J.W.; Brewer, G.J. The relationship between red cell 2,3-diphosphoglycerate and levels of hemoglobin in the human. Proc. Nat. Acad. Sci. 61:756-761; 1968.

10. Emmett, B.; Hochachka, P.W. Scaling of oxidative glycolytic enzymes in mammmals. Respir. Physiol. 45:261-272; 1981.

11. Eriksson, B.O. Physical training, oxygen supply, and muscle metabolism in 11-13 year old boys. Acta Physiol. Scand. Suppl. 384:1-48; 1972.

12. Fournier, M.; Ricci, J.; Taylor, A.W.; Ferguson, R.J.; Montpetit, R.R.; Chaitman, B.R. Skeletal muscle adaptation in adolescent boys: sprint and endurance training and detraining. Med. Sci. Sports Exerc. 14:453-456; 1982.

13. Gilliam, T.B.; Sady, S.; Thorland, W.G.; Weltman, A.C. Comparison of peak performance measures in children ages 6 to 8, 9 to 10, and 11 to 13 years. Res. Quart. 48:695-702; 1977.

14. Haralambie, G. Enzyme activities in skeletal muscle of 13-15 year old adolescents. Bull. Europ. Physiopath. Resp. 18:65-74; 1982.

15. Hartley, L.H.; Grimby, G.; Kilbom, A.; Nilsson, N.J.; Åstrand, I.; Bjure, J.; Ekblom, B.; Saltin, B. Physical training in sedentary middle-aged and older men. Scand. J. Clin. Lab. Invest. 24:335-344; 1969.

16. Hochachka, P.W. The biochemical limits of muscle work. In: Taylor, A.W.; Gollnick, P.D.; Green, H.J.; Ianuzzo, C.D.; Noble, E.G.; Métivier, G.; Sutton, J.R., eds. Biochemistry of exercise VII. Champaign, IL: Human Kinetics; 1990:p. 1-8.

17. Johnson, R.L.; Taylor, H.F.; Lawson, W.H. Maximal diffusing capacity of the lung for carbon monoxide. J. Clin. Invest. 44:349-355; 1965.

18. Kalofoutis, A.; Paterakis, S.; Koutselinis, A.; Spanos, V. Relationship between erythrocyte 2, 3—diphosphoglycerate and age in a normal population. Clin. Chem. 22:1918-1919; 1976.

19. Kleiber, M. The fire of life. An introduction to animal energetics. New York: Wiley; 1961:p. 177-230.

20. Koch, G. Muscle blood flow after ischemic work and during bicycle ergometry work in boys aged 12 years. Acta Paediatr. Belg. 28 Suppl:29-39; 1974.

21. Koch, G. Muscle blood flow in prepubertal boys. Med. Sport 11:39-46; 1978.

22. Koch, G.; Rocker, L. Plasma volume and intravascular protein masses in trained boys and fit young men. J. Appl. Physiol. 43:1085-1088; 1977.

23. Krasilnikoff, P.A.; Weeks, B. The intravascular mass of 21 serum proteins in normal mature and premature children. Protides Biol. Fluids Proc. Colloq. 18:169-171; 1971.

24. Krebs, H.A. Body size and tissue respiration. Biochim. Biophys. Acta 4:249-269; 1950.

25. Krogh, A. The anatomy and physiology of capillaries. 2nd ed. New Haven, CT: Yale University Press; 1929.

26. Krovetz, L.J.; McLoughlin, T.G.; Mitchell, M.B.; Schiebler, G.L. Hemodynamic findings in normal children. Pediatr. Res. 1:122-130; 1967.

27. Kunkel, H.O.; Spalding, J.F.; de Franciscis, G.; Futrell, M.F. Cytochrome oxidase activity and body weight in rats and in three species of large animals. Amer. J. Physiol. 186:203-206; 1956.

28. Lehmann, M.; Keul, J.; Korsten-Reck, U. The influence of graduated treadmill exercise on plasma catecholamines; aerobic and anaerobic capacity in boys and adults. Eur. J. Appl. Physiol. 47:301-311; 1981.

29. Lexell, J.; Sjostrom, M.; Nordlund, A.; Taylor, C.C. Growth and development of human muscle: a quantitative morphological study of whole vastus lateralis from childhood to adult age. Muscle Nerve 15:404-409; 1992.

30. Lundberg, A.; Eriksson, B.O.; Mellgren, G. Metabolic substrates, muscle fibre composition, and fibre size in late walking and normal children. Eur. J. Pediatr. 130:79-92; 1979.

31. Mácek, M. Aerobic and anaerobic energy output in children. In: Rutenfranz, J.; Mocellin, R.; Klimt, F., eds. Children and exercise XII. Champaign, IL: Human Kinetics; 1986:p. 3-11.

32. Mácek, M.; Vavra, J.; Novosadova, J. Prolonged exercise in prepubertal boys. Europ. J. Appl. Physiol. 35:299-303; 1976.

33. Martin, A.W.; Fuhrman, F.A. The relationship between summated tissue respiration and metabolic rate in the mouse and dog. Physiol. Zool. 28:18-34; 1955.

34. Mathieu, O.; Krauer, R.; Hoppeler, H.; Gehr, P.; Lindstedt, S.L.; Alexander, R.; Taylor, C.R.; Weibel, E.R. Design of the mammalian respiratory system. VII. Scaling mitochondrial volume in skeletal muscle to body mass. Resp. Physiol. 44:113-128; 1981.

35. McArdle, W.D.; Katch, F.I.; Katch, V.L. Exercise physiology. Energy, nutrition, and human performance. Philadelphia: Lea & Febiger; 1981:p. 228-229.

36. Miyamura, M.; Honda, Y. Maximum cardiac output related to sex and age. Jap. J. Physiol. 23:645-656; 1973.

37. Oertel, G. Morphometric analysis of normal skeletal muscles in infancy, childhood and adolescence. An autopsy study. J. Neurol. Sci. 88:303-313; 1988.
38. Rowell, L.B. Human cardiovascular adjustments to exercise and thermal stress. Physiol. Rev. 54:75-159; 1974.
39. Rowell, L.B. Human circulation. Regulation during physical stress. Oxford: Oxford University Press; 1986:p. 213-287.
40. Rowland, T.W.; Staab, J.; Unnithan, V.; Siconolfi, S. Maximal cardiac responses in prepubertal and adult males [abstract]. Med. Sci. Sports Exerc. 20 Suppl:S332; 1988.
41. Rowland, T.W., Stagg, L.; Kelleher, J.F. Iron deficiency in adolescent girls. Are athletes at increased risk? J. Adol. Health 12:22-25; 1991.
42. Saltin, B. Physiological effects of physical conditioning. Med. Sci. Sports 1:50-56; 1969.
43. Saltin, B.; Blomqvist, G.; Mitchell, J.H.; Johnson, R.L.; Wildenthal, K.; Chapman, C.B. Response to exercise after bed rest and after training. Circulation 38 Suppl 7:1-78; 1968.
44. Saltin, B.; Hartley, L.H.; Kilbom, A.; Åstrand, I. Physical training in sedentary middle-aged and older men. II. Oxygen uptake, heart rate, and blood lactate concentrations at submaximal and maximal exercise. Scand. J. Clin. Lab. Invest. 24:323-334; 1969.
45. Schmidt-Nielsen, K. Scaling. Why is animal size so important? Cambridge: Cambridge University Press; 1984.
46. Smith, C.H. Blood diseases of infancy and childhood. St. Louis: Mosby; 1972:p. 13-22.
47. Smith, R.E. Quantitative relations between liver mitochondria and total body weight in mammals. Ann. N.Y. Acad. Sci. 62:403-422; 1956.
48. Sproul, A.; Simpson, E. Stroke volume and related hemodynamic data in normal children. Pediatrics 33:912-918; 1964.
49. Stahl, W.R. Scaling of respiratory variables in mammals. J. Appl. Physiol. 22:453-460; 1967.
50. Sundberg, S.; Elovainio, R. Cardiorespiratory function in competitive endurance runners aged 12-16 years compared with ordinary boys. Acta Paediatr. Scand. 71:987-992; 1982.
51. Yamaji, K.; Miyashita, M. Oxygen transport system during exhaustive exercise in Japanese boys. Europ. J. Appl. Physiol. 36:93-99; 1977.

CHAPTER 11

SUBMAXIMAL ENERGY EXPENDITURE

It might be assumed that physiological processes will always operate at a minimal energy cost. Nature is not wasteful, and one should expect that animals will accomplish locomotion in the most energy-efficient manner—performing the greatest amount of work at the least energy cost. It is intriguing, then, that one of the most consistent findings in developmental exercise physiology is the progressive improvement in energy economy during weight-bearing exercise as children grow. These differences are more than minimal. For instance, if a 6-year-old child and a young adult are walking at the same speed, the metabolic cost to the child of moving a kilogram of body mass may be 30% greater than for the young adult (86).

Why are children so apparently wasteful in energy expenditure compared to adults? What factors are responsible for the progressive improvement in efficiency of locomotion during childhood? Can changes in submaximal exercise economy in children be translated into improvements in physical performance? Can energy economy of locomotion be manipulated in children through physical training? These are questions this chapter will address.

The study of submaximal exercise economy bears importance for both children and adults for a number of reasons. Our typical daily activities, of course, are rarely maximal, and the efficiency with which we perform these submaximal physical tasks may influence our capacity for both recreational and occupational work. Some studies in adult athletes suggest that performance in distance events is directly related to economy of submaximal motion.

Understanding economy may also help people with chronic illnesses. For example, some children with muscle diseases display poor exercise economy (3); learning more about the causes of this inefficiency may provide insight into the reasons for their poor muscle function as well as means of improving their work capacity.

DEFINITIONS OF EFFICIENCY AND ECONOMY

In the interest of preventing confusion, certain definitions are in order at the start of this chapter on changes in energy costs of locomotion during childhood. *Muscular efficiency* is the work accomplished during exercise divided by the energy expended. On the cycle ergometer, the numerator is readily determined by the load applied, while the denominator is established by measurement of the O_2 uptake demand, converted to its caloric equivalent with the respiratory exchange ratio taken into account.

A large number of variables, both biochemical and mechanical, contribute to muscular efficiency. Some, such as efficiency of contraction coupling and the fraction of energy released from adenosine triphosphate in the muscle cell, relate directly to external work production. Others, particularly those contributing to the energy requirements of resting metabolism, do not. To minimize the influence of these latter factors, efficiency during exercise is often expressed as *net efficiency* (work accomplished divided by energy expended above that at rest), *work efficiency* (work accomplished divided by energy expended above that in unloaded cycling), or *delta efficiency* (change in work accomplished between two loads divided by the energy expended between the same two loads) (8).

In contrast to cycle exercise, actual work performed is difficult to determine during treadmill running or walking. For this reason "efficiency" of performance is usually assessed with treadmill exercise by the measurement of *economy*, the O_2 uptake per kg body mass at a given treadmill speed and/or slope. Economy has been expressed also as the slope of the linear regression equation relating several treadmill speeds (or gradients) with O_2 uptake or, alternatively, as the O_2 uptake demand of moving 1 kg body mass a given distance.

MEASUREMENT OF ECONOMY

Economy must be measured during steady state exercise and, for greatest accuracy, at intensities beneath those that enlist a significant degree of anaerobic metabolism (i.e., below the anaerobic threshold). Some of the studies of economy in children described in this chapter have utilized protocols in which O_2 uptake is recorded at the end of 6 min of steady-load exercise to assure steady state. As noted in chapter 4, steady state appears to be effectively achieved in children by 3 min, at least at low and moderate work intensities, and several investigations have determined economy during progressive protocols with stage durations of 3-4 min.

Studies in adults have indicated that a period of practice in treadmill running or walking is necessary before stability of metabolic costs is observed. These data suggest the importance of having subjects habituated to treadmill exercise before measuring submaximal economy. There is little information about the influence of habituation on energy costs of treadmill exercise in children. Frost et al. had 24 treadmill-naive children ages 7 to 11 years perform six 6 min bouts of running or walking on two separate occasions less than 5 days apart (27). Steady state was observed by 4 min in both walking and running groups. No significant differences in between-day or between-trial values for $\dot{V}O_2$ were observed, suggesting that habituation is not necessary in this age group.

The study by Frost et al. also indicates a high reliability of economy measurements in children (27). Rogers et al. found that the coefficient of variation (sample variation relative to the sample mean) for running economy was 7-8% in a group of 7- to 9-year-old children tested on two occasions (63). These values are somewhat greater than the 1-4% values described in adults (53). Because of this evidence of greater biological variability in children, the authors concluded that (a) two measurements will provide a more reliable estimate of running economy in children than a single value, and (b) a greater accommodation time may be necessary for children than for adults.

Unnithan assessed the stability of $\dot{V}O_2$ in 10 boys ages 9-11 years during three 6 min runs at three speeds (7.2, 8.0, and 8.8 km/hr) on two separate days 2-4 weeks apart (84). The subjects had been previously fully habit-

uated to treadmill exercise. The mean differences in economy at the three speeds on the two visits were 4.2%, 5.6%, and 5.9%, respectively. Wide intersubject differences were observed, however; the range at the fastest speed, for instance, was 0.3% to 17.3%. The author concluded that "single economy testing sessions are valid for estimating group stability of running economy in non-elite active boys. If individual profiles are required then multiple submaximal and maximal testing will be necessary" (p. 49).

ANIMAL STUDIES

The energy costs of locomotion have long occupied the attention of comparative biologists. In the late 1800s, Zuntz exercised dogs, horses, and humans on a treadmill and reported that metabolic expenditure was not related to the weight of the subject but rather to weight raised to the 2/3 power (92). A long series of subsequent investigations has consistently supported this concept: at a given running speed, larger animals are more economical in their energy expenditure than smaller ones (74, 83).

Figure 11.1 illustrates what happens when the metabolic expenditures of animals of a wide diversity of size are measured at increasing running speeds (80). First, the relationship between running velocity and energy cost is linear for all species, and this holds true whether the subject is a pygmy mouse or a horse. But the smaller the animal, the greater the energy expenditure (per body weight) for any given velocity. Moreover, the line relating $\dot{V}O_2$ per kg with speed is increasingly steeper in the smaller animals. That is, the smaller animal is faced

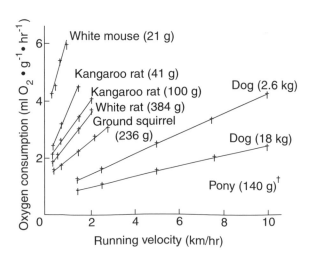

Figure 11.1 Smaller animals have a steeper increase in O_2 uptake with increasing speed of running than larger animals. Reprinted from Schmidt-Nielsen 1984.

with a higher weight-relative energy cost than a larger animal when increasing its speed of running.

Figure 11.2 indicates the cost of running, expressed as the O_2 cost of transporting 1 kg of body mass over a distance of 1 km, relative to animal weight (80). The larger the animal, the more economical is its running. Studying 11 mammalian species varying in mass from 0.5 to 254 kg, Taylor et al. (79) reported that the energy cost of locomotion per kg body mass ($\dot{V}O_2/Mb$) could be expressed relative to body mass as

$$\dot{V}O_2/Mb = 0.533Mb^{-0.32}.$$

Dividing both sides of this equation by body mass, one finds that the scaling exponent for absolute energy cost relative to body mass is 0.68. The similarity of this exponent for submaximal locomotion with the one relating $\dot{V}O_2$ to body mass at both rest and maximal exercise in animals cannot be ignored (see chapter 6).

It is important to recognize that this allometric equation is based on energy expenditure of animals during horizontal locomotion. We can expect that the mass-O_2 uptake relationship will be altered in people who are running or walking uphill (or on a graded treadmill). This occurs because the energy expenditure required to move 1 kg body mass a given vertical distance is independent of body size (74, 78).

From this relationship, Schmidt-Nielsen (74) presented an interesting concept supported by the experimental work of Taylor et al. (78): it is easier for a small animal to run uphill than for a large animal. The explanation: "At rest, a mouse has a specific metabolic rate about 15 times higher than a 1000-kg horse. Because the vertical component of moving one unit of body weight uphill is the same for the two animals, the increase in metabolic rate attributable to the vertical component, relative to the resting rate, will be only 1/15 as

great in the mouse as in the horse" (p. 175). Taylor et al. found that mice running on a 15° treadmill did not significantly increase their energy expenditure over that during level running (78). Chimpanzees (17 kg body weight) showed a twofold increase over horizontal running, while in horses the increase was greater (depending on speed). Similar comparisons have not yet been done in children and adults, but these animal studies suggest that uphill running would be better tolerated by smaller subjects.

Why should these issues interest the developmental exercise physiologist? Differences in running economy observed in various animal species may, in fact, provide important insights concerning the cause of changes in economy during childhood. That's because the trends in economy in animals can be presumed to reflect principally differences in *body size* rather than dimension-independent factors such as substrate utilization, elastic recoil, or biomechanical patterns. The improvements in submaximal running economy in bigger adult animals tell us that the basis for enhanced economy of motion as the child ages is likely to be influenced largely by mechanisms linked to increases in body dimensions. We will return to this animal model of size and economy in discussions later in this chapter that deal with economy changes during childhood.

EXERCISE ECONOMY DURING CHILDHOOD

Changes in treadmill running and walking economy in the growing child were initially indicated by cross-sectional studies, and these patterns have since been confirmed by longitudinal investigations. The finding in these studies of a progressive decline in weight-relative

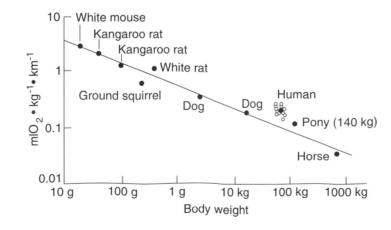

Figure 11.2   The energy cost of running (O_2 demand for transporting 1 kg over 1 km) falls with increasing animal size. Reprinted from Schmidt-Nielsen 1984.

metabolic demand for a given submaximal exercise with increasing age has been remarkably consistent.

Cross-Sectional Studies

The first data indicating an increased energy cost of locomotion in children came from Robinson's studies in the Harvard Fatigue Laboratory in the 1930s (61). Six-year-old boys walking on a treadmill for 15 min at 5.6 km/hr at an 8.6% grade demonstrated an average $\dot{V}O_2$ of 33.0 ml $\cdot$ kg^{-1} $\cdot$ min^{-1}, while the metabolic demand for young men (mean age 24.9 years) was 27.1 ml $\cdot$ kg^{-1} $\cdot$ min^{-1}. Using the same protocol a decade later at the University of Chicago, Morse et al. found that $\dot{V}O_2$ during steady state exercise fell with increasing age from an average of 28.1 ml $\cdot$ kg^{-1} $\cdot$ min^{-1} at age 10 years to 25.7 ml $\cdot$ kg^{-1} $\cdot$ min^{-1} at 17 years (55).

The 4-18-year-old subjects studied by Åstrand ran on a horizontal treadmill at varying speeds up to 16 km/hr (2). His data clearly show that $\dot{V}O_2$ increases linearly with running speed at all ages. Weight-relative O_2 uptake at a treadmill speed of 10 km/hr fell with age, from 47 ml $\cdot$ kg^{-1} $\cdot$ min^{-1} at age 4-6 years to 39 ml $\cdot$ kg^{-1} $\cdot$ min^{-1} at age 16-18. Freedson et al. reported that economy was lower compared to previously reported values in adults in four boys and four girls during treadmill walking at three different speeds (26). A curvilinear response was observed, with poorer economy at higher speeds.

More recent cross-sectional studies comparing treadmill economy between children and adults have indicated similar maturity-related differences (20, 33, 66, 70, 85). Rowland et al. measured economy during horizontal running at four speeds in 20 boys 9-13 years old and 20 young men ages 23-33 years (66). Mean values for $\dot{V}O_2$ per kg at 9.6 km/hr were 49.5 and 40.0 for the two groups, respectively (23.8% greater in the children). In a similar study involving premenarcheal girls and young women, the premenarcheal girls demonstrated a 15.8% greater weight-relative $\dot{V}O_2$ during horizontal running at 7.3 km/hr (70).

Unnithan and Eston compared treadmill running economy between boys ages 9-10 who were involved in cross-country running and trained men ages 18-25 years (85). Mean $\dot{V}O_2$max values were 63.0 and 65.3 ml $\cdot$ kg^{-1} $\cdot$ min^{-1} for the two groups, respectively. Weight-relative O_2 cost was 15-20% greater in the boys at each of four submaximal horizontal speeds (see fig. 11.3).

Ebbeling et al. examined submaximal energy costs during flat treadmill walking in 10 prepubertal boys and 10 male college students (20). This study was different in that the investigators selected three walking speeds corresponding to 50%, 75%, and 100% of average speeds previously reported for the 1-mile walk test in the two age groups. Subjects were therefore presumably

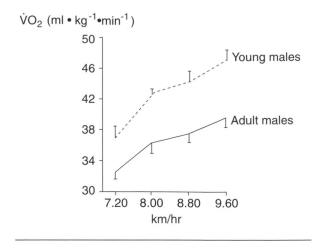

Figure 11.3 Submaximal treadmill running economy in boys and men.

exercising at similar relative intensities (percentage of $\dot{V}O_2$max) rather than the same absolute workload. Age-related economy differences persisted. Average $\dot{V}O_2$ per kg values for the children at the three speeds were 14.3, 19.7, and 30.0 ml $\cdot$ kg^{-1} $\cdot$ min^{-1} compared to 10.9, 15.0, and 24.7 ml $\cdot$ kg^{-1} $\cdot$ min^{-1} in the adults.

Three large-scale studies have provided a broad cross-sectional look at exercise economy across the pediatric age group. Kanaley et al. examined submaximal energy cost of treadmill walking in 298 boys ages 7-15 years (33). In this study the treadmill speed remained constant at 5.8 km/hr while slope started at 10% and increased 2.5% every 3 min. At all exercise stages, the average weight-relative O_2 uptake fell as the age of the subjects increased. The differences were less than those previously reported with use of flat treadmill protocols, however; this possibly related to variations in the effect of weight on energy cost of vertical versus horizontal exercise (reviewed earlier). In the third stage, for instance, the metabolic cost for the 7-8-year-olds was only 7.4% greater than for those 13-15 years old.

Waters et al. collected gas exchange data on 114 children and adolescents, ages 6 to 19 years, while they walked around an outdoor track "at their customary speed" (86, p. 185). To enable age group comparisons, the investigators determined economy independent of speed by expressing O_2 cost as $\dot{V}O_2$ per meter walked. By this measure, economy progressively improved with increasing age, expressed as $\dot{V}O_2$ (ml $\cdot$ kg^{-1} $\cdot$ meter^{-1}) = 0.269 – .0058 (age) (see fig. 11.4). Average values for the youngest children were approximately 50% higher than for the young adults.

MacDougall et al. presented regression lines of weight-relative O_2 uptake versus flat treadmill running speed in 134 subjects ages 7-16 years (42). When sub-

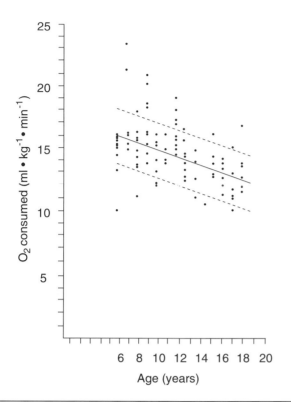

Figure 11.4 Energy cost of walking with increasing age. Reprinted from Waters et al. 1983.

jects were grouped into four age categories, the findings showed a progressive improvement in economy with age. The younger and the shorter the child, the higher was the energy cost of running at any speed.

The cross-sectional data, gathered by different methodologies and protocols, are thus uncharacteristically consistent. Submaximal exercise economy, measured as $\dot{V}O_2$ per kg, steadily improves as the child grows. However, Eston et al. have challenged the conclusion that locomotion in small children is "inefficient," citing the weakness of the ratio standard in comparing O_2 uptake between groups of subjects of different size (see chapter 3) (21). They utilized the alternative approach of comparing the regression lines of mass versus O_2 uptake while covarying for body mass. Reexamining the data of Unnithan and Eston referred to previously, they found that analysis of covariance showed no difference in the gradient or elevation of the regression lines between groups. In other words, when the influence of body mass was removed, the two groups, which were significantly different in submaximal $\dot{V}O_2$ per kg, showed no differences in exercise energy cost. The authors concluded that "it is questionable whether the 'hypermetabolic' response in children is real, or whether it is really attributable to the confounding and uncontrollable factor of body size and the latter's relationships to the body mass:oxygen uptake ratio" (p. 6).

It might be argued that the findings of Eston et al. could also be interpreted to indicate that the factor or factors responsible for changes in economy as children grow simply covary with body weight (which might include any determinant—such as biomechanical efficiency or stride frequency—that changes with maturation).

Longitudinal Studies

Serial testing of the same subjects over time have confirmed the trends in exercise economy during childhood indicated by the cross-sectional studies. Krahenbuhl et al. evaluated running economy in six physically active boys at a mean age of 9.9 years and then again at age 16.8 years (36). Subjects ran on a flat treadmill for 6 min at speeds of 134, 154, and 174 m/min in the initial testing and 161, 188, and 214 m/min in the follow-up session. Expressed as aerobic cost per kilometer of distance run, economy improved 13% during the 7-year age span (234 vs. 203 ml $\cdot$ kg^{-1} $\cdot$ km^{-1}).

Three more extensive longitudinal studies have provided a picture of economy changes across the entire age range of childhood and adolescence. Forster et al. measured treadmill walking economy (10% grade, 4 km/hr) in 19 children at a mean age of 5.2 years and then 4 years later at age 9.3 years (23). Initial average aerobic demand was 29.0 ml $\cdot$ kg^{-1} $\cdot$ min^{-1}. At age 9 the value fell to 22.6 ml $\cdot$ kg^{-1} $\cdot$ min^{-1}, an average decline of 1.6 ml $\cdot$ kg^{-1} $\cdot$ min^{-1} per year.

Rowland and Cunningham obtained similar findings during annual testing of 20 boys and girls between the mean ages of 9 and 13 years (unpublished data). Submaximal treadmill economy was determined during the final minute of a 4 min walk at 3.25 mph at an 8% grade. Weight-relative O_2 uptake fell progressively during the 5 years, from a mean initial value of 31.0 ml $\cdot$ kg^{-1} $\cdot$ min^{-1} to a final value of 26.5 ml $\cdot$ kg^{-1} $\cdot$ min^{-1} (0.9 ml $\cdot$ kg^{-1} $\cdot$ min^{-1} decrease per year) (see fig. 11.5).

In the longitudinal Amsterdam Growth, Health, and Fitness Study, 84 males and 98 females performed the same three-stage submaximal running treadmill test at ages 13, 14, 15, 16, 21, and 27 years (52). Stages consisted of running for 2 min in duration at 8 km/hr while slope was increased from 0% to 2.5% to 5%. Between ages 13 and 27 years, the submaximal O_2 demand of horizontal running fell in the males from 37.6 to 30.3 ml $\cdot$ kg^{-1} $\cdot$ min^{-1} and in the females from 36.5 to 29.8 ml $\cdot$ kg^{-1} $\cdot$ min^{-1} (an average decline of 1.0 and 0.96 ml $\cdot$ kg^{-1} $\cdot$ min^{-1} per year, respectively). Only small changes were observed in each sex between ages 21 and 27 years.

These data allow us to conclude that the O_2 cost per kg body mass for a given exercise workload steadily declines in a continuum throughout childhood and adolescence. $\dot{V}O_2$ per kg can be expected to fall by an average

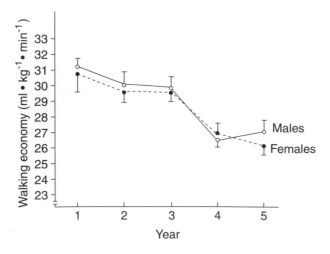

Figure 11.5 Longitudinal changes in treadmill walking economy in boys and girls (Rowland and Cunningham, unpublished data).

of about $1.0 \, ml \cdot kg^{-1} \cdot min^{-1}$ for each increasing year of age until late adolescence.

Allometric Scaling Exponents

Efforts have been made to identify allometric scaling exponents for exercise economy. Bergh et al. measured economy during submaximal horizontal treadmill running in several groups of adult endurance athletes (5). For the equation $\dot{V}O_2 = aM^b$, the exponent b for mass (M) ranged from 0.60 to 0.83. These findings indicate that submaximal economy improved ($\dot{V}O_2$ per kg decreased) with increasing body mass. This trend mimics that described earlier in comparisons of adult animals of different species of varying size.

An examination of mass-related scaling exponents for economy in children is helpful, since (1) if such exponents are similar to those in adults, changes in economy as children grow could be assumed to relate to body dimensions rather than developmental changes in size-independent factors such as biomechanics, substrate utilization, and elastic recoil, and (2) an identified exponent could serve as a useful means of comparing economy in children of different ages and sizes.

Sjodin and Svedenhag measured treadmill running economy (15 km/hr for 4 min) every 6 months for 8 years in eight male trained runners and four ex-runners, beginning at an average age of 12.5 years (76). Serial values for absolute $\dot{V}O_2$ were related allometrically to the increase in body mass for each individual. The average scaling factor for both groups was 0.75, but the intersubject range was wide. Values varied from 0.64 to 0.80 in the trained group and from 0.56 to 0.99 in the nontraining boys. Bergh et al. reported that when Åstrand's data (2) on children were

analyzed by the equation $\log \dot{V}O_2 = I + b_1 (\log M) + b_2 A$—the standard allometric equation for O_2 uptake and mass with added consideration for age (A)—the exponent b_1 was 0.74 (5).

Rogers et al. examined economy at level treadmill speeds of 5 and 6 mph in 42 children (21 boys and 21 girls) ages 7 to 9 years (64). The mean body mass exponents for the two speeds were both 0.65, regardless of gender.

From the limited information now available on allometric scaling factors relative to body mass for the metabolic costs of submaximal exercise in children, one can infer exponents similar to those relating mass and $\dot{V}O_2$ at rest both in children and in adult animals (see chapter 6). This suggests that the factor(s) responsible for weight-relative $\dot{V}O_2$ variations in respect to body mass in these conditions might be similar. In this connection it is worthwhile noting that four studies in children have shown that age differences disappear when submaximal $\dot{V}O_2$ is related to body surface area rather than body mass (20, 64, 66, 70). Whether this finding represents simply a coincident allometric relationship of both submaximal $\dot{V}O_2$ and surface area to weight, or whether there might be a causal link between surface area and energy expenditure during exercise, is unknown.

Gender Differences

Most studies in adult subjects show no differences in exercise economy between males and females. There are reports, however, that males have both better and inferior economy compared to women (see Morgan et al. [53] for review). It is interesting, then, that of the eight studies that have examined gender differences in economy in children, four have demonstrated lower energy cost for submaximal exercise in girls (2, 52, 62, 86) while the other four indicated no sex-related differences (17, 23, 39, 42). This author is not aware of any study in children that has reported greater economy in boys.

Why might girls have better exercise economy during submaximal exercise? The difference could stem from the fact that females have a lower basal metabolic rate in relation to body size than males (35). Åstrand computed net economy (submaximal $\dot{V}O_2$ per kg minus estimated basal metabolic rate) in 6- to 18-year-olds running at three speeds, and could find no statistically significant gender differences (2). However, the O_2 demand was greater for the boys at virtually all ages and speeds. Females possess greater body fat than males, particularly after puberty, but adiposity does not appear to affect treadmill economy (45, 65). Biomechanical factors have been suggested as an explanation of gender differences in economy in adults (53), but these have not been evaluated in children.

WHY DO SMALLER CHILDREN HAVE INFERIOR ECONOMY?

The list of metabolic, biomechanical, psychological, and environmental factors that influence energy cost during exercise is a long one, and many of these factors have been suspected of contributing to maturity-related differences in economy. The issue remains far from resolved, and there is no reason to exclude the possibility that more than one determinant may be responsible for improvements in economy as children grow. In this section, the potential candidates will be reviewed.

In this analysis the developmental physiologist is confronted with a conundrum: since economy improves with age, *any* factor that changes as children grow can be expected to show a statistically significant correlation with submaximal energy expenditure. That includes not only variables such as stride frequency and distance running performance but also features such as hat size, vocabulary, and food consumption! Differentiating association from causality remains a difficult challenge.

Resting Energy Expenditure

Basal or resting energy expenditure related to body size steadily diminishes throughout childhood (see chapter 6). Could the similar fall in weight-relative submaximal $\dot{V}O_2$ be simply a reflection of this pattern in resting O_2 uptake? In other words, does *net* $\dot{V}O_2$ remain stable in children?

While intuitively attractive, this concept does not appear to hold up when one does the required arithmetic. Subtraction of resting from submaximal $\dot{V}O_2$ reduces the differences in economy with age in children, but the trend remains unaltered.

Robinson described a mean resting $\dot{V}O_2$ of 7.35 and 3.56 ml $\cdot$ kg^{-1} $\cdot$ min^{-1} in subjects 6 and 25 years old, respectively, while metabolic costs of walking 15 min at 5.6 km/hr at 8.6% grade were 33.0 ml $\cdot$ kg^{-1} $\cdot$ min^{-1} for the boys and 27.1 ml $\cdot$ kg^{-1} $\cdot$ min^{-1} for the men (61). Net $\dot{V}O_2$ for the two groups was thus 25.7 and 23.5 ml $\cdot$ kg^{-1} $\cdot$ min^{-1}, respectively.

Åstrand examined net O_2 uptake per kg values for males and females ages 4 to 18 years (based on literature values of basal metabolic rate) and found a persistent improvement in economy with age for both genders (2). MacDougall et al. studied resting and submaximal O_2 uptake in 27 subjects ages 7-37 years (42). They found that "there was a tendency for resting $\dot{V}O_2$ per kg to be inversely related to age [but] the differences were relatively small (1-2 ml/kg over the age range) and could only account for a small portion of the difference in gross $\dot{V}O_2$ while running" (p. 197).

Cooke et al. performed the same analysis in groups of eight children and eight adults, both well trained, who ran at four horizontal treadmill speeds (10). $\dot{V}O_2$ demands for the children averaged approximately 7 ml $\cdot$ kg^{-1} $\cdot$ min^{-1} greater in the boys. When the estimated resting metabolic rate was subtracted from values for each group, the difference between mean energy expenditure was reduced by only about 1.8 ml $\cdot$ kg^{-1} $\cdot$ min^{-1}. Thorstensson obtained similar findings when comparing gross and net weight-relative $\dot{V}O_2$ during submaximal exercise in 10-year-old boys and 29-37-year-old men (82).

Net $\dot{V}O_2$ does not, therefore, seem to be the answer to age differences in economy in children. But as noted earlier, initial investigations have yielded allometric scaling exponents for submaximal $\dot{V}O_2$ in children that are similar to those described for basal metabolism (0.67-0.75). When Cooke et al. expressed energy costs of treadmill running in boys and men as $\dot{V}O_2$ per kg$^{0.75}$ instead of $\dot{V}O_2$ per kg$^{1.00}$, they saw no significant differences in economy between the two groups (10). As mentioned previously, a potential link between changes in resting and submaximal metabolic rate in growing children is intriguing. However, in considering this possibility, it is of interest to remember that the determinants of energy cost at rest (approximately 80% by brain, heart, kidney, liver, and lung) are very different from those with activity, altered as the latter are by the predominance of skeletal muscle energy expenditure during exercise.

A connection between resting and exercise rates of energy expenditure in growing children was suggested by the findings of Silverman and Anderson (75). These authors studied the metabolic cost of treadmill exercise in four children (22-53 kg) 6 to 11 years old. Multiple speeds and gradients were employed such that a total of 46 walking loads and 52 running loads were included in the assessment. A constant correction factor for $\dot{V}O_2$ of 90 ml/min was subtracted from the exercise values because the relationship between O_2 uptake in ml/min and body weight (W) at rest was found to be $\dot{V}O_2 = 2.5W + 90$. With use of this correction factor, no significant difference in the weight-relative cost of treadmill exercise was found between small and large children.

Muscular Efficiency

Studies of muscular efficiency during cycle ergometry (i.e., non-weight-bearing exercise) provide no evidence that children differ from adults in the efficiency of intracellular energy transfer or contraction coupling. In other words, the energetics of muscular contraction appear to be independent of subject maturity. Changes in economy as children grow are therefore not explainable on the basis of metabolic differences in the muscle contractile process.

Cooper et al. found that mean delta efficiency during cycle exercise was 28% and 29% in 6-year-old and

18-year-old boys, respectively (13). Over that age span a gradual increase in efficiency was seen in girls, however, reaching statistical significance between the youngest (29%) and oldest (33%) (p < .05). Rowland et al. studied energy expenditure of 19 prepubertal boys (mean age 10.5 years) and 21 male college students (mean age 21.3 years) during a progressive cycle protocol (72). Delta efficiency was determined at two identical absolute and two relative workloads. Net efficiency was estimated from gross efficiency by published norms for basal metabolic rate. Net efficiency improved with increasing work intensity, reaching a plateau at approximately 40% $\dot{V}O_2$max in the adults and 60% $\dot{V}O_2$max in the boys (see fig. 11.6). Beyond these points, net efficiency was similar in the two groups (about 19%). Mean delta efficiency between workloads of similar relative intensity was 23.2% for the prepubertal subjects and 22.5% for the adults. Between equal absolute workloads the values were 23.2% and 26.5%, respectively (p > .05). These values are comparable to the average delta efficiency of 23.6% described by Klausen et al. in 53 children ages 9-14 years (34).

Values for net efficiency in studies of adults have ranged from 13.8% to 23.0% (77). In comparison, a mean net efficiency of 19.7% was described by Taylor et al. in boys 7 to 15 years (77), and Bal et al. reported a mean value in 6-14-year-old girls of 17.3% (3). Thompson compared net efficiency in six women ages 21-28 and six girls ages 9-11 years and reported values of 19.2% and 19.3%, respectively (81).

Stride Frequency

The fact that at a given treadmill speed children need to run or walk with a greater stride frequency has often been cited to explain age-related differences in economy. Indeed there is abundant experimental evidence indicating an association between stride frequency and energy cost of exercise in children, but whether this represents a true causal relationship is uncertain.

Studies in children and adults have documented the obvious: children utilize a shorter stride length and greater stride frequency for any particular treadmill speed. The 20 prepubertal boys studied by Rowland et al. ran on a horizontal treadmill at speeds of 7.2, 8.0, 8.8, and 9.6 km/hr while young adult males ran at 8.0, 8.8, 9.0, and 10.4 km/hr (66). With increasing treadmill speed, both groups progressively increased stride length with virtually constant stride frequency. Frequency at 8.8 km/hr was 75 and 88 strides/min in the men and boys, respectively. Between the slowest and fastest speeds, the stride length increased from 1.35 to 1.73 m (28% rise) in the boys and from 1.80 to 2.30 m (28% increase) in the men. The ratio of stride length to leg length was virtually identical in the two groups.

Waters et al. asked children ages 6-12 years and adolescents 13-19 years to walk around an outdoor track "at their customary walking speed" (86, p. 185). Velocity was 70 and 73 m/min for the two groups, respectively. The cadence among the children was 120 steps/min as compared to 104 steps/min in the adolescents. In a 5-

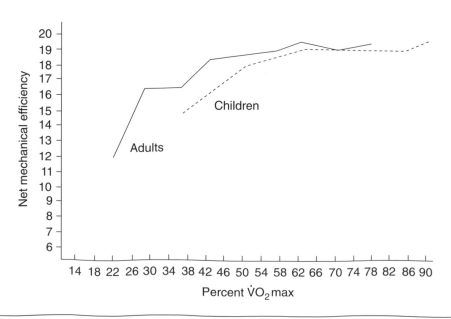

Figure 11.6 Estimated net efficiency during cycle exercise relative to work intensity in boys and men. Reprinted from Rowland et al. 1990.

year longitudinal study of 20 children beginning at age 9, Rowland and Cunningham found a decline in stride frequency during inclined treadmill walking (3.25 mph at 8%) from 67 strides/min at the beginning of the study to 58 strides/min at its conclusion (unpublished data).

Biologists have traditionally used these differences in stride frequency associated with body size to explain concomitant changes in energy costs of locomotion. Hill concluded that energy cost per stride per kg at equivalent speeds should be the same, regardless of animal size (31). He arrived at this concept on the basis of the following line of reasoning:

1. All mammalian muscles generate the same force per cross-sectional area, independent of animal size.
2. Muscle mass is, in general, proportional to body mass.
3. Vertebrate muscles shorten by the same fraction of their resting length.
4. Efficiency of muscular contraction is independent of animal size.
5. Dimensionality theory holds that the steps an animal takes to cover a certain distance (n) is inversely related to its linear dimension (height), which is proportional to the one-third power of its mass (M). That is, $n = kM^{-0.33}$. This scaling exponent for stride frequency turns out to be almost exactly that determined experimentally by Taylor et al. for energy cost during running ($\dot{V}O_2$ per kg = $0.533 M^{-0.32}$).

As summarized by Taylor et al., "Each gram of muscle performs the same work and consumes the same energy during a step, but the small animals have to take many more steps to cover the same distance because of their shorter legs. Therefore when running at the same speed small animals should have higher stride frequencies and consume energy at higher rates" (79, p. 2).

If such an analysis holds true as a means of explaining economy differences in growing children, the amount of O_2 uptake per kg for each stride should be similar, regardless of body size. In fact, each of the five studies that have examined this question have shown this to be the case. The children and adolescents studied by Waters et al. exhibited a cost per stride during free level walking of .128 and .129 ml · kg^{-1} · min^{-1}, respectively (86). When $\dot{V}O_2$ per stride was calculated at three treadmill speeds, Rowland et al. could find no differences between boys and young men (66). In this study, no significant relationship was observed between stride frequency and running economy within either the child or adult groups. The authors hypothesized that homogeneity within the groups might have obscured such a relationship. In a subsequent study encompassing a broader range of fitness, there was a significant correlation in children between stride frequency and economy defined as the $\dot{V}O_2$ demands of increasing treadmill speed by 1 mph (r = .39, p < .05) (67).

Unnithan and Eston found no significant differences in $\dot{V}O_2$ per kg per stride in prepubertal and adult athletes during treadmill running at three speeds (85), and Ebbeling et al. duplicated this finding when comparing treadmill walking energy costs between children and adults (20). In the boys and men studied by Thorstensson, average values of $\dot{V}O_2$ per kg per stride during running at 8, 10, and 11 km/hr were 0.15, 0.19, and 0.21 (boys) and 0.16, 0.20, and 0.21 (men), respectively (82). As reviewed earlier, all these studies revealed significant differences in running economy between younger and older subjects.

Rowland and Cunningham examined stride frequency and submaximal energy costs for boys and girls annually between the ages of 9 and 13 years (unpublished data). While submaximal walking $\dot{V}O_2$ per kg fell progressively over the 5 years, no significant changes were observed in $\dot{V}O_2$ per kg per stride (except for a decline in the girls in the final 2 years) (see fig. 11.7).

This information supports the concept that the obligatory greater stride frequency in small children contributes to their lower submaximal running and walking economy. It should be reemphasized, however, that the available data reflect only a strong association between the two; a cause-and-effect relationship remains to be established.

Mass-Speed Imbalance

Research in both animals and humans indicates that the force applied to a muscle must be kinetically balanced with the speed of its shortening for the optimal conversion of energy into mechanical work (30, 88). Since at a given treadmill speed children move smaller body mass, it has been hypothesized that this mass-speed mismatch might contribute to changes in economy during childhood. Three studies have investigated this premise using measurements of metabolic cost to submaximal exercise with external loading (10, 17, 82). The results only partially support the importance of mass (independent of body size) in determining treadmill economy.

Davies investigated the effect on running economy of adding weighted jackets, equal to 5% and 10% of body weight, in 15 children 12-13 years old (17). In the unloaded condition, economy was poorer than that of adults who had been previously studied. With weights applied, the energy cost ($\dot{V}O_2$ per kg) of running decreased at high velocities and was comparable to data for adults, but at the slower speeds no changes were observed.

Thorstensson performed a similar loading study in which he measured effects on economy in adult men

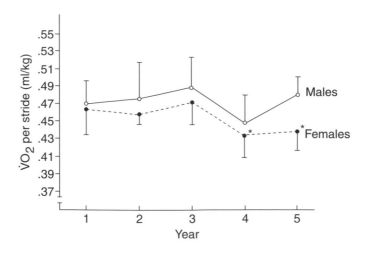

Figure 11.7   Longitudinal changes in $\dot{V}O_2$ per kg per stride during treadmill walking in boys and girls (Rowland and Cunningham, unpublished data).

(ages 29-37 years) and 10-year-old boys (82). The boys demonstrated the expected higher energy cost in the unloaded condition at each of the 8, 10, and 11 km/hr speeds. With application of an external load equal to 10% body weight, a small but consistent decline in net $\dot{V}O_2$ per kg was seen in both groups, but the fall was greater in the boys. The decrease in the boys tended to be greater at higher speeds, and the difference in economy between the boys and men in the loaded condition was significant only at the highest speed. These changes in energy expenditure with loading could not be correlated with changes in step frequency.

These two studies support the idea that the relationship of mass to velocity could help explain age-related economy differences, particularly at high speeds. However, Cooke et al. found no changes in $\dot{V}O_2$ with 5% and 10% vertical loading when comparing treadmill running economy in 10-12-year-old children and 19-16-year-old adults (10). In this study both groups showed a significant increase in stride frequency in the loaded condition, which the authors surmised could have been responsible for the limited changes in O_2 uptake.

Gait Kinematics

It is not difficult to create a mental picture of a person with an "awkward" gait and suspect that such a running style would be "inefficient" compared to that of a highly coordinated athlete. In fact, however, biomechanical studies have demonstrated no clear-cut economy advantages to any particular running style (89). Indeed, some of the world's greatest runners have competed with seemingly ungainly "unique" gaits (8).

Common observational experience tells us that the fluidity of running style improves as children grow, and this

has been quantitated by several investigators (7, 22, 28, 87). Younger children typically show a greater vertical displacement with each stride. They have an increased hip, knee, and ankle extension at takeoff, increased time in the nonsupport phase of the stride, and a decrease in the relative distance of the support foot ahead of the body's center of gravity (87). Many of these differences are restricted largely to early childhood, and by the ages of 6 to 13 the adult patterns of running style are evident (28). The range of joint angles in this age group has been reported to be similar to that in adults, but linear displacements, velocities, and acceleration of body segments are greater in the children (22).

Fortney reported surprisingly high peak vertical ground forces in 2-6-year old children running at maximal speed (24). Cavagna et al. reported that for a 2-year-old child, the muscle power per kg needed to move the center of mass at a walking speed of 4.5 km/hr was more than twice that for an adult (7).

Considering these age-related differences in running mechanics, it would not be unreasonable to consider that the evolution of running style might contribute to energy requirements of locomotion in growing children. Little research has been conducted on this point, however. Ebbeling et al. evaluated the contribution of kinematic parameters to economy in 10 boys ages 8-10 years and 10 young men ages 17 to 23 years who walked at three treadmill speeds of similar relative intensities (20). The expected significant differences in economy were observed between the two groups, with $\dot{V}O_2$ per kg values of 19.7 and 15.0 for the children and men, respectively, at 75% maximal speed. Angles at touchdown, maximum flexion, and total range of motion of the hip, knee, and ankle were measured. Increased walking speed resulted in patterns of change in the joint angles that were similar for the children and adults, but the children showed greater range of motion at the knee and hip. The authors concluded that although children and adults do display biomechanical differences, the magnitude of these alone cannot account for differences in submaximal energy expenditure between the two groups.

Elastic Recoil Forces

When a kangaroo is exercising on a treadmill (don't try this at home), it moves at slow speeds not by hopping but by utilizing all four limbs and its tail in an awkward "pentapedal" locomotion (18). With increasing speeds up to about 5 km/hr, O_2 uptake increases steeply and linearly. At this point, the kangaroo begins to hop, with progressively increasing stride lengths as speed rises. At the time of transition to hopping, the $\dot{V}O_2$ ceases to rise and actually slightly declines, even as treadmill speeds reach 20 km/hr. Treadmill energy demands for the hopping kangaroo are actually less at 20 km/hr than at 5 km/hr (see fig. 11.8)!

This phenomenon is explainable by the greater storage and recovery of energy in the elastic elements of the kangaroo's hopping apparatus. It's an example that illustrates rather dramatically the degree of influence that elastic recoil forces, acting like a spring, can have on energy requirements during locomotion. Differences in such forces have been suggested to contribute to economy variations in humans. However, clarification of this question has been hampered by the lack of a precise method of determining the contribution of elastic energy during walking or running.

In a study of adult runners and jumpers, Williams et al. examined elastic contributions using measures of stiffness, ground reaction forces to jumping, and O_2 uptake with knee bends (90). No important differences

were observed between the two groups, and the authors concluded that differences in running economy and jumping ability in the groups in this study could not be attributed to significant differences in use of elastic energy.

There is some evidence, however, for differences in the elastic contribution to exercise between adults and children. Moritani et al. compared myoelectric activity in lower extremity muscles in 9-year-old boys and adult men during hopping (54). During maximal-height hopping, the adults showed greater utilization of the medial gastrocnemius muscle, particularly in the eccentric phase. The authors noted that "the lesser degree of activation during the eccentric phase will influence the stiffness and thus the ability to utilize elastic energy stored in the triceps surae muscle complex. A lower stiffness in the boys could explain part of the lower performance in the maximal hopping trials" (p. 354).

The study of Bosco and Komi suggested that enhancement of elastic energy potentiation was dependent upon a particular threshold during maximal-tolerable stretch loading (6). Their findings indicated that this threshold was lower for children. Moritani et al. suggested that limited performance in stretch-shortening exercises in children might be accounted for by such age-related changes, as well as by the possibility that children have "less-developed elastic components, qualitatively and/or quantitatively, and thereby a limited possibility of storing elasticity" (p. 355).

Other Factors

A number of additional factors have been identified that might influence the expression of energy expenditure during exercise in children. It is unclear whether their collective magnitude is sufficient to contribute significantly to economy changes during growth.

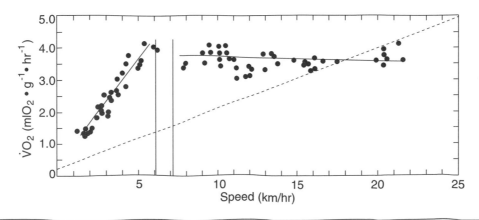

Figure 11.8 Oxygen uptake in the kangaroo with increased speed shows a decrease once the animal begins hopping (see text). Reprinted from Dawson and Taylor 1973.

Body Composition.

Waters et al. suggested that differences in body composition might partially explain the relatively higher metabolic demands of exercise in children (86). As children grow, the muscle mass of the lower extremities constitutes a progressively larger percentage of body mass; in other words, the size of the "motor" relative to the load steadily increases. Malina summarized estimates of muscle mass relative to body weight based on creatinine excretion from several sources (46). In males, total skeletal muscle composes a progressively increasing percentage of body weight during the growing years, rising from about 42% at age 5 years to 50% at age 15. A similar change is not seen in females, whose percentage remains relatively constant at approximately 43%. This presumably reflects their greater accumulation of body fat compared to males.

At the same time, the distribution of muscle mass changes with growth. It has been estimated that the muscles of the lower extremity compose 40% of total muscle mass at birth but 55% at the time of puberty (47). This reflects the observation that leg length makes up about 45% of the height of an 8-year-old but 50% in the 13-year-old (41). How these alterations might affect the calculation of exercise economy is not certain.

Less Efficient Ventilation.

As reviewed in chapter 9, children ventilate more than adults for each liter of O_2 consumed during both submaximal and maximal exercise. This extra cost of breathing is relatively small at low-intensity exercise. At higher workloads, however, the greater $\dot{V}_E/\dot{V}O_2$ in children could adversely influence economy, since at maximal exercise the energy cost of ventilation may reach 14-19% of total body $\dot{V}O_2$ (56).

Substrate Utilization.

There is sufficient research data to indicate that children may rely to a greater extent than adults on fats as an energy source during submaximal exercise (49). This could contribute to the higher weight-relative $\dot{V}O_2$ values in younger subjects, since greater O_2 consumption is required for oxidation of fats than of carbohydrates. This information will be examined in detail in chapter 14.

Anaerobic Energy.

The measurement of exercise economy includes only that energy expenditure that is derived from aerobic metabolic sources. Since total energy demands might include contributions from anaerobic metabolism, it is important to recognize that children appear to be less able to generate anaerobic energy during exercise than adults (see chapter 12). The extent of the contribution of anaerobic metabolism to energy expenditure during treadmill walking and running is unclear, but presumably the input is significant at intensity levels above the anaerobic threshold (about 60%

$\dot{V}O_2$max). How much these observations explain economy differences in children and adults is equally uncertain. But they do suggest the importance of comparing economy between subject groups at relatively low exercise intensities.

ECONOMY AND AEROBIC FITNESS

Intuitively, lower energy demands during submaximal locomotion would be expected to "pay off" in higher levels of aerobic fitness, expressed as either $\dot{V}O_2$max or field performance. It makes sense that the economical runner should be able to conserve energy stores for greater endurance, or should be able to run a distance at a greater speed, than the runner with poor submaximal economy. Studies in adults, however, have not clearly supported these expectations. When differences between $\dot{V}O_2$max are narrow, economy has been shown to correlate closely with distance running performance (9). Others have found that economy is not an important determinant of performance in adults (14), while Pate et al. demonstrated that submaximal economy was inversely related to $\dot{V}O_2$max in runners (57).

Studies of groups of children of similar age have failed to provide convincing evidence that economy relates to either endurance performance or $\dot{V}O_2$max. Similarly, economy has not been found to differ in nonathletic and endurance-trained children, and little or no change in economy has been observed with aerobic training. At the same time, changes in economy during childhood serve as the foundation for the concept that a progressive decrease in fractional utilization (percentage $\dot{V}O_2$max at a given speed) may be responsible for the improvements in endurance performance as children age.

Economy and $\dot{V}O_2$ max

Studies of children and adolescents have revealed no evidence that economy optimizes maximal aerobic power. Indeed, Cunningham's study of female high school runners indicated the reverse. Mimicking the findings of Pate et al. in older subjects (57), the girls with a higher $\dot{V}O_2$max tended to run less economically ($r = 0.45$ for submaximal $\dot{V}O_2$ per kg and $\dot{V}O_2$max, $p < .05$) (15). Rowland and Boyajian obtained similar findings in a cross-sectional study of 38 sixth-grade boys and girls (68). Submaximal economy, measured at 3.25 mph at 8% grade, was inversely related to $\dot{V}O_2$max per kg, with a correlation coefficient between maximal and submaximal O_2 uptake of $r = 0.34$ ($p < .05$).

Rowland et al. measured economy as (a) $\dot{V}O_2$ per kg at 9.6 km/hr and (b) $\dot{V}O_2$ expenditure for increasing treadmill running speed by 1.6 km/hr (delta economy) in 28 prepubertal boys ages 9-14 years with diverse athletic abilities (67). No correlation was seen between energy cost at 9.6 km/hr and $\dot{V}O_2$max (r = –0.01), while a weak relationship was observed between delta economy and maximal aerobic power (r = 0.33, p = .09). In a subsequent study, Rowland and Cunningham could find no association between economy and $\dot{V}O_2$max during graded treadmill walking in 20 children 10 years of age (r = 0.21, p > .05) (69).

Economy and Endurance Performance

On the basis of current information, submaximal economy cannot be expected to serve as a predictor of field endurance performance in any group of children of similar ages. Krahenbuhl et al. studied aerobic demands of submaximal exercise in 8-year-old boys who were divided into groups of good and poor runners based on distance run times (38). The good runners had values for submaximal O_2 uptake that were 1-2 ml · kg^{-1} · min^{-1} lower than those of the poor runners, but the differences were not statistically significant. The authors concluded that $\dot{V}O_2$ (ml · kg^{-1} · min^{-1}) at submaximal speeds is "of little value in differentiating distance running ability" (p. 419).

In a subsequent investigation, Krahenbuhl and Pangrazi studied groups of 10-year-old boys who had placed above the 55th percentile and below the 45th percentile on a 1.6 km run (37). No significant differences were observed in submaximal running economy at three speeds (5.0, 5.75, and 6.5 mph) at 0% grade.

Within groups of endurance athletes, both pre- and postpubertal, a similar lack of association between performance and economy has been reported. Unnithan et al. examined physiological correlates to running performance in 13 trained prepubertal distance runners (mean age 11.7 years) (84). Submaximal demands during treadmill running at 8, 9.6, 11.2, and 12.8 km/hr were related to performance on a 3000 m time trial on an indoor track. Correlation coefficients ranged from –0.59 to –0.24 across the four speeds for submaximal O_2 uptake and 3000 m run time. The only significant correlation between the two was at the 8 km/hr speed (r = –0.59), indicating that better performance (i.e., lower finish time) was associated with poorer economy (higher submaximal weight-relative O_2 uptake).

Cunningham investigated the relationship between treadmill running economy and performance on a 5K race in a group of female high school cross-country runners (15). Economy was defined as the $\dot{V}O_2$ demand of running on a horizontal treadmill at 8 mph, which amounted to a mean of 77% $\dot{V}O_2$max. No significant association was observed between economy and race time (r = –0.05).

Failure to demonstrate an economy-performance relationship in these studies does not necessarily imply

that changes in submaximal O_2 demands as children grow do not influence the development of endurance capacity. It has been reasoned (a) that $\dot{V}O_2$max per kg remains relatively stable during childhood, particularly in boys, and (b) that during this time, a steady decline is observed in the submaximal energy cost of exercise. It therefore follows that as children grow, they will exercise at the same submaximal speed at a progressively lower percentage of $\dot{V}O_2$max (i.e., at a lessened relative exercise intensity) (39). As a result one could anticipate an improvement in endurance performance, since it might be expected that (a) a child running at 75% of $\dot{V}O_2$max at 6 mph will be able to endure that exercise longer than a child running at 85% of $\dot{V}O_2$max at the same speed, and (b) on a field test (such as a 1-mile run) a child running at 7 mph at 85% $\dot{V}O_2$max will outperform the child who is running 6 mph at 85% $\dot{V}O_2$max.

According to this line of reasoning, then, the improvements in endurance performance typically observed in growing children reflect whatever factors are responsible for their progressive decline in weight-relative energy expenditure. As will be described in the paragraphs to follow, some research data support this construct. However, issues of association versus causality remain clouded.

Krahenbuhl et al. evaluated performance on a 9 min run test as well as maximal and submaximal $\dot{V}O_2$ in six males at a mean age of 9.9 years and then again 7 years later (36). No significant change in $\dot{V}O_2$max occurred between the two testing sessions (48.9 vs. 47.8 ml · kg^{-1} · min^{-1}). The average aerobic demands of submaximal running decreased 13% (234 vs. 203 ml · kg^{-1} · km^{-1}, p < 0.001), while the distance covered on the 9 min run was 29% greater on the second test (1637 vs. 2115 m). Similar findings were described by Daniels et al., who showed stable $\dot{V}O_2$max per kg, improved economy, and better endurance performance in run-trained boys over 2-5 years (16).

In a cross-sectional study, Krahenbuhl et al. investigated the relationship between changes in $\dot{V}O_2$max and submaximal $\dot{V}O_2$ in children 6, 7, and 8 years of age (39). No significant change was observed in weight-relative $\dot{V}O_2$max in the three groups. Aerobic demands per kg measured during a horizontal treadmill run at a speed of 115 m/min fell with increasing age (from approximately 32 to 30 ml · kg^{-1} · min^{-1}), but the differences did not reach statistical significance. Submaximal O_2 uptake represented 77%, 71%, and 69% of $\dot{V}O_2$max in the 6-, 7-, and 8-year-old groups, respectively.

Rowland and Cunningham investigated longitudinal changes in maximal and submaximal $\dot{V}O_2$ and mile walk times in 20 children studied annually for 5 years beginning at age 9 (unpublished data). $\dot{V}O_2$max per kg did not change significantly over the 5-year period, while values during a 3.25 mph treadmill walk at 8%

incline progressively improved from a mean of 31.0 ml · kg^{-1} · min^{-1} at the beginning of the study to 26.4 ml · kg^{-1} · min^{-1} at its conclusion. This translated into a decline in fractional utilization (percentage $\dot{V}O_2$max) from 64.2% to 53.5% (see fig. 6.14, page 89). Meanwhile, average 1-mile walk time fell from 14:36 to 13:30 (a 10% improvement).

Effects of Training

Two cross-sectional studies comparing economy in child runners and controls have provided conflicting results. Mayers and Gutin demonstrated greater economy in eight elite cross-country runners ages 8-11 years compared to normal active control subjects (50). Submaximal $\dot{V}O_2$ per kg was approximately 3 ml · kg^{-1} · min^{-1} greater in the controls running at 5, 6, and 7 mph. However, when analysis of covariance was performed with height as the covariate, submaximal $\dot{V}O_2$ differences between the two groups disappeared.

Unnithan compared submaximal running economy in 15 run-trained boys and 18 control children matched for age, height, and weight (84). Average $\dot{V}O_2$max values were 60.5 and 51.1 ml · kg^{-1} · min^{-1} for the runners and nonrunners, respectively. The two groups ran at 8.0 and 9.6 km/hr for 3 min. No significant differences in economy were found at either speed. At 8.0 km/hr, $\dot{V}O_2$ was 38.4 and 36.9 ml · kg^{-1} · min^{-1} for the runners and controls, respectively.

Longitudinal training studies, of course, provide greater information regarding the malleability of exercise economy with increased physical activity. Petray and Krahenbuhl measured economy during overground running in a group of 10-year-old children to determine the effects of an 11-week running training program on submaximal aerobic costs (58). A portion of the run-trained group also received specific instruction on running form. No statistically significant changes in running economy or technique were observed in training versus control nontraining children.

Sjodin and Svedenhag tested eight runners and four control subjects every 6 months for 8 years, beginning at age 12 (76). $\dot{V}O_2$max per kg declined with growth in the controls but remained essentially unchanged in the training runners. The runners had a lower mean O_2 cost of running at 15 km/hr than controls at all ages, but economy declined similarly with age in both groups. No changes in the rate of this decrease were observed in either group at the age of peak height velocity (i.e., puberty). These findings would appear to support the conclusion that intensive run training (36-81 km/week in this study) does not influence the rate of normal decline in submaximal aerobic demands with age.

Unnithan, on the other hand, was able to demonstrate small but significant improvements in submaximal O_2

cost in 10 child runners after a 10-week training program (84). The subjects, who had a pretraining $\dot{V}O_2$max of 60.1 ml · kg^{-1} · min^{-1}, had already been involved in run training for an average of a year before the start of the study. The training regimen included endurance, interval, and speed work. No changes in $\dot{V}O_2$max were observed with training, but improvements in submaximal economy were 7.6%, 5.9%, and 7.2% at speeds of 9.6, 11.5, and 13.1 km/hr. No significant change in economy was observed in nontraining controls running at 9.6 km/hr. The training subjects demonstrated a significantly greater increase in mean body mass (1.44 kg) and decrease in mean skinfold thickness measurements (−0.71 mm) over the 10-week period. The author suggested that these findings, indicative of an increase in muscle mass resulting from the training, may have influenced energy expenditure relative to body mass.

OXYGEN UPTAKE KINETICS

Examining the *rate* of change of $\dot{V}O_2$ both at the onset of exercise and during sustained activities may provide further information on age-related differences in submaximal energy utilization. The speed of rise of $\dot{V}O_2$ at the onset of exercise is an indication of the performance of O_2 delivery mechanisms versus anaerobic metabolic capabilities. The slow rise of O_2 uptake observed during prolonged submaximal exercise, or *aerobic drift,* is an inadequately understood phenomenon that may relate to temperature regulation, intravascular volume, or changes in muscle fiber recruitment.

$\dot{V}O_2$ Dynamics at Onset of Exercise

When a subject begins constant-load exercise, $\dot{V}O_2$ rises to reach steady state by 2-3 min. Since the energy required to perform the work remains constant from the start, alternative energy sources (i.e., from stored phosphates and anaerobic glycolysis) are called upon to meet the energy demands of exercise before $\dot{V}O_2$ steady state is achieved (51). The rate of the $\dot{V}O_2$ rise, and the difference between energy requirements in the initial phase of exercise and those supplied by $\dot{V}O_2$, serve to indicate the relative functional capacities of aerobic and anaerobic energy systems.

Cooper hypothesized that the rate of $\dot{V}O_2$ rise at onset of exercise should be independent of age during childhood (11). He reasoned that "gas exchange measured at the mouth represents the organism's response to events occurring at the cellular level. Because these requirements are the same in adults and children (viz., biological similarity), then the response of the whole organism should reflect this similarity" (p. 86).

Cooper et al. measured $\dot{V}O_2$ transients between rest and a workload at the same relative intensity (75% of anaerobic threshold) in 10 children 7-9 years old and 10 adolescents ages 15-18 years (12). No differences in characteristics of the curve of $\dot{V}O_2$ rise were observed in the two groups (see fig. 11.9). However, Mácek and Vavra (43) as well as Sady (73) found different $\dot{V}O_2$ dynamics at onset of high-intensity exercise in children and young adults. Mácek and Vavra had 21 boys ages 10-11 years cycle against a load equivalent to the load that elicited $\dot{V}O_2$max on a previous test (43). The half-time to the maximal O_2 uptake (time to reach 1/2 $\dot{V}O_2$max, or $t_{1/2}$) was approximately 20 s, a "value lower than that previously reported in adults." The authors considered two possible explanations for their findings: either (1) lower glycolytic capacity in children impairs the generation of anaerobic energy during early exercise, or (2) "it can be postulated that the ability for rapid mobilization of aerobic metabolism in the initial phase of exercise in children makes the high capacity of glycolysis unnecessary" (p. 67).

Sady also found that children have quicker $\dot{V}O_2$ responses to onset of exercise than adults (73). Ten-year-old boys and adult men (mean age 30 years) pedaled a cycle ergometer at 103% and 105% $\dot{V}O_2$max, respectively. The children demonstrated an average $t_{1/2}$ of 17.2 s compared to 28.5 s in the adults (p < .05).

Freedson et al. reported O_2 uptake response during the initial phase of exercise in 28 children (mean age 10.2 years) (25). Subjects cycled at a constant load of 59 W, which represented an average of 60.8% $\dot{V}O_2$max for the entire group. The overall mean $t_{1/2}$ was 34.8 s; this was considered "similar to other data for adults working at similar relative intensities" (p. 171). However, there was a strong correlation in the children between $t_{1/2}$ and age (r = 0.77).

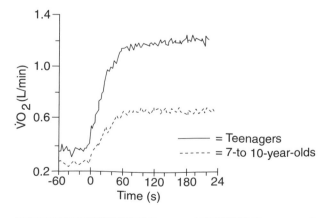

Figure 11.9 $\dot{V}O_2$ response at onset of exercise in teenagers (upper curve) and 7-10-year-old children (lower curve). Reprinted from Cooper et al. 1985.

Zanconato et al. recorded $\dot{V}O_2$ dynamics to onset of exercise in 10 children (7-11 years old) and 13 adults (26-42 years old) (91). Patterns of change were observed at multiple intensities: 50% of anaerobic threshold (AT), 80% AT, 50% of the difference between AT and $\dot{V}O_2$max, and 100% and 125% $\dot{V}O_2$max. The $t_{1/2}$ was not altered by work intensity in either group. No significant differences were observed in average $t_{1/2}$ values between the children and adults (23.0 and 24.8 s, respectively).

These studies have not yet provided a clear picture of maturity-related variations in $\dot{V}O_2$ kinetics at the onset of exercise. Additional information will be important, too, in unraveling the physiological implications of any such differences.

Aerobic Drift

The phenomenon of *aerobic drift,* which occurs when an adult subject performs prolonged constant-load exercise, is well characterized: sustained cycle pedaling for 45-60 min at an intensity of 60% $\dot{V}O_2$max typically produces a progressive rise in metabolic rate, manifest as a 10-15% rise in $\dot{V}O_2$ (60). Termed the *slow component* of O_2 uptake kinetics, this increase in $\dot{V}O_2$ is most evident at high exercise intensities (above the anaerobic threshold). Changes in cardiac function (stroke volume, heart rate) and ventilation (breathing frequency, tidal volume) accompany those of O_2 uptake (60); these have been addressed in chapters 8 and 9.

Factors responsible for aerobic drift remain uncertain. The rise in metabolic rate with sustained exercise parallels that expected from increases in body temperature; however, recent experimental data have cast doubt on this relationship (48, 59). Since aerobic drift occurs largely at exercise intensities above the anaerobic threshold, the role of factors linked to high-intensity work has been investigated. Levels of blood lactate, as well as catecholamines, parallel increases in $\dot{V}O_2$, but evidence that either of these rises is causal is lacking (29, 59). The rise in metabolic rate with sustained exercise may reflect recruitment of less efficient fast-twitch muscle fibers, but there is no direct proof for this hypothesis (59).

Considering these proposed mechanisms, there is reason to suspect that the degree of aerobic drift might be different in children. Compared to adults, children are less tolerant of sustained exercise in the heat (4, 19). Anaerobic threshold in prepubertal subjects typically occurs at a higher relative exercise intensity than with adults (32). Also, lactate and catecholamine responses to both maximal and submaximal exercise have been reported to be lower in children (40). Nonetheless, three studies that have measured aerobic drift in children have shown no qualitative or quantitative differences from adult subjects in changes in $\dot{V}O_2$ during sustained exercise (1, 44, 71). These findings indicate that the mechanisms responsible for the rise in metabolic rate are not related to maturity.

Asano and Hirakoba measured $\dot{V}O_2$ in 11 boys ages 10-12 years and 12 men ages 20-34 years during 60 min of cycling at approximately 60% $\dot{V}O_2$max (1). Mean $\dot{V}O_2$max values for the two groups were 45.6 and 47.2 ml · kg^{-1} · min^{-1}, respectively. Between minutes 10 and 60 of exercise, $\dot{V}O_2$ rose by 11% in the children and 8% in the adults (p > .05). Mácek et al. performed a similar study with 10 boys ages 11.6 to 14 years working under the same exercise conditions (1). Mean $\dot{V}O_2$ per kg rose from 28.5 to 31.5 ml · kg^{-1} · min^{-1} (10.5%) between minutes 10 and 60.

Rowland and Rimany compared physiological responses to sustained cycle exercise in 11 premenarcheal girls (mean age 11.4 years) and 13 women ages 21 to 32 years (71). Subjects pedaled at a constant load equivalent to 63% $\dot{V}O_2$max for 40 min. Between minutes 10 and 40, mean $\dot{V}O_2$ rose by 8.6% and 8.3% in the girls and women, respectively (see fig. 11.10). Supporting the etiologic role of increased temperature, no significant differences were observed in average rise in body temperature between the two groups (0.9 and 1.2 °F for the girls and women, respectively). This study did not support the importance of factors related to anaerobic metabolism (lactate, catecholamines, fast-twitch fiber recruitment), since 45% of the girls were cycling above their ventilatory anaerobic threshold compared to 77% of the women. No significant difference was observed in average change in $\dot{V}O_2$ in children exercising above and below the ventilatory anaerobic threshold.

SUMMARY

The research data have provided a consistent descriptive picture of changes in submaximal energy expenditure during the course of childhood. Other issues, particularly those related to causality, are not so clear.

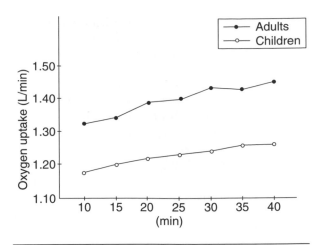

Figure 11.10   Changes in $\dot{V}O_2$ during 40 min of steady state cycling at 60% $\dot{V}O_2$max in children and adults. Reprinted from Rowland and Rimany 1995.

Walking or running economy has been shown in all studies to improve during the course of childhood. The cause of these improvements in economy is unclear. Much information—including data on the similarity of allometric scaling factors for weight relative to submaximal $\dot{V}O_2$ in children, adults, and animals—suggests that differences in energy expenditure with exercise are linked to body size. Determinants independent of body dimension (coordination of gait, substrate utilization, elastic recoil forces) may also contribute to the evolution of economy during childhood.

Fractional utilization, the percentage $\dot{V}O_2$max utilized at a given treadmill speed, declines with age during childhood. At the same time, endurance performance improves. Whether the former is responsible for the latter represents an intriguing but as yet unproven possibility.

Studies comparing the rise of $\dot{V}O_2$ at the onset of exercise between children and adults have provided conflicting results. The significance of any observed differences in terms of relative capacities of aerobic and anaerobic metabolism remains clouded.

What We Know

1. The aerobic cost of weight-bearing exercise, measured as $\dot{V}O_2$ per kg, steadily declines as children age.
2. The improvements in economy are not related to the energy efficiency of muscle contraction itself, which is age-independent.
3. Submaximal $\dot{V}O_2$ per stride does not change with age, suggesting that greater stride frequency is associated with poorer economy in smaller children.

4. At the same speed, children exercise at a progressively lower intensity (percentage of $\dot{V}O_2$max) as they grow.
5. Within groups of children of similar age, submaximal economy is not associated with either $\dot{V}O_2$max or endurance performance.

What We Would Like to Know

1. What causes the improvements in submaximal economy as children grow?
2. Is there a means of identifying a single anthropometric factor that will "normalize" submaximal energy expenditure for size?
3. Are there gender differences in economy? If so, why?
4. Does the decreased fractional utilization of $\dot{V}O_2$max during submaximal exercise as children grow explain their progressive improvement in endurance performance?

References

1. Asano, K.; Hirakoba, K. Respiratory and circulatory adaptation during prolonged exercise in 10-12 year old children and in adults. In: Ilmarinen, J.; Valimaki, I., eds. Child and sport. Berlin: Springer-Verlag; 1984:p. 119-128.
2. Åstrand, P.O. Experimental studies of physical working capacity in relation to sex and age. Copenhagen: Munksgaard; 1952.
3. Bal, M.E.R.; Thompson, E.M.; McIntosh, E.M.; Taylor, C.M.; MacLeod, G. Mechanical efficiency in cycling of girls six to fourteen years of age. J. Appl. Physiol. 6:185-188; 1953.
4. Bar-Or, O. Sports medicine for the practitioner. New York: Springer-Verlag; 1983:p. 227-228.
5. Bergh, U.; Sjodin, B.; Forsberg, A.; Svedenhag, J. The relationship between body mass and oxygen uptake during running in humans. Med. Sci. Sports Exerc. 23:205-211; 1991.
6. Bosco, C.; Komi, P.V. Influence of aging on the mechanical behavior of leg extensor muscles. Eur. J. Appl. Physiol. 45:200-219; 1980.
7. Cavagna, G.A.; Franzetti, P.; Fuchimoto, T. The mechanics of walking in children. J. Physiol. 343:323-339; 1983.
8. Cavanagh, P.R.; Kram, R. The efficiency of human movement—a statement of the problem. Med. Sci. Sports Exerc. 17:304-308; 1985.
9. Conley, D.; Krahenbuhl, G. Running economy and distance running performance of highly trained athletes. Med. Sci. Sports Exerc. 12:357-360; 1980.
10. Cooke, C.B.; McDonagh, M.J.N.; Nevill, A.M.; Davies, C.T.M. Effects of load on oxygen intake in trained boys and men during treadmill running. J. Appl. Physiol. 71.1237-1244; 1991.
11. Cooper, D.M. Development of the oxygen transport system in normal children. In: Advances in pediatric sport sciences. Vol. 3, Bar-Or, O., ed. Biological issues. Champaign, IL: Human Kinetics; 1989:p. 67-100.
12. Cooper, D.M.; Berry, C.; Lamarra, L.; Wasserman, K. Kinetics of oxygen uptake at the onset of exercise as a function of growth in children. J. Appl. Physiol. 59:211-217; 1985.
13. Cooper, D.M.; Weiler-Ravell, D.; Whipp, B.J.; Wasserman, K. Aerobic parameters of exercise as a function of body size during growth in children. J. Appl. Physiol. 56:628-634; 1984.
14. Costill, D.L.; Thomason, H.; Roberts, E. Fractional utilization of the aerobic capacity during distance running. Med. Sci. Sports 5:248-252; 1973.
15. Cunningham, L.N. Relationship of running economy, ventilatory threshold, and maximal oxygen consumption to running performance in high school females. Res. Q. Exerc. Sport 61:369-374; 1990.
16. Daniels, J.; Oldridge, N.; Nagle, F.; White, B. Differences and changes in $\dot{V}O_2$ among young runners 10 to 18 years of age. Med. Sci. Sports Exerc. 10:200-203; 1978.
17. Davies, C.T.M. Metabolic cost of exercise and physical performance in children with some observations on external loading. Eur. J. Appl. Physiol. 45:95-102; 1980.
18. Dawson, T.J.; Taylor, C.R. Energetic cost of locomotion in kangaroos. Nature 246:313-314; 1973.
19. Drinkwater, B.L.; Kupprat, I.C.; Denton, J.E.; Crist, J.L.; Horvath, S.M. Response of prepubertal girls and college women to work in the heat. J. Appl. Physiol. 43:1046-1053; 1977.
20. Ebbeling, C.J.; Hamill, J.; Freedson, P.S.; Rowland, T.W. An examination of efficiency during walking in children and adults. Pediatr. Exerc. Science 4:36-49; 1992.
21. Eston, R.G.; Robson, S.; Winter, E.M. A comparison of oxygen uptake during running in children and adults. In: Kinanthropometry IV. Duquet, J.W.; Day, J.A.P., eds. London: E & FN Spon, in press.
22. Foley, C.D.; Quanbury, A.O.; Steinke, T. Kinematics of normal child locomotion—a statistical study based on TV data. Biomechanics 12:1-6; 1979.

23. Forster, M.A.; Hunter, G.R.; Hester, D.J.; Dunaway, D.; Shuleva, K. Aerobic capacity and grade-walking economy of children 5-9 years old: a longitudinal study. Pediatr. Exerc. Sci. 6:31-38; 1994.

24. Fortney, V.L. The kinematics and kinetics of the running pattern of two-, four-, and six-year old children. Res. Q. Exerc. Sport 54:126-135; 1983.

25. Freedson, P.S.; Gilliam, T.B.; Sady, S.P.; Katch, V.L. Transient $\dot{V}O_2$ characteristics in children at the onset of steady-rate exercise. Res. Q. 52:167-173; 1981.

26. Freedson, P.S.; Katch, V.L.; Gilliam, T.B.; MacConnie, S. Energy expenditure in prepubescent children: influence of sex and age. Am. J. Clin. Nutr. 34:1827-1830; 1981.

27. Frost, G.; Bar-Or, O.; Dowling, J.; White, C. Habituation of children to treadmill walking and running: metabolic and kinematic criteria. Pediatr. Exerc. Science 7:162-175; 1995.

28. Grieve, D.W.; Gear, R.J. The relationships between length of stride, step frequency, time of swing, and speed of walking for children and adults. Ergonomics 5:379-399; 1966.

29. Hagberg, J.M.; Mullin, J.P.; Nagle, F.J. Oxygen consumption during constant-load exercise. J. Appl. Physiol. 45:381-384; 1978.

30. Hill, A.V. The mechanical efficiency of frog's muscle. Proc. Roy. Soc. Lond. 127:434-451; 1939.

31. Hill, A.V. The dimensions of animals and their muscular dynamics. Sci. Progr. Lond. 38:209-230; 1950.

32. Kanaley, J.A.; Boileau, R.A. The onset of the anaerobic threshold at three stages of physical maturity. J. Sports Med. 28:367-374; 1988.

33. Kanaley, J.A.; Boileau, R.A.; Massey, B.H.; Misner, J.E. Muscular efficiency during treadmill walking: the effects of age and workload. Pediatr. Exerc. Science 1:155-162; 1989.

34. Klausen, K.; Rasmussen, B.; Glensgaard, L.K.; Jensen, O.V. Work efficiency of children during submaximal bicycle exercise. In: Binkhorst, R.A.; Kemper, H.C.G.; Saris, W.H.M., eds. Children and exercise XI. Champaign, IL: Human Kinetics; 1985:p. 210-217.

35. Kneobel, L.K. Energy metabolism. In: Selkurt, E.E., ed. Physiology. Boston: Little, Brown; 1963:p. 564-579.

36. Krahenbuhl, G.S.; Morgan, D.W.; Pangrazi, R.P. Longitudinal changes in distance-running performance of young males. Int. J. Sports Med. 10:92-96; 1989.

37. Krahenbuhl, G.; Pangrazi, R. Characteristics associated with running performance in young boys. Med. Sci. Sports Exerc. 15:486-490; 1983.

38. Krahenbuhl, G.S.; Pangrazi, R.P.; Chomokas, E.A. Aerobic responses of young boys to submaximal running. Res. Q. Exerc. Sport 50:413-421; 1979.

39. Krahenbuhl, G.S.; Pangrazi, R.P.; Stone, W.J.; Morgan, D.W.; Williams, T. Fractional utilization of maximal aerobic capacity in children 6 to 8 years of age. Pediatr. Exerc. Science 1:271-277; 1989.

40. Lehmann, M.; Keul, J.; Korsten-Reck, U. The influence of graduated treadmill exercise on plasma catecholamines, aerobic, and anaerobic capacity in boys and adults. Eur. J. Appl. Physiol. 47:301-311; 1981.

41. Lowrey, G.H. Growth and development of children. 8th ed. Chicago: Year Book Medical; 1986:p. 80.

42. MacDougall, J.D.; Roche, P.D.; Bar-Or, O.; Moroz, J.R. Maximal aerobic capacity of Canadian schoolchildren: prediction based on age-related oxygen cost of running. Int. J. Sports Med. 4:194-198; 1983.

43. Mácek, M.; Vavra, J. Oxygen uptake and heart rate with transition from rest to maximal exercise in prepubertal boys. In: Berg, K., ed. Children and exercise IX. Baltimore: University Park Press; 1980:p. 64-68.

44. Mácek, M.; Vavra, J.; Novosadova, J. Prolonged exercise in prepubertal boys. I. Cardiovascular and metabolic adjustment. Eur. J. Appl. Physiol. 35:291-298; 1976.

45. Maffeis, C.; Schutz, Y.; Schena, F.; Zaffanello, M.; Pinelli, L. Energy expenditure during walking and running in obese and non-obese prepubertal children. J. Pediatr. 123:193-199; 1993.

46. Malina, R.M. Quantification of fat, muscle, and bone in man. Clin. Orthop. Rel. Res. 65:9-20; 1969.

47. Malina, R.M. Growth of muscle tissue and muscle mass. In: Falkner, F.; Tanner, J.M., eds. Human growth. 2. Postnatal growth. New York: Plenum Press; 1978:p. 273-294.

48. Martin, B.J.; Morgan, E.J.; Zwillich, C.W.; Weil, J.V. Control of breathing during prolonged exercise. J. Appl. Physiol. 50:27-31; 1981.

49. Martinez, L.R.; Haymes, E.M. Substrate utilization during treadmill running in prepubertal girls and women. Med. Sci. Sports Exerc. 24:975-983; 1992.

50. Mayers, N.; Gutin, B. Physiological characteristics of elite prepubertal cross country runners. Med. Sci. Sports Exerc. 11:172-176; 1979.

51. McArdle, W.D.; Katch, F.I.; Katch, V.L. Exercise physiology. Philadelphia: Lea & Febiger; 1981:p. 83-84.

52. Mechelen, W.V.; Kemper, H.C.G.; Twisk, J. The development of running economy from 13-27 years of age [abstract]. Med. Sci. Sports Exerc. 26:S205; 1994.

53. Morgan, D.W.; Martin, P.E.; Krahenbuhl, G.S. Factors affecting running economy. Sports Med. 7:310-330; 1989.

54. Moritani, T.; Oddson, L.; Thorstensson, A.; Åstrand, P.O. Neural and biomechanical differences between men and young boys during a variety of motor tasks. Acta Physiol. Scand. 137:347-355; 1989.

55. Morse, M.; Schlutz, F.W.; Cassels, D.E. Relation of age to physiological responses of the older boy (10-17 years) to exercise. J. Appl. Physiol. 1:683-709; 1949.

56. Pardy, R.L.; Hussain, S.N.A.; MacKlem, P.T. The ventilatory pump in exercise. Clin. Chest Med. 5:35-49; 1984.

57. Pate, R.R.; Macera, C.A.; Bailey, S.P.; Bartoli, W.P.; Powell, K.E. Physiological, anthropometric, and training correlates of running economy. Med. Sci. Sports Exerc. 24:1128-1133; 1992.

58. Petray, C.K.; Krahenbuhl, G.S. Running training, instruction on running technique, and running economy in 10-year old males. Res. Q. Exerc. Sport 56:251-255; 1985.

59. Poole, D.C.; Schaffartzik, W.; Knight, D.R.; Derion, T.; Kennedy, B.; Guy, H.J.; Preduketto, R.; Wagner, P.D. Contribution of exercising legs to the slow component of oxygen uptake kinetics in humans. J. Appl. Physiol. 71:1245-1253; 1991.

60. Raven, P.B.; Stevens, G.H.J. Cardiovascular function and prolonged exercise. In: Perspectives in exercise science and sports medicine. Vol. 1, Lamb, D.R.; Murray, R., eds. Prolonged exercise. Indianapolis: Benchmark Press; 1988:p. 43-74.

61. Robinson, S. Experimental studies of physical fitness in relation to age. Arbeitsphysiologie 10:251-323; 1938.

62. Rogers, D.M.; Turley, K.R.; Kujawa, K.I.; Harper, K.M.; Wilmore, J.H. Gender differences in running economy in 7, 8, and 9 year old children [abstract]. Med. Sci. Sports Exerc. 26:S206; 1994.

63. Rogers, D.M.; Turley, K.R.; Kujawa, K.I.; Harper, K.M.; Wilmore, J.H. The reliability and variability of running economy in 7, 8, and 9 year old children. Pediatr. Exerc. Science 6:287-296; 1994.

64. Rogers, D.M.; Turley, K.R.; Kujawa, K.I.; Harper, K.M.; Wilmore, J.H. Allometric scaling factors for oxygen uptake during exercise in children. Ped. Exerc. Science 7:12-25; 1995.

65. Rowland, T.W. Effects of obesity on aerobic fitness in adolescent females. Am. J. Dis. Child. 145:764-768; 1991.

66. Rowland, T.W.; Auchinachie, J.A.; Keenan, T.J.; Green, G.M. Physiological responses to treadmill running in adult and prepubertal males. Int. J. Sports Med. 8:292-297; 1987.

67. Rowland, T.W.; Auchinachie, J.A.; Keenan, T.J.; Green, G.M. Submaximal aerobic running economy and treadmill performance in prepubertal boys. Int. J. Sports Med. 9:201-204; 1988.

68. Rowland, T.W.; Boyajian, A. Aerobic response to endurance training in children [abstract]. Med. Sci. Sports Exerc. 26:S83; 1994.

69. Rowland, T.W.; Cunningham, L.N. Oxygen uptake plateau during maximal treadmill exercise in children. Chest 101:485-489; 1992.

70. Rowland, T.W.; Green, G.M. Physiological responses to treadmill exercise in females: adult-child differences. Med. Sci. Sports Exerc. 20:474-478; 1988.

71. Rowland, T.W.; Rimany, T.A. Physiological responses to prolonged exercise in premenarcheal and adult females. Pediatr. Exerc. Science 7:183-191; 1995.

72. Rowland, T.W.; Staab, J.S.; Unnithan, V.B.; Rambusch, J.M.; Siconolfi, S.F. Mechanical efficiency during cycling in prepubertal and adult males. Int. J. Sports Med. 11:452-455; 1990.

73. Sady, S. Transient oxygen uptake and heart rate responses at the onset of relative endurance exercise in prepubertal boys and adult men. Int. J. Sports Med. 2:240-244; 1981.

74. Schmidt-Nielsen, K. Scaling. Why is animal size so important? Cambridge: Cambridge University Press; 1984:p.165-181.

75. Silverman, M.; Anderson, S.D. Metabolic cost of treadmill exercise in children. J. Appl. Physiol. 33:696-698; 1972.

76. Sjodin, B.; Svedenhag, J. Oxygen uptake during running as related to body mass in circumpubertal boys: a longitudinal study. Eur. J. Appl. Physiol. 65:150-157; 1992.

77. Taylor, C.M.; Bal, M.E.R.; Lamb, M.W.; MacLeod, G. Mechanical efficiency in cycling of boys seven to fifteen years of age. J. Appl. Physiol. 2:563-570; 1950.

78. Taylor, C.R.; Caldwell, S.L.; Rountree, V.J. Running up and down hills: some consequences of size. Science 178:1096-1097; 1972.

79. Taylor, C.R.; Heglund, N.C.; Maloiy, G.M.O. Energetics and mechanics of terrestrial locomotion. J. Exp. Biol. 97:1-21; 1982.

80. Taylor, C.R.; Schmidt-Nielsen, K.; Raab, J.L. Scaling of energetic costs of running to body size in mammals. Amer. J. Physiol. 218:1104-1107; 1970.

81. Thompson, E.M. A study of the energy expenditure and mchanical efficiency of young girls and adult women [dissertation]. New York: Columbia University Press; 1940.

82. Thorstensson, A. Effects of moderate external loading on the aerobic demand of submaximal running in men and 10 year old boys. Eur. J. Appl. Physiol. 55:569-574; 1986.

83. Tucker, V.A. Energetic cost of locomotion in animals. Comp. Biochem. Physiol. 34:841-846; 1970.

84. Unnithan, V.B. Factors affecting submaximal running economy in children [doctoral thesis]. Glasgow: University of Glasgow; 1993.

85. Unnithan, V.B.; Eston, R.G. Stride frequency and submaximal treadmill running economy in adults and children. Pediatr. Exerc. Science 2:149-155; 1990.

86. Waters, R.L.; Hislop, H.J.; Thomas, L.; Campbell, J. Energy cost of walking in normal children and teenagers. Develop. Med. Child. Neurol. 25:184-188; 1983.

87. Wickstrom, R.L. Fundamental motor patterns. Philadelphia: Lea & Febiger; 1983.

88. Wilkie, D.R. The relation between force and velocity in human muscle. J. Physiol. 110:249-280; 1950.

89. Williams, K.R. The relationship between mechanical and physiological energy estimates. Med. Sci. Sports Exerc. 17:317-325; 1985.

90. Williams, K.R.; Agruss, C.D.; Snow, R.E.; Jones, J.E. Elastic contributions to running economy and jumping performance [abstract]. Med. Sci. Sports Exerc. 22:S41; 1990.

91. Zanconato, S.; Cooper, D.M.; Armon, Y. Oxygen cost and oxygen uptake dynamics and recovery with 1 min of exercise in children and adults. J. Appl. Physiol. 71:993-998; 1991.

92. Zuntz, N. Ueber den Stoffverbrauch des Hundes bei Muskelarbeit. Arch. Ges. Physiol. 68:191-211; 1897.

CHAPTER 12

SHORT-BURST ACTIVITIES AND THE DEVELOPMENT OF ANAEROBIC FITNESS

Research attention in developmental exercise physiology has focused primarily on endurance, or aerobic fitness. The reasons have been outlined in chapter 6: (a) aerobic activities are linked to long-term cardiovascular health, (b) there is concern regarding the safety of highly intensive athletic training in endurance sports in prepubertal children, and (c) augmenting aerobic fitness may prove beneficial to children with chronic cardiac and pulmonary diseases. Researchers interested in these issues benefit from the ability to safely and easily measure a subject's O_2 uptake, an accurate index of the contribution of aerobic metabolism to physical activity.

The physical exercise usually performed in daily living (climbing stairs, moving objects), however, is rarely sustained. We rely principally on anaerobic metabolic pathways to carry out these habitual activities that last less than 1 to 2 min. This is particularly true in the short-burst activities characteristic of small children, who are perhaps best described as in perpetual brownian motion. For example, recording of heart rates during daily activities of the typical 7-year-old child reveals multiple short peaks, with values rarely over 120-130 bpm (34). Children therefore spend most of their lives fueled by anaerobic rather than aerobic metabolism.

Despite its obvious importance, the development of anaerobic fitness in children has received less research attention. As a result, our understanding of the maturation of a child's capability to perform short-burst, high-intensity exercise is limited. The constraining factor here is the lack of an accurate, noninvasive method of measuring the participation of anaerobic metabolism during exercise. There is no "$\dot{V}O_2max$" for the investigation of anaerobic fitness; instead the researcher is left

with attempting to glimpse the contributions of anaerobic metabolism through a group of measures that at best provide only an estimate of nonaerobic metabolic work.

During the growing years, the performance of children on short-burst activities such as the 50 yd dash or serial sit-ups progressively improves. When youngsters are brought into the exercise laboratory, results on Wingate and force-velocity testing (see chapter 3) reveal the same thing, but with an interesting twist. Not only does anaerobic fitness increase with age, but a similar pattern of improvement emerges when findings such as maximal or mean anaerobic power are related to body size. That is, *anaerobic fitness improves in children at a faster rate than can be ascribed to growth alone.* There appear to be qualitative changes in the factors that determine performance on short-burst activities—changes that occur quite independently of increase in body dimensions. This, we will recall, is very different from the development of aerobic fitness in children; in that case, improvement in the laboratory measure (maximal O_2 uptake) with age approximates the increase in body mass (i.e., $\dot{V}O_2max$ per kg is stable across age groups in males, while values in females slowly decline). At the same time, dramatic improvements are seen in endurance fitness (as seen in the mile run).

What factor or factors are responsible for the development of fitness in short-burst activities in children? Among the many potential candidates: contributions to neuromuscular fatigue (differences in neurotransmitter release and uptake, alterations in calcium accumulation in the sarcoplasmic reticulum); muscle architecture, fiber type, and recruitment pattern; central neurological factors (psychological issues such as level of perceived exertion); and the capacity for energy production (rate of anaerobic glycolysis). In the latter category, maturation of triggering factors (testosterone, catecholamines), substrate utilization (glycogen storage and breakdown), or activities of enzymes of glycolytic metabolic pathways might all play a role.

Investigation into the developmental changes in these factors has effectively extended only as far as the area of anaerobic energy production. And here there are clues from divergent sources that the rate of anaerobic glycolysis in exercising muscle does, in fact, improve as the child grows. To summarize this evidence:

1. Blood lactate levels at both submaximal and maximal exercise increase with age throughout childhood.
2. The scant data from muscle biopsies in children suggest that the activity of enzymes critical for glycolysis (particularly phosphofructokinase) is less in children than in adults.
3. The ventilatory anaerobic threshold, expressed as percentage of $\dot{V}O_2$max, is higher in children than in adults, perhaps reflecting differences in anaerobic capacity.
4. Recovery $\dot{V}O_2$, or O_2 debt, increases with age during childhood.
5. Blood pH after maximal exercise declines as the child grows.

It should be reemphasized that none of these variables, by itself, can be counted on to serve as a reliable marker of anaerobic metabolic rate. Still, the collective consistency of this evidence supports the concept of a progressive improvement in ability to generate anaerobic energy during exercise throughout the course of childhood. The extent to which this pattern might be responsible for improvements in performance in short-burst activities in the growing child remains problematic.

This chapter will describe the literature that supports—or in some cases, refutes—the concept of such a progressive improvement. In addition, the influence of sexual development on anaerobic capacity, the capacity of anaerobic fitness to improve with training, and the evidence linking developmental changes in glycolytic metabolism with serum catecholamines will be reviewed.

PERFORMANCE ON SHORT-BURST ACTIVITIES

Field performance in virtually any short-burst exercise activity improves during childhood. In general, average performance is superior in males, even well before puberty, and the rate of improvement with age also is greater in males. This was well demonstrated in the various AAHPERD cross-sectional testing results in the 50 yd dash between 1958 and 1975. In 1958 and again in 1965, girls 10 to 17 years old showed small changes in finish times, with an overall average of about 8.5 s (42). Males, on the other hand, improved in all years, with a mean time of approximately 8.5 s at age 10 years falling to 7.0 s at age 17 years (see fig. 12.1). Similar gender-related time differences were observed when children performed a shuttle run of 30 ft four times.

In a 5-year longitudinal study of 10 boys and 8 girls, Rowland and Cunningham found progressive improvement in the 50 yd dash in both sexes (unpublished data). Finish times were faster, however, in the boys at most ages. Improvement in sprint time over the 5 years was 14.2% for the boys and 10.5% for the girls. Similar findings have been reported in cross-sectional studies of sprint times in boys and girls in Canada (40), Bavaria (2), Israel (72), and the United Kingdom (14).

Lariviere and Godbout described cross-sectional differences in an ice skating test in boys between the ages of 6 and 16 years (49, cited by Malina and Bouchard [52]). Subjects were asked to skate 60 ft as rapidly as possible 12 times. Performance times declined almost linearly with age, from an average of 69 s at age 6-8 years to 52 s at age 15-16 years.

From these limited data we can conclude that improvements of approximately 25% in performance on short-burst activities can be expected in boys over a 10-year age span. Average finish times and improvement with age are somewhat less in females.

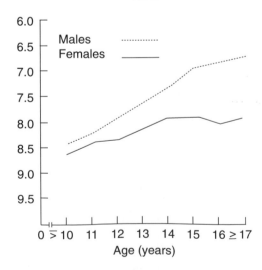

Figure 12.1   Changes in 50 yd dash times in boys and girls. Cross-sectional data from Hunsicker and Reiff (42). Reprinted from American Alliance for Health, Physical Education, Recreation and Dance 1976.

LABORATORY TESTS OF ANAEROBIC FITNESS

Laboratory testing of mean and peak anaerobic power in children reveals a progressive improvement with age, regardless of how these values are expressed relative to body size. As with aerobic power, males tend to have greater values than females, and this is particularly true after the age of puberty. Since weight-relative maximal aerobic power remains stable or declines during childhood, the ratio of anaerobic to aerobic fitness increases with age. Laboratory measures of anaerobic fitness may be reflected in short-burst exercise performance, but the finding of only moderately high correlation coefficients between the two suggests that other factors may play a significant role.

Cross-Sectional Studies

Bar-Or has provided cross-sectional data from his laboratory on Wingate test results in normal healthy children (5) (see figs. 12.2 through 12.5). Absolute values for mean and peak anaerobic power more than double between the ages of 8 and 14 years, with higher values for males. When normalized for body mass, mean anaerobic power rises from 5.5 to 6.5 W/kg over the same time span in the girls (18.2% increase) and from 5.6 to 8.0 W/kg (42.9% rise) in the boys. Peak power per kg increased from 6 to 9 W/kg in the girls and from 6.8 to 9.7 W/kg in the boys (50% and 43% increase, respectively).

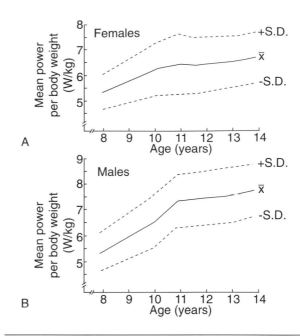

Figure 12.3 Changes in anaerobic capacity relative to body mass in children and adolescents measured by Wingate testing. Reprinted from Bar-Or 1983.

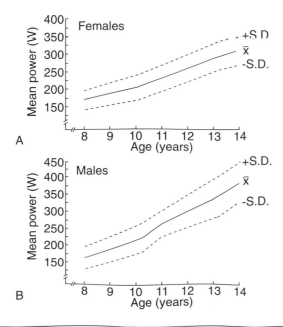

Figure 12.2 Changes in anaerobic capacity in children and adolescents measured by Wingate testing. Reprinted from Bar-Or 1983.

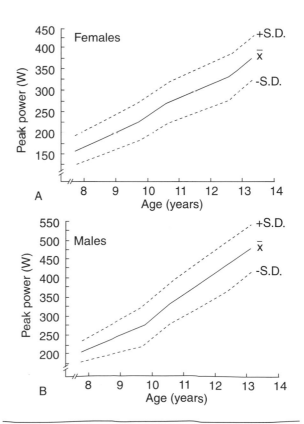

Figure 12.4 Changes in peak anaerobic power in children and adolescents measured by Wingate testing. Reprinted from Bar-Or 1983.

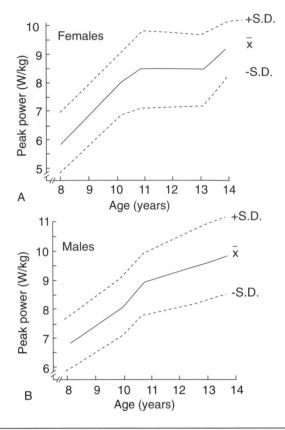

A

B

Figure 12.5   Changes in peak anaerobic power relative to body mass in children and adolescents measured by Wingate testing. Reprinted from Bar-Or 1983.

power. A progressive rise in both measures related to body weight was observed with age. Mean peak power rose from 6.2 W/kg at age 6-8 to 10.8 W/kg at age 14-15 years (74.2% increase), while average mean power rose from 4.7 to 7.6 W/kg (61.7% increase). Mean $\dot{V}O_2$max per kg on cycle testing did not change from 6 to 15 years (about 49 ml · kg^{-1} · min^{-1}); therefore the ratio of anaerobic to aerobic fitness, as indicated by mean power:$\dot{V}O_2$max and peak power:$\dot{V}O_2$max, increased with age (r = 0.71 and 0.73, respectively).

Blimkie et al. studied the anaerobic:aerobic power ratio in 24 boys and 27 girls between the ages of 14 and 18 years to assess the relative importance of these energy systems in growing children (11). Anaerobic power was measured by Wingate testing, while $\dot{V}O_2$max was determined on a progressive cycling protocol. Figure 12.6 illustrates the ratio of the two expressed per kg body mass, with added values from Bar-Or (5) and Cumming (16) for aerobic fitness in the age range 8-14 years. The data show a progressive increase during childhood with a plateau in adolescence.

Mercier et al. found that maximal anaerobic power in 69 males ages 11 to 19 years related closely to leg volume (r = 0.84) and lean body mass (r = 0.94) (56). However, when maximal anaerobic power was normalized to lean body mass, values still increased progressively between 11 and 19 years.

Saavedra et al. used tests of all-out knee extension work over 10, 30, and 90 s to assess anaerobic fitness in 84 girls and 83 boys ages 9 to 16 years (73). Anaerobic performance improved with increasing age in all tests, whether or not results were related to body weight, fat-free mass, or thigh cross-sectional area. The authors concluded that "factors other than muscle mass must be involved in order to explain the differences in maximal anaerobic working capacity between children and

Falgairette et al. reported findings on a cross-sectional study of 144 boys ages 6-15 years (28). Maximal anaerobic power was determined by force-velocity test, while the Wingate test was used to establish mean

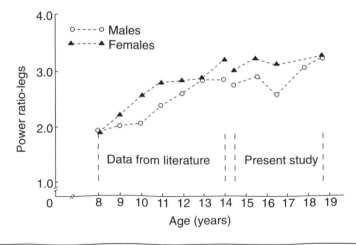

Figure 12.6   Changes in the anaerobic:aerobic power ratio during childhood and adolescence. Reprinted from Blimkie, Roche, and Bar-Or 1986.

adults" (p. 1087). In this study, males tended to have greater values for anaerobic power relative to the different anthropometric indices, most prominently after puberty. For instance, maximal work output for 90 s expressed as a function of body mass or fat-free mass was significantly greater in the males from age 13 on but not in younger age groups.

Sargeant and Dolan hypothesized that the reason for adult-child differences in anaerobic power might be that "measurements of power output may not be made at the optimal velocity for maximal power output because of systematic differences between the groups" (75, p. 39). They studied power output over a wide range of contraction velocities in 30 adults and 25 children using an isokinetic cycle ergometer. Contrary to their theory, crank velocity was not different between the groups at maximal power (about 125 rpm). When normalized for the size of the active muscle mass, power output in the children was about 17% less than in the adults.

Van Praagh et al. compared the anaerobic characteristics of the legs in 12-year-old boys and girls (88). Maximal power, measured with the force-velocity test, was 33% greater in the males. This difference fell to 31% and 15% when peak power was expressed relative to body mass and fat-free mass, respectively. This same pattern of gender differences was observed with mean power.

Sargeant et al. showed lower levels of peak power in 13-year-olds compared to adults (76). Using a 20 s all-out test during isokinetic work at four different pedaling speeds, the authors found that peak power relative to upper leg volume was 40% greater in the adults.

Longitudinal Studies

Duche et al. reported longitudinal data on anaerobic fitness in 13 boys from age 9 to 11 years and in 11 additional subjects from 12 to 14 years (22). Mean and maximal power were determined by Wingate and force-velocity testing, respectively. $\dot{V}O_2$max was established by cycle testing. Results normalized to body mass indicated a steady rise in both measures of anaerobic fitness (see fig. 12.7). When values of peak and mean power were related to $\dot{V}O_2$max, the increase in ratios with age mimicked those described by Blimkie et al. (11).

These findings were duplicated in the mixed cross-sectional longitudinal study of Falk and Bar-Or (30). Prepubertal (n = 16), midpubertal (n = 15), and late pubertal (n = 5) boys were studied via measurements of $\dot{V}O_2$max and peak and mean anaerobic power (by Wingate testing) at 6-month intervals for 18 months. No changes were observed in $\dot{V}O_2$max per kg, but peak and mean anaerobic power expressed per kg body mass increased progressively across the age groups. Thus this

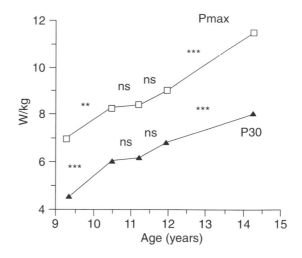

Figure 12.7 Longitudinal development of maximal anaerobic power (Pmax) and mean anaerobic power (P30) during childhood and early adolescence. Reprinted from Duche et al. 1992.

study confirmed a rise in the anaerobic:aerobic power ratio between ages 10 and 14, with a plateau thereafter.

Two additional pieces of information arose from this study. First, a high degree of tracking, or maintenance of relative position in the groups, was reported over the 18-month period. This short-term stability was indicated by rank order correlation coefficients between sessions 1 and 4 of 0.92 and 0.97 for absolute peak and mean anaerobic power, respectively, and 0.56 and 0.85 when these values were expressed relative to body weight. Secondly, a high correlation between peak mechanical aerobic power and peak and mean anaerobic power was observed in the pre- and circumpubertal boys but not in the late pubertal group. This finding supports the concept proposed by Bar-Or (5) that children, in contrast to adults, are "metabolic non-specialists" (p. 16). That is, children who are skilled in aerobic activities tend to do well in short-burst anaerobic activities as well.

Arm Exercise

Studies investigating anaerobic fitness with arm exercise have been limited to adolescents. In general, these have demonstrated the same findings as the studies involving leg exercise reviewed earlier. Blimkie et al. evaluated the anaerobic capacities of the upper arms in 50 girls and 50 boys 14 to 19 years of age (12). Peak as well as mean power by Wingate testing increased with age in the boys but not the girls, and both power values were greater in the boys at comparable ages. When corrected for arm volume, both power values were still greater in the older than in the younger boys, but, again, the values did not vary with age in the girls. Gender differences in powers related to arm volume were significant only in the older age groups. This study reinforced the concept that factors other than muscle mass are important in the development of anaerobic fitness in the teenage years, but this pattern was evident only in males.

Vandewalle et al. explored age-related differences in peak anaerobic power in adolescent athletes using the force-velocity test (86). They tested 28 male swimmers who ranked within the top 40 swimmers in France in their age groups. Between the ages of 12 and 15 years, there was a progressive increase in peak power with age (from 6.3 to 9.0 W/kg), but values subsequently remained stable through to age 18 years.

Studies During Exercise Recovery

Further evidence for a limitation of anaerobic fitness in younger children comes from an examination of (1) age-related changes in the O_2 debt during recovery from maximal exercise, and (2) the rapidity of recovery of anaerobic power after Wingate testing.

The total $\dot{V}O_2$ during recovery from maximal exercise (the O_2 debt) has been considered an indicator of anaerobic energy contribution to the preceding exercise bout. Paterson et al. reported longitudinal changes in recovery $\dot{V}O_2$ in 19 boys studied yearly from ages 11 to 15 years (63). Oxygen debt was estimated from the total recovery $\dot{V}O_2$ after maximal treadmill testing minus the value of pre-exercise $\dot{V}O_2$. Absolute recovery $\dot{V}O_2$ increased 98% over the five testing sessions while weight-relative values rose 80%. The improvement was

virtually linear when values were expressed relative to either chronological age or biological maturation (peak height velocity) (see fig. 12.8). Average annual increment was 0.8 L or 9 ml/kg.

Hebestreit et al. showed that prepubertal males experience a more rapid recovery of muscle power after high-intensity short-term exercise than adults (41). Eight boys ages 9-12 years and eight young men ages 19-23 years performed two consecutive 30 s Wingate cycling tests separated by 1, 2, and 3 min recovery periods. Average values for mean power for the boys were 89% of the initial value after 1 min of recovery, 96% after 2 min, and 103% after 10 min. Respective values for the men were 71%, 77%, and 94%. The authors suggested that lower blood lactate and less acidosis at maximal exercise (discussed later in this chapter) in the boys might explain these findings.

Relationship of Laboratory Testing to Field Performance

Moderately strong correlations are observed when performance on short-burst exercise activities is related to findings on anaerobic laboratory testing. As with other comparisons of physiologic variables in children, however, cause and effect are difficult to prove: any such correlation may simply reflect a "linkage" of two factors that independently increase with growth, age, or biological maturation. The observation, too, that the correlation between field and laboratory performance is not high indicates that even if the association is causal, other factors (e.g., skill, motor coordination) are important in short-burst activities.

Van Praagh et al. compared the results of maximal anaerobic power (force-velocity test) and mean aerobic power (Wingate test) with sprint performance in 7-year-old boys (87). Maximal power was significantly correlated with velocity on a 30 m dash (r = 0.45, p < .05). A stronger relationship was observed between velocity on a 30 s shuttle run and mean anaerobic power (r = 0.60, p < .001).

In another report cited previously, Van Praagh et al. described 31% higher maximal power per kg in 12-year-old boys than in girls (88). The authors noted that these laboratory differences were also manifest in field performance on short-burst events: velocity on a 30 m dash was 5.8 and 5.4 m/s for the boys and girls, respectively (p < .05), and the boys covered a greater distance on the 30 s shuttle run (142 vs. 132 m, p < .001). The field test results were moderately linked to findings in the laboratory. Correlation coefficients between peak power per kg and the 30 m dash were r = 0.23 (p > .05) and 0.71 (p < .001) in the girls and boys, respectively. For mean power per kg the coefficients were r = 0.58 and 0.62 (p < .05 for both).

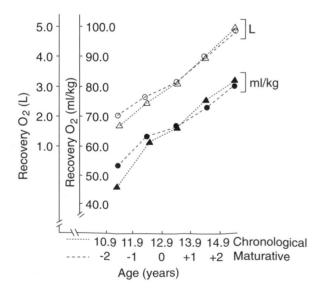

Figure 12.8 Longitudinal increases in postexercise O_2 debt during childhood relative to chronological and biological age. Reprinted from Paterson et al. 1986.

Tharp et al. found correlations of r = −0.69 with 50 yd dash times and peak power per kg on Wingate testing in 10-15-year-old children (84), and Bar-Or and Inbar reported a coefficient between 40 m run speed and absolute peak power of 0.84 in the same age group (7). In reviewing these data, Bar-Or stated, "One may conclude that the correlation between the Wingate anaerobic test power indices and 'anaerobic performance' is quite high, but not high enough for using the Wingate anaerobic test as a predictor of success in these specific tasks" (6, p. 388).

BLOOD LACTATE LEVELS

Lactic acid is a by-product of anaerobic glycolysis. It would seem logical, then, that the amount of lactate released from exercising muscle cells should serve as an accurate gauge of anaerobic energy expenditure. On the basis of this reasoning, blood lactate level during exercise has been utilized as a marker of both aerobic and anaerobic fitness. In the former case, lactate levels are interpreted as an expression of the limits of aerobic fitness before anaerobiosis ensues as a "default" energy source; in the latter, lactate concentrations serve as an indicator of the capability of the anaerobic metabolic machinery to generate energy.

But serious questions have arisen about the validity of blood lactate levels during exercise as an accurate indicator of glycolysis occurring within the muscle cell. Most importantly, blood lactate levels reflect not only lactate production but also clearance; indeed, lactate levels might be best interpreted as an index of the balance between the two processes. Other factors may significantly influence lactate levels as well, including rate of release from the muscle cell, rate of lactate utilization by organs such as the liver and heart, and volume of distribution within the body fluids.

A number of methodological issues regarding lactate determination can significantly influence blood levels. These problems, reviewed by Armstrong and Welsman (1), make comparisons between studies difficult. Lactate levels can be profoundly influenced by mode of exercise (e.g., cycle vs. running), site of blood sampling (arterial vs. venous, upper vs. lower extremity), test protocol, timing of the determination, and method of assay.

With these caveats in mind, reports of the patterns of lactate response to exercise in growing children can be reviewed. The research data in this case are remarkably consistent: both submaximal and maximal exercise lactate levels rise progressively during the course of childhood and adolescence. Limited biopsy information suggests that this is a direct reflection of changes in muscle lactate concentration. The literature shows that girls tend to have slightly higher levels than boys. The anaerobic threshold, estimated noninvasively by ventilatory responses to exercise, rises in age in absolute terms but decreases when expressed as percentage of $\dot{V}O_2max$. This has been interpreted as indicative of improved glycolytic function or, alternatively, of diminished aerobic fitness with biological maturation.

Cross-Sectional Studies

Robinson was the first to describe cross-sectional peak exercise lactate levels related to age (68). He reported a progressive increase in values at exhaustion from treadmill exercise from ages 6 to 19, with lactate levels more than doubling in that age span (from 25.1 to 65.7 grams percent). Morse et al. performed a similar study with 80 boys ages 12 to 17 years (59). Again, a progressive increase in peak lactate levels was seen with age; this was expressed by the formula $Y = -10.1 + 5.0X$ (where Y = maximal lactate in milligrams percent and X = age). Difference between the mean values for the youngest and oldest subjects was again more than twofold (32 and 68 milligrams percent, respectively).

Åstrand was the first to compare boys and girls in his lactate responses to exercise (3). His 1952 study confirmed a steady rise with age in peak lactate values during cycling. Levels in boys rose from an average of 56.3 milligrams percent at age 4-6 years to 104.9 milligrams percent in the 16-18-year-old group. Values were somewhat higher at all ages compared to the data of Robinson (68) and Morse et al. (59), perhaps reflecting the fact that Åstrand obtained blood specimens "when intensity of work was close to maximum" instead of at 5 min postexercise as in both of the earlier studies (p. 21). Åstrand found no significant differences between peak lactate concentrations in boys and girls before the time of puberty, but in the 12-18-year-old age range the girls had higher values.

Eriksson et al. provided additional insights into maturity-related differences in lactate responses to exercise (27). These authors studied eight circumpubertal 13-year-old boys during progressive maximal cycle exercise, using serial quadriceps biopsies and blood lactate levels. Muscle lactate rose little until an intensity of approximately 50% $\dot{V}O_2max$ was reached. Beyond this point there was a curvilinear rise to a maximal value of 11.3 mm/kg. Blood lactate concentration paralleled that of muscle lactate. These patterns were similar to those observed in adults, but the values were lower (see fig. 12.9). The authors concluded, "It seems likely that the reason for the lower blood lactate concentration in young subjects after exercise is due to a lower production of lactate" (p. 156). That study showed a moderate correlation (r = 0.67) between maximal muscle lactate and testicular volume, suggesting that sexual maturity may influence lactate production.

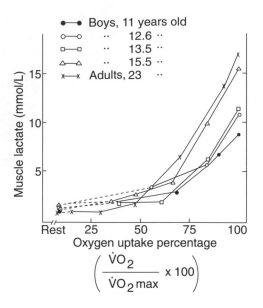

Figure 12.9 Maturational effects on muscle lactate at different work intensities. Reprinted from Eriksson et al. 1971.

Several cross-sectional studies have subsequently confirmed the pattern of progressively increasing peak blood lactate levels as children grow (3, 17, 18, 20, 28, 78, 100). These data are presented in figures 12.10 and 12.11. The question of gender differences in lactate production, however, has not been so neatly delineated. In their study of 100 boys and 91 girls ages 11 to 16 years, Williams and Armstrong found that mean peak blood lactate values were significantly greater in the girls than in the boys (6.1 vs. 5.8 mmol/L, p < .01) (95). The authors noted that such discrepancies might be explained by variations in sexual maturation. For any particular chronological age, girls can be expected to be ahead of boys in level of biological maturation by about 2 years; hence, the higher peak lactates in the girls might reflect their more advanced biological age. However, in this particular study, no relationship was observed between level of sexual maturation and peak lactate levels.

Others have described no gender effects on peak lactate levels (17, 20, 79, 88). Van Praagh et al. found no significant differences in peak lactate between 12-year-old boys and girls with Wingate testing or after a 30 s shuttle run (88). Shephard et al. reported no significant differences between boys and girls in mean arterial lac-

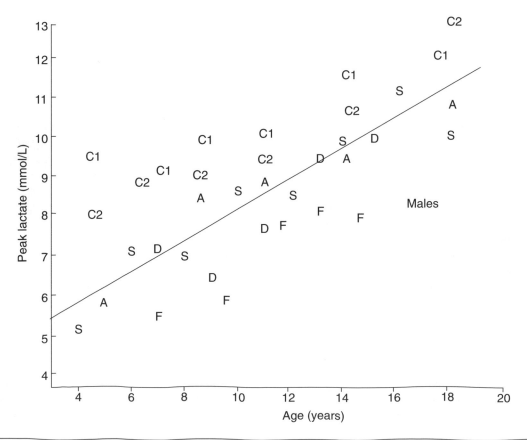

Figure 12.10 Cross-sectional studies of maximal blood lactate level with age in boys. Data are from various sources: A (3), C1 (18), C2 (19), D (20), F (28), S (78).

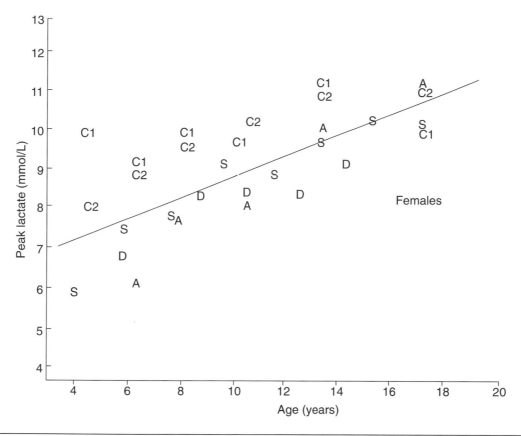

Figure 12.11   Cross-sectional studies of maximal blood lactate levels with age in girls. Reference abbreviations are the same as for figure 12.10.

tate concentrations after a maximal treadmill test (78.7 vs. 77.1 milligrams percent, respectively) (79). Likewise, no gender differences in peak lactate values were reported by Davies et al. (20) in children 7-15 years (determined immediately at peak cycling) or by Cumming et al. (17) in subjects 4 to 20 years old 2 min after maximal treadmill exercise.

Consistent with the progressively higher peak blood lactate levels observed with age, blood pH at maximal exercise also declines as children grow. Bar-Or (5) compiled data from three studies in the German literature indicating a steady decline in maximal pH with age after maximal cycle exercise as well as after a 300 m run (45, 53, 91) (see fig. 12.12).

Cumming et al. found higher postexercise lactate levels in children than others had obtained, and suggested that "previous investigators emphasizing low serum lactate levels in young children may not have had their children perform enough anaerobic work" (18, p. 66). Still, the data of Cumming et al. show a progressive rise in peak exercise lactate levels in boys, with a mean of 9.5 mmol/L at ages 4-5 years and 12.1 mmol/L at ages 16-20 years. While overall there were no gender influences seen in peak lactate concentrations, the girls

showed no clear-cut trend for increase with age. In fact, mean values at ages 4-5 and 16-20 were identical (10.4 mmol/L). Williams and Armstrong also could find no significant differences in peak lactate values relative to age in their study of boys and girls 11 to 16 years (95).

Submaximal blood lactate levels are lower in children than in adults, too, and this is true even when values are obtained at the same relative work load. Wirth et al. measured blood lactate immediately after a 15 min bout of cycling at 70% $\dot{V}O_2$max in 41 swimmers ages 8 to 18 years (98). Mean values for pre-, circum-, and postpubertal boys were 2.03, 2.45, and 3.40 mmol/L, respectively. Levels for female swimmers in the same pubertal groups were 2.41, 2.72, and 3.33 mmol/L. No significant differences in submaximal lactate values were found between the boys and girls.

Longitudinal Studies

Paterson et al. described the rate of development of maximal lactate production during treadmill exercise in 19 boys (63). Subjects were tested annually for 5 years beginning at age 11. Maximal lactate levels increased with chronological age, rising from 7.8 mmol/L at age

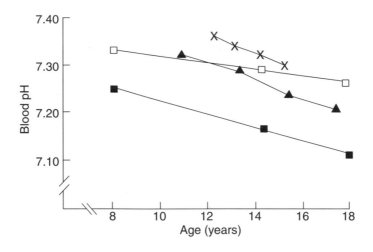

Figure 12.12   Blood pH at finish of maximal cycle and run exercise relative to age. Reprinted from Bar-Or 1983.

11 to 11.0 mmol/L at age 15 (see fig. 12.13). Increases were similar from year to year, averaging 0.9 mmol/L per year. A similar pattern was observed when the peak lactate concentrations were analyzed relative to biological maturation (peak height velocity, PHV). That is, there was no evidence that puberty influenced the capacity for lactate production.

Sjodin and Svedenhag could not confirm this finding in a small number of subjects (80). They tested four healthy, nontraining boys every 6 months for 8 years beginning at age 12. Blood lactate levels measured within 1 min after maximal treadmill running remained almost constant with no observable upward trend (mean about 9.5 mmol/L).

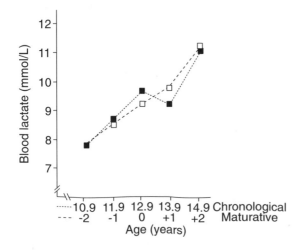

Figure 12.13   Longitudinal changes in maximal blood lactate relative to chronological and biological age. Reprinted from Paterson et al. 1986.

ANAEROBIC THRESHOLD

During a progressive exercise test, little change is typically observed in blood lactate levels until work intensity reaches 50-60% $\dot{V}O_2$max. Beyond this point, lactate levels rise in a curvilinear fashion to maximum. The point at which lactate begins to rise has been termed the *anaerobic threshold* (AT). According to the traditional paradigm, AT marks the point when O_2 supply to exercise muscle begins to be limited, triggering the onset of anaerobic metabolism as a backup energy source. There is, however, a great deal of controversy surrounding the measurement and interpretation of the AT, and this has been reviewed elsewhere (13, 21). In reviewing the current research information, Armstrong and Welsman concluded, "The majority view now appears to be that the level of lactate measured in the blood reflects the balance between lactate production and elimination. The first increase in lactate levels observed during incremental exercise therefore reflects the intensity at which processes of production and diffusion from muscle to blood exceed those of elimination and metabolism rather than indicating the onset of anaerobiosis in the muscle cell" (1, p. 458).

Uncertainties regarding its meaning notwithstanding, the AT has been utilized to (1) establish a target heart rate for aerobic training and rehabilitation exercise programs (71); (2) estimate aerobic fitness in subjects who may not tolerate maximal testing (67); (3) distinguish the pathophysiological basis for exercise limitation (92); (4) provide training guidelines for competitive athletes (43); (5) indicate an individual's capacity to exercise "aerobically" without triggering anaerobic metabolism (91); and (6) assess capability of generating energy by glycolytic pathways during exercise (65).

In most studies, AT has been estimated noninvasively by alterations in gas exchange parameters during exercise rather than by determination of lactate concentrations. This is based on the concept that at AT, the buffering of lactic acid generates excessive CO_2 production beyond that produced by exercising muscles. The increase in ventilation triggered by this extra CO_2 results in a divergence of $\dot{V}_E$ from its linear relationship to $\dot{V}O_2$ and a subsequent rise in the ventilatory equivalent for O_2. These markers of the *ventilatory anaerobic threshold* (VAT) presumably relate to AT, but studies attempting to verify this linkage (all in adult subjects) have proven conflicting (90). The noninvasive ease of determining VAT, however, has led to its almost exclusive use in the pediatric age group.

The pattern of changes in ventilation relative to $\dot{V}O_2$ during a progressive exercise test are similar in children and adults. But there are differences in VAT in the two groups that appear to relate directly with increasing age during childhood. Absolute $\dot{V}O_2$ at VAT increases as expected during childhood, reflecting increasing body size. But most studies have indicated that when expressed per kg, VAT falls with age. With a relatively stable $\dot{V}O_2$max per kg, this results in a progressive decline in VAT as percentage of $\dot{V}O_2$max. This finding has been interpreted as indicating an increase in anaerobic capacity during growth (65).

The following results of studies investigating VAT in children must be considered with the potential influences of testing methodology in mind. Little is known about the effects on VAT of test protocol (i.e., stage duration), testing modality (treadmill vs. cycle), measurement techniques (1 min Douglas bag collection vs. breath-by-breath analysis), test to test reproducibility, and intraobserver reliability. For instance, in their investigation of AT in children (reviewed further on), Kanaley and Boileau showed that AT as percentage of $\dot{V}O_2$max was significantly greater on a walk/run protocol than with a continuous walk (71% vs. 57%) (44).

Cross-Sectional Studies

Reybrouck et al. investigated the influence of age on VAT in a cross-sectional study of 257 children between the ages of 5 and 18 years (66) (see fig. 12.14). $\dot{V}O_2$max per kg showed a slight upward trend over this age span in the boys, while values in the girls were essentially stable. $\dot{V}O_2$ per kg at AT declined in both groups, more so in the males. Consequently, for both boys and girls a significant decline in VAT as a percentage of $\dot{V}O_2$max was observed. Ventilatory anaerobic threshold at age 5-6 years was 74.4% and 69.2% of $\dot{V}O_2$max in the boys and girls, respectively, while values at age 15-16 years were 61.0% and 53.8%.

Cooper et al. studied 109 healthy children using breath-by-breath analysis with a ramp cycle protocol (15). Subjects were divided into four groups by gender and age: younger girls (6-11 years), younger boys (6-13 years), older girls (12-17 years), and older boys (14-17 years). Absolute AT correlated closely with body weight, with an overall allometric scaling factor of 0.92. When AT was normalized for body weight there was no significant correlation with age (r = 0.30). Anaerobic threshold as a percentage of $\dot{V}O_2$max decreased slightly as weight increased (r = –0.28, p < .05), with a mean overall value of 60%. In the older boys, average AT was 55% $\dot{V}O_2$max, while mean value in the younger boys was 64%. Values for the older and younger girls followed the same pattern (58% and 61%, respectively).

Fifty-two children ages 6, 11, and 14 years, studied by Weymans et al., performed a graded progressive walking treadmill test (94). Expired air was collected every minute in Douglas bags. Ventilatory anaerobic threshold was determined as "the starting point of the

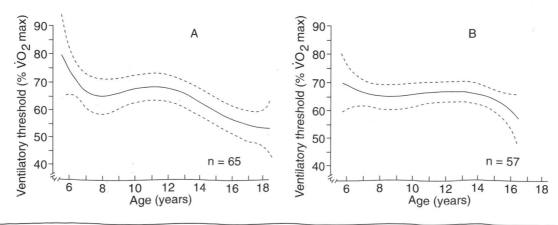

Figure 12.14 Cross-sectional values for ventilatory anaerobic threshold expressed as percentage $\dot{V}O_2$max in A) boys and B) girls. Reprinted from Reybrouck et al. 1985.

nonlinear change in $\dot{V}_E$ with increasing $\dot{V}O_2$" (p. 114). Overall VAT mean was 66% $\dot{V}O_2$max for both boys and girls. Ventilatory anaerobic threshold expressed either as ml $\cdot$ kg^{-1} $\cdot$ min^{-1} or percentage of $\dot{V}O_2$max declined progressively with increasing age group in both sexes.

Kanaley and Boileau studied the effects of biological maturity on AT in groups of males who were prepubertal (age 8.7 to 11.8 years), pubertal (age 13.1 to 14.6 years), and postpubertal (age 18.7 to 24.4 years) (44). When expressed as percentage of $\dot{V}O_2$max, AT declined with increasing age, with mean values of 68.8%, 65.4%, and 58.5% in the three groups, respectively. The authors suggested that these findings reflected an increase in anaerobic capacity with growth.

Girandola et al. described mean VAT values of 66% and 54% $\dot{V}O_2$max in girls 11 and 16 years old, respectively, during treadmill testing (35). Rowland and Green found higher average VAT values in 13 premenarcheal girls and 13 young adult females (71% vs. 67% $\dot{V}O_2$max), but the difference was not statistically significant (70).

Longitudinal Study

Vanden Eynde et al. measured physiological responses to maximal cycle exercise in 30 healthy Flemish boys once a year for a period of six consecutive years (85). Values for $\dot{V}O_2$max, percentage of $\dot{V}O_2$max at AT, and sport participation are depicted in figure 12.15 relative to the age of PHV. The mean value for percentage $\dot{V}O_2$max at AT decreased from 68.4% at 1.5 years prior to PHV to 59.4% at 1.5 years after PHV. The decrease was relatively linear and showed no clear change at PHV itself.

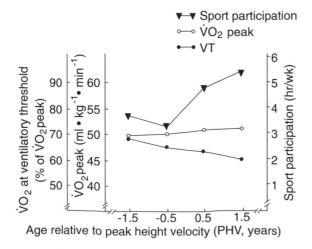

Figure 12.15 Longitudinal changes in $\dot{V}O_2$max and ventilatory anaerobic threshold expressed as percentage $\dot{V}O_2$max relative to age at peak height velocity in 30 boys. Reprinted from Vanden Eynde et al. 1989.

Effects of Physical Training

The issue of anaerobic trainability will be considered later in this chapter, but an examination of changes in AT with training at this point may be useful in clarifying the physiological significance of this measurement. It will be recalled that the higher AT as percentage of $\dot{V}O_2$max in children as compared to adults has been ascribed to an inferior anaerobic capacity in prepubertal subjects. Still, elite child endurance athletes typically have even higher AT values, suggesting that AT as percentage of $\dot{V}O_2$max is an index of aerobic rather than anaerobic fitness. Supporting this idea, VAT as a percentage of $\dot{V}O_2$max has been shown to rise following both endurance (aerobic) and interval (anaerobic) training. It might be reasonable to conclude from these data that VAT as percentage of $\dot{V}O_2$max can serve as an index of either anaerobic or aerobic fitness.

Several studies have indicated higher AT values in child athletes. Nudel et al. studied 16 well-trained runners 8-17 years old (61). Subjects had been running competitively for an average of 8.4 years and were currently training 30-105 miles weekly. Mean $\dot{V}O_2$max values were 61.0 and 43.2 ml $\cdot$ kg^{-1} $\cdot$ min^{-1} in runners and nonathletic control subjects, with VAT of 48.8 and 25.0 ml $\cdot$ kg^{-1} $\cdot$ min^{-1}, respectively. Percentage of $\dot{V}O_2$max at VAT averaged 80.6% for the runners and 57.8% for the controls.

Faria et al. reported VAT in 15 highly trained adolescent road racing cyclists (mean age 15.0 years) (31). $\dot{V}O_2$max averaged 75.5 ml $\cdot$ kg^{-1} $\cdot$ min^{-1} for the group, and mean VAT was 83% of $\dot{V}O_2$max. Wolfe et al. found a mean VAT of 70.1% $\dot{V}O_2$max in female cross-country runners 10-13 years old (99). The 24 female cross-country runners (mean age 15.9 years) studied by Cunningham had an average VAT of 78.8% (19).

In a rare study of lactate AT in children, Atomi et al. compared AT during treadmill running in athletic and nonathletic boys ages 11-12 years (4). Eleven subjects had trained 3 hr daily, 6 days a week, for more than 3 years, while 13 were untrained controls. Mean $\dot{V}O_2$max values in the two groups were 58.0 and 51.2 ml $\cdot$ kg^{-1} $\cdot$ min^{-1}, respectively. Average AT of the athletic boys was significantly greater than that of the nontraining subjects in both absolute values (45.5 vs. 33.2 ml $\cdot$ kg^{-1} $\cdot$ min^{-1}) and relative values (78.9% vs. 63.7% $\dot{V}O_2$max).

Studies of changes in AT after physical training of nonathletic children have produced mixed results. Mahon and Vaccaro found that run training produced significant increases in VAT, both in absolute terms and relative to $\dot{V}O_2$max (51). After 8 weeks of training, a 19.4% rise in VAT from 30.5 to 36.4 ml $\cdot$ kg^{-1} $\cdot$ min^{-1} was observed in 8 boys 10-14 years of age. Ventilatory anaerobic threshold as percentage of $\dot{V}O_2$max rose from a mean of 67% to 74%. Similar changes were not seen in nontraining controls.

Haffor et al. trained five 11-year old boys with interval work (intensities above AT) five times a week for 6 weeks (38). $\dot{V}O_2$max did not change significantly, but the training resulted in an average increase in VAT from 59.0% to 72% $\dot{V}O_2$max. There were no nontraining control subjects in this study, however; the importance of this is illustrated by the following report.

Becker and Vaccaro trained 11 boys ages 9-11 years with cycle exercise for 8 weeks (9). Subjects pedaled at an intensity halfway between heart rate at AT and heart rate at $\dot{V}O_2$max for 40 min, 3 days/week. $\dot{V}O_2$max rose from 39.0 to 47.0 ml $\cdot$ kg^{-1} $\cdot$ min^{-1} in the training subjects and from 41.7 to 44 ml $\cdot$ kg^{-1} $\cdot$ min^{-1} in nontraining controls. Respective changes for VAT were 26.0 to 33.2 ml $\cdot$ kg^{-1} $\cdot$ min^{-1} and 28.5 to 32.3 ml $\cdot$ kg^{-1} $\cdot$ min^{-1}. Thus the rise in VAT as percentage of $\dot{V}O_2$max was similar in the two groups (66.6% to 70.7% and 68.3% to 73.4% in trained and control subjects, respectively). The authors commented that "the increase in AT demonstrated by the control group cannot be readily explained. One can only speculate that it might be at least in part due to a high physical activity level in this group which could not be practically controlled" (p. 447).

The report of Paterson et al. suggests that sport training can reverse the expected fall in AT as percentage of $\dot{V}O_2$max as children grow (64). These investigators determined VAT during maximal treadmill testing yearly in 18 highly fit boys between the ages of 10.8 and 14.8 years. The boys, who had an initial mean $\dot{V}O_2$max value of 60.8 ml $\cdot$ kg^{-1} $\cdot$ min^{-1}, were actively training in a variety of sports, including hockey, basketball, football, and track and field. Both weight-relative $\dot{V}O_2$max and VAT increased with age, but the relative greater rise in the latter resulted in an increase in percentage of $\dot{V}O_2$max at AT from 56.0% to 61.6% over the 5 years.

Rotstein et al. studied the effects of a 9-week interval training program on aerobic and anaerobic fitness of 28 nonathletic boys ages 10.2 to 11.6 years (69). Mean $\dot{V}O_2$max improved by 8.9% with training, a significant rise over the control value. Anaerobic threshold, determined during treadmill running at 1% grade, was evaluated by four different indices: (a) running velocity when blood lactate reached 4 mmol/L; (b) running velocity at the point of upward deflection of the lactate curve; (c) percentage of $\dot{V}O_2$max when (a) occurred; and (d) percentage of $\dot{V}O_2$max when (b) occurred. The experimental group demonstrated a small but significant increase in (a), while significant decreases in (c) and (d) of 4.4% and 4.3%, respectively, "may reflect the increase in $\dot{V}O_2$max" (p. 285). No changes in any of the indices were observed in the control subjects. The authors concluded that "the absolute and rel-

ative AT are less responsive to such a training regimen than is the $\dot{V}O_2$max" (p. 285).

Relationship to Performance

The cross-sectional data reviewed indicate that higher AT values are associated with superior athletic performance. When the relationship of field performance to AT is examined within homogeneous fitness groups, however, the relationship is weakened.

Wolfe et al. reported no significant relationship between performance scores (cumulative order of finish during a competitive season) and AT as percentage of $\dot{V}O_2$max in their study of 10-13-year-old female cross-country runners (99). In a similar group of female runners, Cunningham found that $\dot{V}O_2$ at VAT correlated with 5K race time (r = −.66, p < .001), but there was no such relationship with VAT as percentage of $\dot{V}O_2$max (r = .08) (19). However, Tanaka reported that the start of blood lactate accumulation was significantly related to performance in a 5 min run in 14-year-old boys (82).

Maximal Lactate Steady State

Another approach to the evaluation of aerobic and anaerobic fitness is to assess physiological parameters relative to a fixed blood lactate value. In adults, a value of 4.0 mmol/L has been often utilized, since this level typically corresponds to the greatest submaximal exercise intensity that can be sustained without a rise in lactate (the maximal lactate steady state). That is, an exercise intensity eliciting a lactate level of 4.0 mmol/L is a reasonable approximation for mean AT within a group of adult subjects. Of course, there is significant interindividual variability around this value.

Lactate levels are lower in children than in adults at the same relative exercise intensity. Therefore a value of 4.0 mmol/L is too high as an estimate of maximal lactate steady state in children. Williams et al. evaluated the 4 mmol/L lactate levels as an indicator of exercise performance in 103 children ages 11-13 years (97). Mean $\dot{V}O_2$max values were 48 and 42 ml $\cdot$ kg^{-1} $\cdot$ min^{-1} for boys (n = 53) and girls (n = 50), respectively. The exercise intensity corresponding to a blood lactate concentration of 4 mmol/L averaged 91% of $\dot{V}O_2$max in both boys and girls. This intensity was considered too high to permit use of this lactate threshold (LT) for evaluating exercise performance in children of this age.

In a subsequent study, Williams and Armstrong demonstrated that maximal lactate steady state occurred at mean lactate levels of 2.1 and 2.3 mmol/L in 13-year-old untrained boys and girls, respectively (96). They proposed a 2.5 mmol/L level as an appropriate means of measuring submaximal fitness in children. In that study the 2.5 mmol/L criterion was established at an average of 84% and 82% $\dot{V}O_2$max in the boys and girls, respectively. Corresponding values at the 4.0 mmol/L level were 93% and 90% $\dot{V}O_2$max, respectively.

Gaisl and Buchberger found lower values in a group of 45 boys ages 10-11 years who had just finished their 3rd month of an 8 hr/week training program (33). Mean percentage of $\dot{V}O_2$max with blood lactate of 2.5 mmol/L was 64.7%, with a value at 4.5 mmol/L of 84.2%.

Tanaka and Shindo reported findings at a blood LT of "just below 2 mmol L^{-1}" in five age groups ranging from 6 to 18 years (83, p. 92). No statistically significant differences in running velocity at LT were seen between the 6- and 15-year-old groups, but velocity was related to bone maturity scores ($r = -0.32$, $p < .05$). Percentage maximal heart rate at LT was inversely related to both chronological and bone age.

ANAEROBIC ENZYME ACTIVITY

The qualitative and quantitative integrity of glycolytic metabolic pathways in children would be ideally studied by in vivo analysis of enzymatic activities during exercise. Instead, methodological and ethical constraints have limited information on this question to a very few studies using in vitro enzyme analysis in a limited number of subjects. Moreover, comparisons between groups is rendered difficult because the physical activity status of the subjects has not been controlled. These concerns notwithstanding, the available data do suggest that activity levels of key enzymes in the gly-

colytic pathway may be depressed in children compared to adults (25).

Animal Studies

Emmett and Hochachka have presented some intriguing scaling information indicating that the activities of enzymes important in anaerobic glycolysis (glycogen phosphorylase, pyruvate kinase, lactic dehydrogenase) increase as the body size of animals increases (24). They examined enzyme activities in the gastrocnemius muscles of 10 mammalian species varying in size by a factor of 10^6. Scaling exponents of these three enzymes relative to body mass ranged from +.09 to +.15. In other words, the larger the animal, the greater the skeletal muscle anaerobic enzyme activity (see fig. 12.16).

Somero and Childress reported similar findings in their study of anaerobic enzyme activities in skeletal muscle of 13 species of fish (81). In most species, a direct relationship was found between animal mass and glycolytic enzyme activity (lactic dehydrogenase, pyruvate kinase). The relationship was not observed in brain tissue, leading the authors to conclude that "the scaling in muscle is probably due to selective factors related to locomotion" (p. 334).

There is some evidence in animals, then, that size per se influences the potential for production of anaerobic energy. The reason for this observation is not readily apparent. Nonetheless, these animal data provide an interesting backdrop to information suggesting an increase in glycolytic capacity and short-burst activity fitness in growing children.

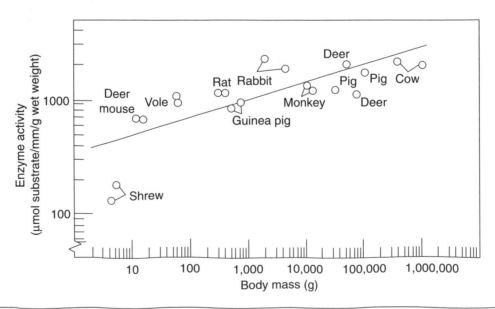

Figure 12.16   Activity of lactic dehydrogenase in samples of gastrocnemius muscle in adult animals of different sizes. Reprinted from Emmett and Hochachka 1986.

Enzyme Activities in Children

In a frequently cited study, Eriksson et al. assessed activity of phosphofructokinase (PFK), a rate-limiting enzyme in the glycolytic chain, in biopsies of vastus lateralis muscle in five boys (mean age 11.2 years) (26). No direct comparisons were made to adult biopsies in this study, but the average PFK activity, 8.4 μmol/(g × min), was "less than 50% of that usually observed in adults" (26, p. 491).

Berg and Keul performed vastus lateralis biopsies for enzyme analysis in three groups of children having mean ages of 6.4 years (n = 8), 13.5 years (n = 12), and 17.1 years (n = 13) (10). Lowest activities of enzymes involved in glycolytic metabolism (aldolase, pyruvate kinase, lactic dehydrogenase) were observed in the youngest group (see fig. 12.9, page 200). The ratio of fumarase to pyruvate kinase activity was examined as an index of the relative capacities of aerobic and anaerobic metabolism. The ratio was almost 100% greater in the young children than in the other two age groups (see fig. 12.10, page 200). This supports findings on laboratory testing reviewed previously in this chapter indicating a progressive increase in the ratio of anaerobic to aerobic power with age in children.

Haralambie measured the activities of 10 glycolytic enzymes, including PFK, in vastus lateralis biopsies of 7 girls ages 13-15 years and 14 adults 22-42 years (39). No significant differences were observed. The author suggested that the 11-13-year-old boys in the study of Eriksson et al. who had low PFK activity (26) were in an "earlier pubertal phase" (p. 491).

Gender differences in glycolytic enzyme activities among children have not been evaluated. Komi and Karlsson described a more pronounced glycolytic enzyme profile in males in an investigation of older adolescents (mean age 17 and 19 years for males and females, respectively) (47). The authors noted that "although hormonal influences are indisputable as contributory factors, adaptation processes due to different physical activity patterns cannot be excluded" (p. 216).

Further insights into maturity-related changes in glycolytic capacity may rely on more noninvasive procedures. Use of nuclear magnetic resonance spectroscopy offers promise for providing understanding of energy substrates during exercise in children. This technique offers a safe means of examining muscle cell glycolytic activity by assessing cellular inorganic phosphate (P_i), phosphocreatine (PCr), and pH.

Zanconato et al. utilized this method to examine maturational aspects of muscle high-energy phosphate metabolism during exercise (101). Ten children (mean age 9.3 years) and eight adults (mean age 34 years) underwent supine exercise inside a nuclear magnetic resonance imager using a treadle ergometer. No differences in resting pH or ratio of intracellular P_i to PCr were seen between the groups. With exercise, however, the adults showed a greater increase in P_i/PCr and a more accentuated fall in pH than the children. These differing kinetics of P_i/PCr and pH during exercise suggest that children are less capable of stimulating adenosine triphosphate rephosphorylation by anaerobic pathways during high-intensity exercise.

ANAEROBIC TRAINABILITY

As discussed in chapter 7, aerobic trainability, or the ability to increase $\dot{V}O_2$max with endurance training, has been considered to be less in children than in adults. The effect of maturation on improvements in anaerobic fitness after a period of exercise-specific training is less clear. As indicated by the research information outlined in the following sections, the different lines of experimental evidence addressing this question are not altogether consistent. The limited available data indicate, for instance, that a dramatic increase in glycolytic enzyme activity can be triggered by training; at the same time, there is little to support the idea that peak lactate levels can be altered by similar programs.

This area of investigation suffers from the lack of recognized guidelines (such as those available for aerobic training) for the duration, frequency, and intensity of anaerobic training that should be expected to stimulate anaerobic changes. Consequently, comparisons between studies are difficult. The quantitative aspects of changes that have been observed with training in children relative to their biological age have not been investigated. Likewise, the influence of maturation on the mechanisms for changes in anaerobic fitness with training is unknown.

Field Performance

Mosher et al. studied the effects of high-speed activities, 15-20 min three times a week for 12 weeks, on the anaerobic fitness of 10-11-year-old elite-level soccer players (60). Anaerobic fitness was assessed by duration sustained on a treadmill run at 7 mph at 18% grade as well as 40 yd dash time. Compared to nontraining control soccer players, the experimental subjects improved treadmill endurance by 20%, but no significant change was observed in mean 40 yd dash times in either group.

Cross-Sectional Studies of Anaerobic Power

Comparisons of anaerobic characteristics of trained and untrained children allow only tentative insight into the effects of training, since genetic preselection as well as differences in biological maturation can also influence anaerobic profiles.

Falgairette et al. found no differences in maximal anaerobic power (force-velocity test) or mean power (Wingate test) in three groups of 11-year-old boys: swimmers (n = 26, training an average of 8 hr weekly), active boys (n = 16), and nonactive boys (n = 12) (29). Mero et al. evaluated anaerobic fitness with a modified Wingate test in 10-13-year-old males involved in different sports (58). The number of subjects, however, was small (four each of weight lifters, endurance runners, and sprinters, with nine control subjects). The athletes on the whole had significantly greater biological maturation by bone age than controls. Nonetheless, no significant differences were seen in peak or mean anaerobic power between athletic groups or between these groups and the nonathletic controls.

It is interesting to note that greater anaerobic fitness has been demonstrated in trained child endurance athletes. Mayers and Gutin studied competitive distance runners ages 8.3 to 11.8 years with a modified Wingate test (54). Anaerobic capacity was expressed as number of revolutions performed in 30 s. These runners scored significantly better than nontraining controls (54 vs. 44, $p < .05$).

Sady et al. found that prepubertal wrestlers had greater anaerobic fitness on a modified Wingate test than nonathletic control subjects (74). The 15 athletes were participants in other sports as well (track, baseball, soccer). Anaerobic power was 225 and 187 W for the athletes and nonathletes, respectively ($p < .01$). Body composition may have influenced these comparisons. The average weight of the controls was 39.0 kg compared to the wrestlers' 34.2 kg (a difference that would increase the difference between the groups when values of power are expressed per kg), but the wrestlers had less body fat (4.4 vs. 9.1 kg, $p < .01$).

Anaerobic Power Changes With Training

Grodjinovsky et al. divided 50 boys 11-13 years old into two anaerobic training groups (high-intensity cycling and sprint) and a control group (37). Wingate testing was performed in each group before and after a 6-week training period. Small but significant improvements were seen in mean anaerobic power in both testing groups (3.4% and 3.7%) but not in the controls. A significant increase in peak anaerobic power was observed only in those who trained on the cycle.

Sargeant et al. studied the effect of doubling physical education time over 8 weeks (amounting to an extra 150 min/week) in 13-year-old boys (77). Training consisted of a balanced mixture of short-term power and endurance training plus some weight training. Anaerobic

power was assessed with an isokinetic cycle test. Maximal power increased 3.7% in the controls, paralleling a 3% increase in upper leg muscle mass. The training group showed a significantly greater increase in upper leg mass (9.7%) with a rise in peak power of 8.5%. These results were interpreted as showing (a) that changes in short-term power were related to the size of the active muscle in the two groups and (b) that such changes occur over a relatively short time.

Rotstein et al. reported significant improvements in anaerobic fitness of 28 nonathletic boys ages 10-11 years after a 9-week interval training program (69). By Wingate testing, mean anaerobic power increased by 10% and peak power by 14%.

Blood Lactate Responses to Exercise

Studies of peak lactate responses to exercise have shown no apparent changes relative to athletic training. This has been a consistent finding in both cross-sectional and longitudinal studies.

Sjodin and Svedenhag found differences in blood lactate after a maximal treadmill run in trained and detrained 12-year-old distance runners (80). The eight distance runners were tested every 6 months as they trained over the next 8 years. Lactate levels determined 1 min after maximal treadmill tests showed no significant changes over the years (mean about 10.5 mmol/L).

Mero reported no significant differences in peak blood lactate levels in 19 trained and 6 untrained prepubertal boys during a 60 s maximal cycle test (57). Koch performed annual maximal cycle testing in 7 boys who were training for 5 years beginning at a mean age of 11.9 years (46). The boys, who had a mean $\dot{V}O_2max$ of 59.5 ml · kg^{-1} · min^{-1}, participated in soccer, running, badminton, and ice hockey. No significant differences in peak lactate were seen over the 5 years of training. With the exception of the last year, there was, in fact, a downward trend in mean values (7.0, 6.3, 5.6, 5.1, and 6.0 mmol/L in successive years). The authors suggested three possible explanations for this unexpected result: with age there may have been (a) a greater extraction of lactate by other tissues, (b) different rates of lactate production and utilization by the different fiber types in the working muscle, or (c) disproportionate expansion of plasma volume.

The weight lifters, endurance runners, sprinters, and nonathletic boys (ages 10-13 years) described by Mero et al. showed no significant differences in maximal lactate levels (7.4, 8.3, 6.3, and 6.6 mmol/L, respectively) (58).

Ventilatory Anaerobic Threshold

The research data addressing changes in VAT with training have been reviewed in a previous section (see p.

204). In summary, cross-sectional studies of highly trained child distance runners and cyclists indicate significantly greater VAT (expressed both as $\dot{V}O_2$ per kg and as percentage of $\dot{V}O_2$max) than in nonathletic children. However, longitudinal training studies have not provided a clear picture of the plasticity of AT in nonathletic children.

Enzyme Studies

Eriksson et al. evaluated PFK activity in vastus lateralis muscle biopsy specimens in five boys before, during, and after a 6-week cycle training program (26). Mean age of the subjects was 11.2 years. Phosphofructokinase activity prior to training was 8.4 µmol/(g × min). Activity rose to 12.5 and 15.4 µmol/(g × min) after 2 and 6 weeks of training, "suggesting that training increases the glycolytic potential of skeletal muscle of young boys" (p. 491). Supporting this conclusion, glycogen depletion during exhaustive exercise was greater after training than before.

Fournier et al. studied enzyme responses to training in older subjects (32). They found that an interval training program of 3 months in postpubertal adolescents could improve PFK activity on vastus lateralis biopsies by an average of 21%.

HORMONAL INFLUENCES ON ANAEROBIC FITNESS

Considering the evidence that glycolytic capacity is less in children, it is appropriate to consider maturity-related differences in recognized determinants of anaerobic metabolism. Two have come under research scrutiny: the potential influences of testosterone (i.e., the effect of puberty) and catecholamines, particularly epinephrine.

Testosterone

A prepubescent animal that has been castrated shows a diminished capacity for development of anaerobic metabolism. Testosterone administered to the animal blocks this effect of gonadectomy. In animals, too, a relationship has been observed between the size of fast-twitch muscle fibers, the activity of glycolytic enzymes, and testosterone concentration (8, 23, 48). It is not a surprise, then, that in their 1971 study Eriksson et al. reported a moderate correlation between maximal muscle lactate and testicular volume in 13-year-old boys (r = 0.67) (27). Following the animal model, this finding supports the concept that sexual maturity, specifically a rise in serum testosterone level, is highly influential in the development of glycolytic metabolism.

Subsequent studies have in general failed to support this conclusion. For at least two intuitive reasons this is not surprising. First, a progressive development in maximal lactate levels and anaerobic power is evident throughout childhood, not just at the time of puberty. And, second, if testosterone acts as a potent trigger of glycolytic development, one would expect greater lactate production with exercise in males, particularly at and after puberty. As reviewed earlier, there is no evidence for such a gender-specific pattern.

Welsman et al. showed that testosterone levels were not related to blood lactate responses to submaximal exercise in 12-16-year-old males (93). Likewise during treadmill running, no significant relationship was observed between serum testosterone and percentage of peak $\dot{V}O_2$ at 2.5 and 4.0 mmol/L (r = −.24 and .08, respectively). In the longitudinal study of Paterson et al. of maximal lactate levels in boys between ages 11 and 15 years, a progressive linear rise was seen in lactate levels when related to age at PHV (63). That is, there was no evidence that hormonal changes at puberty influenced the rate of rise in lactate-producing capacity. Falk and Bar-Or showed the same linearity of rise in peak and mean anaerobic power by Wingate testing in pre-, mid-, and postpubertal boys (30).

Paterson and Cunningham reported that there were no significant differences in anaerobic fitness in early- and later-maturing boys (by bone age) at a given chronological age (62). Nineteen boys performed a treadmill run at 20% grade, designed to maximally stress the anaerobic energy system, for five consecutive years beginning at age 10. Anaerobic fitness was defined by O_2 debt (recovery $\dot{V}O_2$) and postexercise lactate levels. For the total group, O_2 debt in liters increased 171% and increased relative to body weight by 64% from age 11 to 15 years. Meanwhile, lactate at maximal exercise rose 38%. No significant differences were observed in values or the rate of change with age in early- or late-maturing boys (defined as 1 year ahead or behind skeletal age for chronological age).

These findings suggest that anaerobic fitness is linked to chronological rather than biological age. They do not support the idea that testosterone plays an important role in the development of glycolytic capacity in growing children. Falgairette et al. did report a moderate correlation of mean and peak anaerobic power with salivary testosterone (r = 0.45 and 0.47, respectively) in their cross-sectional study of 6-15-year old boys (28). The authors noted, however, that anaerobic fitness improved significantly between ages 6 and 12 years, when salivary testosterone levels remained unchanged.

Catecholamines

Evidence exists that catecholamines, particularly epinephrine, play a key role as stimulators of glycogenolysis in muscle. Infusions of epinephrine in animals increase lactate production from contracting muscle, and beta-adrenergic blockade decreases the rates of glycogen breakdown and lactate production in both animals and adult humans (55). It is of interest, then, to examine the potential role of maturity-related variations in epinephrine levels during exercise in the modulation of differences in glycolytic capacity.

Lehmann et al. compared catecholamine levels with blood lactate responses during progressive treadmill exercise in eight boys (mean age 12.8 years) and seven adults (mean age 27.8 years) (50). There was a close correlation between lactate and total plasma catecholamines in the two groups (see fig. 12.17). These findings led Berg and Keul to suggest that reduced maximal sympathetic activity and adrenal catecholamine secretion might be responsible for the reduced anaerobic capacity of children (10).

The children and adults studied by Lehmann et al. exhibited no significant differences in maximal epineph-rine levels (50). However, mean maximal norepinephrine levels were 30% lower in the children. A recent investigation in this author's laboratory failed to reveal evidence of differences in maximal or submaximal norepinephrine values when groups of boys 10-12 years old and young men were compared during maximal cycle exercise (unpublished data).

SUMMARY

The laboratory investigation of short-burst anaerobic fitness is hampered by the lack of an accurate noninvasive means of assessing the contribution of anaerobic metabolism during exercise. The picture of the development of anaerobic fitness during childhood has therefore been drawn from a composite of several indirect lines of evidence. In general, collectively this evidence supports the concept that not only does anaerobic fitness improve with increasing age, but these improvements are greater than can be accounted for by changes in body size alone.

It is uncertain whether size-relative changes in anaerobic fitness in the laboratory can be translated into the improvements observed with age in field performance of short-burst physical activities. Likewise, the extent to which field and laboratory indices of anaerobic fitness of children can be altered by physical training is not clear.

Little is known about the factors that might trigger the development of anaerobic fitness in children. The available research data do not support a role for testosterone in this process. A link is observed between the rise in lactate and catecholamines during a progressive exercise test, but evidence suggesting age-related differences in the influence of epinephrine and norepineph-rine on glycolytic capacity is tenuous.

The investigation of fitness in short-burst activities in children has focused almost exclusively on the developmental aspects of glycolytic energy supply. Future insights await experimental tools that can provide information about the evolution of the neurological, muscular, motor skill, and psychological determinants of high-intensity exercise during childhood.

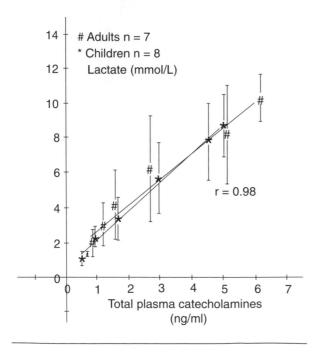

Figure 12.17 Relationship of total plasma catechol-amines and blood lactate during treadmill exercise in boys and men. Reprinted from Berg and Keul 1988.

What We Know

1. By all the different methods of laboratory assessment, peak and mean anaerobic power rise with chronological age, whether expressed in absolute or mass-relative terms.
2. Maximal and submaximal exercise lactate levels rise virtually linearly with age during childhood.
3. Ventilatory anaerobic threshold as percentage of $\dot{V}O_2$max progressively falls as the child grows.

4. Ventilatory anaerobic threshold (as percentage of $\dot{V}O_2$max) is greater in child athletes than in nonathletes.

5. Recovery $\dot{V}O_2$ (O_2 debt) increases through the course of childhood.

What We Would Like to Know

1. What mechanisms explain the size-relative changes in anaerobic fitness as children grow?
2. How do these changes in fitness relate to performance in short-burst activities?
3. Are changes in AT a manifestation of alterations in aerobic or anaerobic fitness, or both?
4. Is the activity of muscle glycolytic enzymes less in children? If so, is this the primary reason for diminished glycolytic capacity in children, or are differences in trigger mechanisms (e.g., catecholamines) instrumental?
5. Are there maturity-related differences in the effect of physical training on anaerobic capacity?

References

1. Armstrong, N.; Welsman, J.R. Assessment and interpretation of aerobic fitness in children and adolescents. Exerc. Sports Sci. Rev. 22:435-476; 1994.
2. Asmussen, E. Growth in muscular strength and power. In: Rarick, G.L., ed. Physical activity, human growth and development. New York: Academic Press; 1973:p. 60-79.
3. Åstrand, P.O. Experimental studies of physical working capacity in relation to sex and age. Copenhagen: Munksgaard; 1952.
4. Atomi, Y.; Fukunaga, T.; Yamamoto, Y.; Hatta, H.H. Lactate threshold and $\dot{V}O_2$max of trained and untrained boys relative to muscle mass and composition. In: Rutenfranz, J.; Mocellin, R.; Klimt, F., eds. Children and exercise XII. Champaign, IL: Human Kinetics; 1986:p. 53-58.
5. Bar-Or, O. Pediatric sports medicine for the practitioner. New York: Springer-Verlag; 1983:p. 311-314.
6. Bar-Or, O. The Wingate anaerobic test. An update on methodology, reliability, and validity. Sports Med. 4:381-394; 1987.
7. Bar-Or, O.; Inbar, O. Relationships among anaerobic capacity, sprint and middle distance running of school children. In: Shephard, R.J.; Lavallee, H., eds. Physical fitness assessment—principles, practice, and application. Springfield, IL: Charles C Thomas; 1978:p. 142-147.
8. Bass, A.; Gutmann, E.; Hanzlikova, V.; Syrovy, I. Sexual differentiation of enzyme pattern and its conversion by testosterone in temporalis muscle of the guinea pig. Physiol. Bohemoslov. 20:423-431; 1971.
9. Becker, D.M.; Vaccaro, P. Anaerobic threshold alterations caused by endurance training in young children. J. Sports Med. 23:445-449; 1983.
10. Berg, A.; Keul, J. Biochemical changes during exercise in children. In: Malina, R.M., ed. Young athletes. A biological, psychological, and educational perspective. Champaign, IL: Human Kinetics; 1988:p. 61-67.
11. Blimkie, C.J.R.; Roche, P.; Bar-Or, O. The anaerobic-to-aerobic power ratio in adolescent boys and girls. In: Rutenfranz, J.; Mocellin, R.; Klimt, F., eds. Children and exercise XII. Champaign, IL: Human Kinetics; 1986:p. 31-37.
12. Blimkie, C.J.R.; Roche, P.; Hoy, J.T.; Bar-Or, O. Anaerobic power of arms in teenage boys and girls: relationship to lean tissue. Eur. J. Appl. Physiol. 57:677-683; 1988.
13. Brooks, G.A. Anaerobic threshold: a review of the concept and directions for future research. Med. Sci. Sports Exerc. 17:22-31; 1985.
14. Campbell, W.R.; Pohndorf, R.H. Physical fitness of British and United States children. In: Health and fitness in the modern world. Washington, DC: Athletic Institute; 1961:p. 161-165.
15. Cooper, D.M.; Weiler-Ravell, D.; Whipp, B.J.; Wasserman, K. Aerobic parameters of exercise as a function of body size during growth in children. J. Appl. Physiol. 56:628-634; 1984.
16. Cumming, G.R. Exercise studies in clinical pediatric cardiology. In: Lavallee, H.; Shephard, R.J., eds. Frontiers of activity and child health. Quebec, PQ: Editions du Pelican; 1977:p. 17-45.
17. Cumming, G.R.; Hastman, L.; McCort, J. Treadmill endurance times, blood lactate, and exercise blood pressures in normal children. In: Binkhorst, R.A.; Kemper, H.C.G.; Saris, W.H., eds. Children and exercise XI. Champaign, IL: Human Kinetics; 1985;p. 140-150.
18. Cumming, G.R.; Hastman, L.; McCort, J.; McCullough, S. High serum lactates do occur in young children after maximal work. Int. J. Sports Med. 1:66-69; 1980.
19. Cunningham, L.N. Relationship of running economy, ventilatory threshold, and maximal O_2 consumption to running performance in high school females. Res. Q. 61:369-374; 1990.

20. Davies, C.T.M.; Barnes, C.; Godfrey, S. Body composition and maximal exercise performance in children. Human Biology 44:195-214; 1972.

21. Davis, J.A. Anaerobic threshold: review of the concept and directions for future research. Med. Sci. Sports Exerc. 17:6-18; 1985.

22. Duche, P.; Falgairette, G.; Bedu, M.; Fellman, N.; Lac, G.; Robert, A.; Coudert, J. Longitudinal approach of bioenergetic profile in boys before and during puberty. In: Coudert, J.; Van Praagh, E., eds. Pediatric work physiology. Methodological, physiological and pathological aspects. Paris: Masson; 1992:p. 43-45.

23. Dux, L.; Dux, E.; Guba, F. Further data on the androgenetic dependency of the skeletal musculature: the effect of pubertal castration on the structural development of the skeletal muscle. Horm. Metab. Res. 14:191-194; 1982.

24. Emmett, B.; Hochachka, P.W. Scaling of oxidative and glycolytic enzymes in mammals. Resp. Phys. 45:261-272; 1986.

25. Eriksson, B.O. Muscle metabolism in children—a review. Acta Paediatr. Scand. Suppl. 283:20-27; 1980.

26. Eriksson, B.O.; Gollnick, P.D.; Saltin, B. Muscle metabolism and enzyme activities after training in boys 11-13 years old. Acta Physiol. Scand. 87:485-497; 1973.

27. Eriksson, B.O.; Karlsson, J.; Saltin, B. Muscle metabolites during exercise in pubertal boys. Acta Paediatr. Scand. Suppl. 217:154-157; 1971.

28. Falgairette, G.; Bedu, M.; Fellman, N.; Van Praagh, E.; Coudert, J. Bio-energetic profile in 144 boys aged from 6 to 15 years. Eur. J. Appl. Physiol. 62:151-156; 1991.

29. Falgairette, G.; Duche, P.; Bedu, M.; Fellman, N.; Coudert, J. Bioenergetic characteristics in prepubertal swimmers. Int. J. Sports Med. 14:444-448; 1993.

30. Falk, B.; Bar-Or, O. Longitudinal changes in peak aerobic and anaerobic mechanical power of circumpubertal boys. Pediatr. Exerc. Science 5:318-331; 1993.

31. Faria, I.E.; Faria, E.W.; Roberts, S.; Yoshimura, D. Comparison of physical and physiological characteristics in elite young and mature cyclists. Res. Q. 60:388-395; 1989.

32. Fournier, M.; Ricci, J.; Taylor, A.W.; Ferguson, R.J.; Montpetit, R.R.; Chaitman, B.R. Skeletal muscle adaptation in adolescent boys: sprint and endurance training and detraining. Med. Sci. Sports Exerc. 14:453-456; 1982.

33. Gaisl, G.; Buchberger, J. Determination of the aerobic and anaerobic thresholds of 10-11 year old boys using blood gas analysis. In: Berg, K.; Eriksson, B.O., eds. Children and exercise IX. Baltimore: University Park Press; 1980:p. 93-98.

34. Gilliam, T.B.; MacConnie, S.E.; Geenen, D.L.; Pels, A.E.; Freedson, P.S. Exercise programs for children: a way to prevent heart disease? Phys. Sportsmed. 10:96-108; 1982.

35. Girandola, R.N.; Wiswell, R.A.; Frisch, F.; Wood, K. $\dot{V}O_2$max and anaerobic threshold in pre- and post-pubescent girls. Med. Sport 14:151-161; 1981.

36. Gollnick, P.D.; Armstrong, R.B.; Saubert, C.W.; Piehl, K.; Saltin, B. Enzyme activity and fiber composition in skeletal muscles of untrained and trained men. J. Appl. Physiol. 33:2312-2319; 1972.

37. Grodjinovsky, A.; Inbar, O.; Dotan, R.; Bar-Or, O. Training effect on the anaerobic performance of children as measured by the Wingate anaerobic test. In: Berg, K.; Eriksson, B.O., eds. Children and exercise IX. Baltimore: University Park Press; 1980:p. 139-145.

38. Haffor, A.A.; Harrison, A.C.; Catledge Kirk, P.A. Anaerobic threshold alterations caused by interval training in 11 year olds. J. Sports Med. Phys. Fit. 30:53-56; 1990.

39. Haralambie, G. Enzyme activities in skeletal muscle of 13-15 year old adolescents. Bull. Europ. Physiopath. 18:65-74; 1982.

40. Hayden, F.; Yuhasz, M. The CAHPER fitness performance test manual for boys and girls 7 to 17 years of age. Toronto, ON: Canadian Association for Physical Health, Education and Recreation; 1965.

41. Hebestreit, H.; Mimura, K.; Bar-Or, O. Recovery of muscle power after high-intensity short-term exercise: comparing boys and men. J. Appl. Physiol. 74:2875-2880; 1993.

42. Hunsicker, P.; Reiff, G.G. AAHPERD youth fitness test manual. Reston, VA: American Alliance for Health, Physical Education, Recreation and Dance; 1976.

43. Jacobs, I. Blood lactate. Implications for training and sports performance. Sports Med. 3:10-25; 1986.

44. Kanaley, J.A.; Boileau, R.A. The onset of the anaerobic threshold at three stages of physical maturity. J. Sports Med. 28:367-374; 1988.

45. Kindermann, V.W.; Keul, J.; Lehmann, M. Ausdauerbelastungen beim Heranwachsenden—metabolische und kardiozirkulatorische Veranderungen. Fortschr. Med. 97:659-665; 1979.

46. Koch, G. Aerobic power, lung dimensions, ventilatory capacity, and muscle blood flow in 12-16 year old boys with high physical activity. In: Berg, K.; Eriksson, B.O., eds. Children and exercise IX. Baltimore: University Park Press; 1980:p. 99-108.

47. Komi, P.V.; Karlsson, J. Skeletal muscle fiber types, enzyme activities and physical performance in young males and females. Acta Physiol. Scand. 103:210-218; 1978.

48. Krotkiewski, M.; Kral, J.G.; Karlsson, J. Effects of castration and testosterone substitution on body composition and muscle metabolism in rats. Acta Physiol. Scand. 109:233-237; 1980.

49. Lariviere, G.; Godbout, P. Mesure de la condition physique et de l'efficacite technique de jouers de hockey sur glace: normes pour differences categories de joueurs. Quebec, PQ: Editions du Pelican; 1976.

50. Lehmann, M.; Keul, J.; Korsten-Reck, U. The influence of graduated treadmill exercise on plasma catecholamines, aerobic, and anaerobic capacity in boys and adults. Eur. J. Appl. Physiol. 47:301-311; 1981.

51. Mahon, A.D.; Vaccaro, P. Ventilatory threshold and $\dot{V}O_2$ max changes in children following endurance training. Med. Sci. Sports Exerc. 21:425-431; 1989.

52. Malina, R.M.; Bouchard, C. Growth, maturation, and physical activity. Champaign, IL: Human Kinetics; 1991:p. 225.
53. Matejkova, J.; Koprivova, Z.; Placheta, Z. Changes in acid base balance after maximal exercise. In: Placheta, Z., ed. Youth and physical activity. Brno: J. E. Purkyne University; 1980:p. 191-199.
54. Mayers, N.; Gutin, B. Physiological characteristics of elite prepubertal cross-country runners. Med. Sci. Sports Exerc. 11:172-176; 1979.
55. Mazzeo, R.S.; Marshall, P. Influence of plasma catecholamines on the lactate threshold during graded exercise. J. Appl. Physiol. 67:1319-1322; 1989.
56. Mercier, J.; Mercier, B.; Granier, P.; LeGallais, D.; Prefaut, C. Maximal anaerobic power: relationship to anthropometric characteristics during growth. Int. J. Sports Med. 13:21-26; 1992.
57. Mero, A. Blood lactate production and recovery from anaerobic exercise in trained and untrained boys. Eur. J. Appl. Physiol. 57:660-666; 1988.
58. Mero, A.; Kauhanen, H.; Peltola, E.; Vuorimaa, T.; Komi, P.V. Physiological performance capacity in different prepubescent athletic groups. J. Sports Med. Phys. Fit. 30:57-66; 1990.
59. Morse, M.; Schlutz, F.W.; Cassels, D.E. Relation of age to physiological responses of the older boy (10-17 years) to exercise. J. Appl. Physiol. 1:683-709; 1949.
60. Mosher, R.E.; Rhodes, E.C.; Wenger, H.A.; Filsinger, B. Interval training: the effects of a 12 week programme on elite prepubertal male soccer players. J. Sports Med. 25:5-9; 1985.
61. Nudel, D.B.; Hasset, I.; Gunian, A.; Diamant, S.; Weinhouse, E.; Gootman, N. Young long distance runners. Physiological and psychological characteristics. Clin. Pediatr. 28:500-505; 1989.
62. Paterson, D.H.; Cunningham, D.A. Development of anaerobic capacity in early and late maturing boys. In: Binkhorst, R.A.; Kemper, H.C.G.; Saris, W.H., eds. Children and exercise XI. Champaign, IL: Human Kinetics; 1985:p. 119-128.
63. Paterson, D.H.; Cunningham, D.A.; Bumstead, L.A. Recovery O$_2$ and blood acid: longitudinal analysis in boys aged 11 to 15 years. Eur. J. Appl. Physiol. 55:93-99; 1986.
64. Paterson, D.H.; McLellan, T.M.; Stella, R.S.; Cunningham, D.A. Longitudinal study of ventilation threshold and maximal O$_2$ uptake in athletic boys. J. Appl. Physiol. 62:2051-2057; 1987.
65. Reybrouck, T.M. The use of the anaerobic threshold in pediatric exercise testing. In: Advances in pediatric sport sciences. Vol. 3, Bar-Or, O., ed. Biological issues. Champaign, IL: Human Kinetics; 1989:p. 131-149.
66. Reybrouck, T.; Weymans, M.; Stijns, H.; Knops, J.; vander Hauwaert, L. Ventilatory anaerobic threshold in healthy children. Age and sex differences. Eur. J. Appl. Physiol. 54:278-284; 1985.
67. Reybrouck, T.; Weymans, M.; Stijns, H.; vander Hauwaert, L. Ventilation anaerobic threshold for evaluating exercise performance in children with congenital left-to-right intracardiac shunt. Pediatr. Cardiol. 7:19-24; 1986.
68. Robinson, S. Experimental studies of physical fitness in relationship to age. Arbeitsphysiologie 10:251-323; 1938.
69. Rotstein, A.; Dotan, R.; Bar-Or, O.; Tenenbaum, G. Effects of training on anaerobic threshold, maximal aerobic power and anaerobic performance of preadolescent boys. Int. J. Sports Med. 7:281-286; 1986.
70. Rowland, T.W.; Green, G.M. Physiological responses to treadmill exercise in females: adult-child differences. Med. Sci. Sports Exerc. 20:474-478; 1988.
71. Rowland, T.W.; Green, G.M. Anaerobic threshold and the determination of training target heart rates in premenarcheal girls. Pediatr. Cardiol. 10:75-79; 1989.
72. Ruskin; H. Physical performance of school children in Israel. In: Shephard, R.J.; Lavallee, H., eds. Physical fitness assessment. Principles, practice, and application. Springfield, IL: Charles C Thomas; 1978:p. 273-320.
73. Saavedra, C.; Lagasse, P.; Bouchard, C.; Simoneau, J. Maximal anaerobic performance of the knee extensor muscles during growth. Med. Sci. Sports Exerc. 23:1083-1089; 1991.
74. Sady, S.P.; Thomson, W.H.; Berg, K.; Savage, M. Physiological characteristics of high-ability prepubescent wrestlers. Med. Sci. Sports Exerc. 16:72-76; 1984.
75. Sargeant, A.J.; Dolan, P. Optimal velocity of muscle contraction for short-term (anaerobic power) output in children and adults. In: Rutenfranz, J.; Mocellin, R.; Klimt, F., eds. Children and exercise XII. Champaign, IL: Human Kinetics; 1986:p. 39-42.
76. Sargeant, A.J.; Dolan, P.; Thorne, A. Isokinetic measurement of maximal leg force and anaerobic power output in children. In: Ilmarinen, J.; Valimaki, I., eds. Children and sport. Berlin: Springer-Verlag, 1984:p. 93-98.
77. Sargeant, A.J.; Dolan, P.; Thorne, A. Effects of supplementary physical activity on body composition, aerobic, and anaerobic power in 13 year old boys. In: Binkhorst, R.A.; Kemper, H.C.G.; Saris, W.H., eds. Children and exercise XI. Champaign, IL: Human Kinetics; 1985:p. 140-150.
78. Saris, W.H.M.; Noordeloos, A.M.; Ringnalda, B.E.M.; Van't Hof, M.A.; Binkhorst, R.A. Reference values for aerobic power of healthy 4- to 18-year-old Dutch children: preliminary results. In: Binkhorst, R.A.; Kemper, H.C.G.; Saris, W.H.M., eds. Children and exercise XI. Champaign, IL: Human Kinetics; 1985:p. 151-160.
79. Shephard, R.J.; Allen, C.; Bar-Or, O.; Davies, C.T.M.; Degre, S.; Hedman, R.; Ishii, K.; Kaneko, M.; La Cour, J.R.; diPrampero, P.E.; Seliger, V. The working capacity of Toronto schoolchildren. Part I. Canad. Med. Ass. J. 100:560-566; 1969.
80. Sjodin, B.; Svedenhag, J. O$_2$ uptake during running as related to body mass in circumpubertal boys: a longitudinal study. Eur. J. Appl. Physiol. 65:150-157; 1992.
81. Somero, G.N.; Childress, J.J. A violation of the metabolism-size scaling paradigm: activities of glycolytic enzymes in muscle increase in larger-size fish. Physiol. Zool. 53:322-337; 1980.
82. Tanaka, H. Predicting running velocity at blood lactate threshold from running performance tests in adolescent boys. Eur. J. Appl. Physiol. 55:344-348; 1986.

83. Tanaka, H.; Shindo, M. Running velocity at blood lactate threshold of boys aged 6-15 years compared with untrained and trained young males. Int. J. Sports Med. 6:90-94; 1985.

84. Tharp, G.D.; Newhouse, R.K.; Uffelman, L.; Thorland, W.G.; Johnson, G.O. Comparison of sprint and run times with performance on the Wingate anaerobic test. Res. Q. Exerc. Sport 56:73-76; 1985.

85. Vanden Eynde, B.; Van Gerven, D.; Vienne, D.; Vuylsteke-Wauters, M.; Ghesquiere, J. Endurance fitness and peak height velocity in Belgian boys. In: Oseid, S.; Carlson, K.-H., eds. Children and exercise XIII. Champaign, IL: Human Kinetics; 1989:p. 19-26.

86. Vandewalle, H.; Peres, G.; Saurabie, B.; Stouvenel, O.; Monod, H. Force-velocity relationship and maximal anaerobic power during cranking exercise in young swimmers. Int. J. Sports Med. 10:439-445; 1989.

87. Van Praagh, E.; Falgairette, G.; Bedu, M.; Fellman, N.; Coudert, J. Laboratory and field tests in 7-year old boys. In: Oseid, S.; Carlson, K.-H., eds. Children and exercise XIII. Champaign, IL: Human Kinetics; 1989:p. 11-17.

88. Van Praagh, E.; Fellman, N.; Bedu, M.; Falgairette, G.; Coudert, J. Gender difference in the relationship of anaerobic power output to body composition in children. Pediatr. Exerc. Science 2:336-348; 1990.

89. Von Ditter, H.; Nowacki, P.; Simai, E.; Winkler, U. Das Verhalten des Saure-Basen-Haushalts nach erschopfender Belastung bei untrainierten und trainierten Jungen und Vergleich zu Leistungssportlern. Sportarzt Sportmed. 28:45-48; 1977.

90. Walsh, M.L.; Bannister, E.W. Possible mechanisms of the anaerobic threshold. A review. Sports Med. 5:269-302; 1988.

91. Washington, R.L. Anaerobic threshold. In: Rowland, T.W., ed. Pediatric laboratory exercise testing. Champaign, IL: Human Kinetics; 1993:p. 115-129.

92. Wasserman, K. The anaerobic threshold measurement to evaluate exercise performance. Am. Rev. Respir. Dis. 129 Suppl:S35-S40; 1984.

93. Welsman, J.R.; Armstrong, N.; Kirby, B.J. Serum testosterone is not related to peak $\dot{V}O_2$ and submaximal blood lactate responses in 12- to 16-year old males. Pediatr. Exerc. Science 6:120-127; 1994.

94. Weymans, M.; Reybrouck, T.; Stijns, H.; Knops, J. Influence of age and sex on the ventilatory anaerobic threshold in children. In: Binkhorst, R.B.; Kemper, H.C.G.; Saris, W.H.M., eds. Children and exercise XI. Champaign, IL: Human Kinetics; 1985;p. 114-118.

95. Williams, J.R.; Armstrong, N. The influence of age and sexual maturation on children's blood lactate responses to exercise. Pediatr. Exerc. Science 3:111-120; 1991.

96. Williams, J.R.; Armstrong, N. Relationship of maximal lactate steady state to performance at fixed blood lactate reference values in children. Pediatr. Exerc. Science 3:333-341; 1991.

97. Williams, J.R.; Armstrong, N.; Kirby, B.J. The 4 mM blood lactate level as an index of exercise performance in 11-13 year old children. J. Sports Sci. 8:139-147; 1990.

98. Wirth, A.; Trager, E.; Scheele, K.; Mayer, D.; Diehm, K.; Reischle, K.; Weicker, H. Cardiopulmonary adjustment and metabolic response to maximal and submaximal physical exercise of boys and girls at different stages of maturity. Eur. J. Appl. Physiol. 39:229-240; 1978.

99. Wolfe, R.R.; Washington, R.; Daberkow, E.; Murphy, J.R.; Brammel, H.L. Anaerobic threshold as a predictor of athletic performance in prepubertal female runners. AJDC 140:922-924; 1986.

100. Yoshizawa, S.; Honda, H.; Urushibara, M.; Nakamura, N. Aerobic-anaerobic energy supply and daily physical activity level in young children. In: Oseid, S.; Carlson, K.-H., eds. Children and exercise. Champaign, IL: Human Kinetics; 1989:p. 11-17.

101. Zanconato; S.; Buchtal, S.; Barstow, T.J.; Cooper, D.M. ^{31}P-magnetic resonance spectroscopy of leg muscle metabolism during exercise in children and adults. J. Appl. Physiol. 74:2214-2218; 1993.

CHAPTER 13

THE DEVELOPMENT OF MUSCULAR STRENGTH

Strength is the amount of force that can be produced by a muscle in a single contraction. Governed by a host of anatomic and physiochemical determinants, strength most directly reflects the tension created from actin sliding past myosin filaments within the muscle fibrils. Neural adaptations, hormonal influences, biochemical flux, and patterns of fiber recruitment all act in concert to control force during muscle contraction. This chapter focuses on the development of muscle strength as children grow, with particular attention to the influence of these determinants. For the most part the discussion will be limited to strength as defined above—differentiated from muscle endurance, or the ability to generate muscle force over time.

In comparison to the situation for aerobic fitness, the link between strength and health is less well documented. Still, the importance of muscular strength in the efficient performance of life's daily physical activities is obvious. Intuitively, too, the development of proper strength should help prevent injuries during both recreational and vocational activities and may be important in preventing the development of lower back disease in adults. For these reasons, the optimization of strength throughout life, beginning in childhood, is deemed important for both well-being and disease prevention.

It comes as no surprise that children become stronger as they grow. Strength is highly dependent on muscle size, and the developing muscle mass during childhood should be expected to be manifest in improving force of muscle contraction. Beyond this straightforward observation a number of intriguing questions surround the development of muscle strength in the childhood years. This chapter will explore each of these issues:

1. What are the factors responsible for making children stronger as they grow? Several lines of evidence suggest that increases in strength do not necessarily parallel those of muscle size. Presumably other determinants, particularly neural influences, are important in the development of strength in children.

2. Can strength be improved by resistance training in prepubertal subjects? Once-traditional dogma held that absence of circulating testosterone precluded the development of strength with resistance training in children. A recent series of studies has quite conclusively proven otherwise: strength can be improved in both boys and girls after a period of resistance training before as well as after the age of puberty. Most studies indicate that these changes occur in children in the absence of muscle hypertrophy, strengthening the argument that neural and other adaptations can have an important bearing on strength development.

3. How influential are the hormonal changes at puberty in the development of strength? Can these endocrine alterations be responsible for gender differences in strength during adolescence? Both cross-sectional and longitudinal studies in children indicate that boys show an acceleration of strength at puberty while the increase in girls remains linear. Before puberty there are minimal sex differences in strength, but once puberty is reached the boys far exceed the girls. This pattern is consistent with a prominent effect of androgenic hormones on muscle size and strength.

4. What are the characteristics of the cardiovascular responses to resistance exercise in children? In adults the data are clear: static exercise causes a significant rise in both systolic and diastolic blood pressure with limited changes in heart rate and cardiac output. The resulting increased afterload work

by the heart may have adverse consequences to individuals with heart disease. Limited studies in children indicate that prepubertal subjects manifest the same cardiovascular responses during resistance exercise as adults.

THE MECHANICS AND MEASUREMENT OF MUSCULAR STRENGTH

A thorough discussion of the mechanics of muscle contraction and assessment of strength is beyond the scope of this chapter. Still, it is important to review certain principles that bear on the interpretation of studies assessing body strength. This becomes particularly critical when one is comparing data between different investigations. Indeed, a review of this information makes it rapidly apparent that the forms of muscle contraction measured and the modes of resistance utilized are sufficiently variable that such comparisons are often difficult.

The muscle fiber is the cell of muscular tissue, each muscle fiber containing up to several thousand thin strands called myofibrils (6). Within the myofibrils are overlapping protein filaments, actin and myosin, and the sliding of these two filaments past each other through interdigitating cross-bridges results in muscle contraction. This process is triggered by electrical impulses from neurological innervation of muscle. Each individual muscle fiber receives innervation from a single motor neuron, but that neuron may be responsible for the contraction of up to several thousand muscle fibers, depending on the muscle's function. The electrical depolarization of the muscle fiber frees calcium ions, which are responsible for initiating contraction of the myofibrils. The result of this entire process is the production of muscle tension, expressed as strength.

During the production of tension, the whole muscle can shorten (concentric contraction), lengthen (eccentric contraction), or remain unchanged (isometric contraction). To accomplish normal daily activities of movement and lifting, all three types of contractions typically occur simultaneously in different muscles. The three different types of contraction vary in their ability to produce strength (e.g., nearly 50% more force can be generated by eccentric than by concentric contractions) and in their strength-velocity relationship (during concentric contractions force is highest at slow velocities—the opposite of what occurs during eccentric contractions).

Laboratory and field testing of strength has usually been limited to measures of concentric or isometric strength. In assessing concentric strength, it is important to realize that the degree of strength produced by the

muscle across a joint (such as flexion at the elbow) depends on the joint angle. That is, within the range of motion of the joint there is one point at which force production will be maximal. Concentric strength is often measured by having someone lift free weights through the range of motion of a joint. The one-repetition maximum (1 RM) is the measure of the maximal weight that can be lifted in a single such contraction. It follows that a 1 RM load is indicative of the strength at the weakest angle in a joint range.

In an isodynamic concentric contraction, the force generated by the muscle remains more similar throughout the joint motion, and this condition is created by isokinetic exercise machines that alter the resistance throughout the joint range (i.e., the resistance is lightest at the weakest joint angles and greatest at the strongest angles). In contrast to what occurs with the 1 RM test of strength, maximal force generated with these devices indicates strength of the muscle at its strongest joint angle (6).

Several devices have been utilized to measure force generated when muscle groups contract isometrically, including the handgrip dynamometer and different forms of cable tensiometers; normative data obtained with these devices are available on a large number of both pediatric and adult populations. Isometric strength scores in different muscle groups tend to be significantly correlated with each other in children and adolescents (6). However, the extent to which handgrip strength can be interpreted as an indicator of strength of other muscle groups is uncertain.

Measures of strength by handgrip are influenced by several factors, including type of dynamometer, hand-arm position, degree of practice, motivation, and hand dominance. For this reason Blimkie cautioned against making direct comparisons of strength among different studies using these techniques (8). In the laboratory, isometric contractions measured by dynamometer have often been studied at a given percentage of a maximal contraction (typically 25-40%) over a given period of minutes to measure associated physiological responses (such as blood pressure elevation).

The test-retest reproducibility of these assessments of strength in children tends to be reasonably high. Variability on repeated tests of 5% to 10% has been reported with isometric strength (5, 8, 22) as well as maximal voluntary isokinetic strength (8, 49). These findings support the validity of these testing modalities. In addition, they suggest that differences in subject motivation do not necessarily contribute in any significant way to changes in test results of strength during childhood.

Strength produced by the various testing techniques is measured independent of body weight, defined as absolute strength. Other forms of exercise that use body weight as the resistance to muscle contraction provide information about relative strength. These tests, such as chin-ups or rope climbing, are often used in field testing of strength in children, particularly in the school setting. In adults, absolute strength is directly related to body weight; on the other hand, relative strength is greater in lighter individuals (6).

A large number of variables influence muscle strength; these can be grouped into two categories:

1. Muscle Tension Development
   • Number of stimulated fibers
   • Frequency of neurological impulses
   • Length of muscle
   • Cross-sectional muscle fiber size
   • Temperature
   • Muscle fiber type
2. Measurement of Strength
   • Type of contraction (eccentric, concentric, isometric)
   • Speed of contraction
   • Joint angle
   • Joint leverage
   • Age
   • Sex
   • Body mass
   • Psychological factors

Obviously the validity of comparing two studies of strength measurement in children is dependent upon a similarity of these determinants. How these factors might be responsible for the evolution of changes in strength during childhood will be addressed in the pages to follow. In certain cases, little information is available. It is recognized, for instance, that temperature regulation during exercise differs in children compared to adults (see chapter 15). Most muscles work in the outer borders, or shell tissue, of the body, and their temperature is not as closely regulated as is core temperature (57). In fact, muscle temperature may vary in warm environments between 25 and 40 °C. At the lower levels of this range, endurance of sustained isometric contractions is significantly shortened in adults. Whether age-related differences in temperature regulation with exercise might alter muscle contractile capacity is unknown.

GROWTH OF MUSCLE SIZE

Since the development of strength is linked to muscle size, it is appropriate to examine the changes in muscle bulk as children grow. This information has been reviewed in detail by Malina and Bouchard (42), who noted that completing the picture of muscle development in children has been hampered by the lack of an

accurate, noninvasive means of assessing muscle size and composition.

Muscle fiber number is fixed at or soon after birth; increases in muscle bulk during childhood and adolescence reflect the process of muscular hypertrophy, or increase in muscle fiber size. Animal studies do suggest that hyperplasia, or increase in fiber number, can occur beyond the immediate postnatal period, particularly with training (3). However, there are no data to indicate that hyperplasia contributes to muscle size during normal growth in children. Lexell et al. studied cross sections of autopsied whole vastus lateralis muscle from 22 males ages 5 to 37 years who had died of accidental causes (35). Despite a wide interindividual variability, the average total number of fibers remained stable across age groups (see fig. 13.1). These findings imply that increase in whole muscle cross-sectional area reflects increases in fiber size rather than cellular hyperplasia.

In a similarly conducted study, Oertel presented data indicating that this process of fiber hypertrophy in both deltoid and vastus lateralis muscle involves an average fivefold increase in diameter from birth to the late adolescent years (54). Other studies suggest that the extent of hypertrophy during childhood differs between muscle groups. Information from Aherne et al. (1) and Bowden and Goyer (11) shows that over the same age span, the fiber diameter of vastus lateralis muscle increases ten times over that at birth while the deltoid increases only about fivefold. Malina and Bouchard speculated that such differences might reflect "function or intensity of work load to which the muscle is exposed during growth" (42, p. 123).

The increase in muscle fiber size with growth is reflected in a rise in total muscle mass. Estimates of total body muscle mass have been derived both from dissection studies and from measurement of excretion of

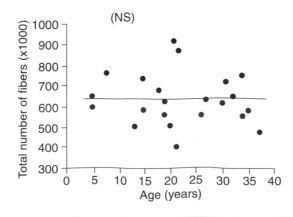

Figure 13.1 Total number of muscle fibers in vastus lateralis muscle with age. Reprinted from Lexell et al. 1992.

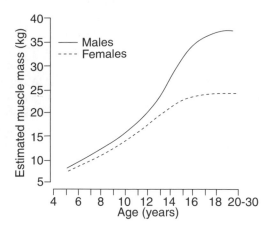

Figure 13.2   Muscle mass estimated from creatinine excretion relative to age in boys and girls. Reprinted from Malina and Bouchard 1991.

urinary creatinine (a muscle metabolite). Information on children is limited largely to the latter. Compiling data from several cross-sectional studies that utilized measures of creatinine excretion, Malina produced age-gender curves for estimated total muscle mass in children (see fig. 13.2) (39). These indicate nearly linear increases, with values for boys slightly greater until the age of puberty. At this time the curves diverge; muscle mass accelerates in males and reaches a plateau in females. We will see in the next section that developmental curves for muscle strength in children and adolescents follow the same sex-related patterns.

On the basis of these estimates, the average muscle mass as percentage body weight in males increases from 42% at age 5 years to 53% at age 17. On the other hand, no appreciable change is seen in females across the same age span (41% and 42%, respectively). Similar magnitude of changes in relative muscularity with growth has been reported. In the longitudinal study of boys by Rasmussen et al., estimated mean muscle mass rose from 10.5 to 25.1 kg between the ages of 10 and 16 years (62). These values represented 33.4% and 41.4% of body mass, respectively. Dissection studies have indicated that the average newborn is about 25% muscle, while the mean value for adults is 40% (42).

MATURATION OF MUSCLE STRENGTH

Many have investigated the changes in strength that occur during the course of childhood. These studies have been extensively reviewed by Blimkie (8) and Pate and Shephard (56). Included are cross-sectional and longitudinal studies of absolute isometric strength (usually by

handgrip), isokinetic strength, and relative strength (by such measures as the flexed arm hang). The picture of the evolution of strength during childhood from these reports is, in general, remarkably consistent: in males, measures of strength typically improve more or less linearly until puberty. At this time strength accelerates dramatically, with smaller increases throughout the remainder of adolescence.

Strength develops linearly with age in prepubertal girls, too, but despite a large overlap in measurements between males and females, mean values for boys are slightly greater at all ages. This small gender difference is apparent in grip strength as early as 3 years of age. At puberty when the strength curve deviates upward in males, the curve for females either continues to rise in a linear fashion or, in some studies, actually plateaus, showing no substantial improvement throughout adolescence.

These changes are shown in figure 13.3, which indicates improvements in grip strength with age in boys and girls (42). It is apparent that there is little gender difference in average scores during the prepubertal years. Puberty clearly influences sex differences in grip strength, as values are almost twice as great in males by the age of 17 years. When handgrip values are expressed relative to body weight, the same age-gender patterns persist.

Blimkie noted that at any given chronological age, girls show a higher proportion of their peak final grip strength (arbitrarily defined as that at age 18 years) compared to boys (8). A 10-year-old girl can be expected to exhibit 50% of her peak final strength, while in males the age at which this occurs is 12.5 years.

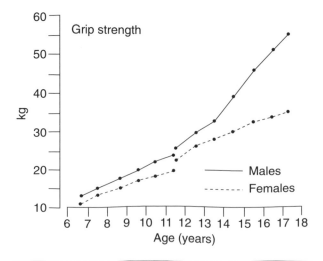

Figure 13.3   Handgrip strength in boys and girls. Reprinted from Malina and Bouchard 1991.

When the combined isometric strength of different muscles is considered (composite strength), the gender-age patterns are virtually identical to those described for grip strength. This led Blimkie to conclude that "the age-associated performance curves for absolute grip strength seem to accurately reflect composite or overall strength development for both sexes during childhood" (8, p. 108).

Only a few studies have provided information on changes in strength as measured by isokinetic dynamometry across the broad range of pediatric years (2, 38, 47, 48). These support the same pubertal influences on strength as studies with other testing modalities, but suggest that some variability may exist between sexes relative to different strength functions in the prepubertal years (8).

Body strength has been considered an important component of all-around health-related fitness. For this reason, some measurement of relative strength has been included in the several field testing batteries of school children. Consequently, a good deal of cross-sectional information is available about changes with growth in relative strength (on specific tests) in both boys and girls. These data confirm the patterns for absolute isometric and isokinetic strength already reviewed.

The development of flexed arm hang time is a good example. In this test, subjects pull the chin to a bar and sustain contraction with an overhand grip. On this measure of relative strength (actually more accurately, muscular endurance), boys have been found to double their mean time between the ages of 7 and 13 years (63). Average time for the girls is always slightly less than for the boys during this age span, and the improvement with age is slower. At puberty the strength of the girls plateaus, while that of the boys accelerates, and strength (relative to body weight) in late adolescence in males is twice that of females.

Alteration in body composition, particularly at puberty, is the most obvious explanation for the consistent gender-age patterns in strength development. Males experience a relatively greater growth of muscle mass as they enter adolescence (secondary to the influence of androgenic hormones), at the same time that girls are accumulating increasing subcutaneous fat (an estrogenic effect).

Experimental data support this conclusion. Davies studied 23 girls and 19 boys (mean ages 12.4 and 12.8 years, respectively) to determine whether or not gender differences in handgrip strength could be attributed to lean arm volume (17). No pubertal assessment was performed, but it was assumed that subjects were prepubertal or in the early stages of puberty. Total forearm volumes were calculated from circumference and length measurements, and the skinfold thickness was taken into account to estimate lean volume. The boys demonstrated superior handgrip strength (mean 234 N compared to 205 N for the girls). However, no significant gender-related differences in grip strength were observed when strength was expressed relative to lean limb volume. Both boys and girls showed a significant linear relationship between strength and lean arm volume (see fig. 13.4). The author suggested that "in children there is no gender difference in muscle performance when differences in muscle mass are allowed for" (p. 142).

As Blimkie pointed out, however, gender differences in habitual physical activity might play a role in sex-related variations in muscular strength and the rate of its

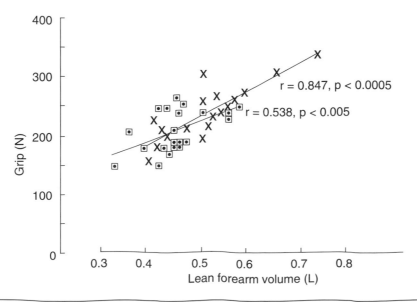

Figure 13.4 Handgrip strength relative to lean forearm volume in 12-year-old boys and girls. Reprinted from Davies 1990.

development (8). Likewise, potential gender differences in neuromuscular, biochemical, and biomechanical factors have not yet been evaluated.

WHAT FACTORS DETERMINE IMPROVEMENTS IN STRENGTH DURING CHILDHOOD?

We have seen that the course of childhood is marked by substantial improvements in muscular strength. Handgrip strength in an 18-year-old male, for instance, is almost four times that of a 7-year-old. What factors are responsible for this improvement? Certainly increase in muscle size concomitant with body growth is a key determinant, and the data reviewed earlier indicate the importance of pubertal hormonal influences in males. But other factors, particularly neurologic, may play important roles as well. This section will review evidence that multifactorial influences may affect strength in the growing child.

The Contractile Process

Could developmental changes in the tension created by the contractile process itself affect strength during childhood? Studies in animals indicate that body size per se does not influence the strength of muscular contraction (relative to the muscle cross-sectional area). When small and large adult animals of different species are compared, the number of filaments per cross-sectional area, the sarcomere length, the maximum overlap between actin and myosin filaments, the degree of muscle fiber shortening, and the maximum force performed in one contraction (calculated per unit volume of muscle) are independent of animal size (66). As Schmidt-Nielsen has pointed out, "The structure of mouse muscle and elephant muscle is so similar that a microscopist would have difficulty identifying them except for a larger number of mitochondria in the muscles of smaller animals" (66, p. 164).

Other animal data suggest, however, that intraspecies maturational status might influence the ability of muscle to generate force. Lodder et al. showed that specific force (force per cross-sectional area) and specific power (power per muscle volume) were about 30% lower in young compared to more mature rats (36). A number of possible explanations for this finding were raised by Sargeant (65), including (a) differences in myofibrillar packing, (b) changes in connective tissue in the muscle, (c) changes in cross-bridge kinetics, and (d) differences in anaerobic energy activity between the younger and older animals.

Limited research information suggests, on the other hand, that similar maturational differences in muscle contractile mechanics do not exist in humans, at least in older children. Davies et al. argued that objective measurement of a muscle's ability to generate force should be independent of subject motivation (18). These investigators used electrically evoked twitch and tetanic tension at supramaximal voltages to measure contractile properties of the triceps surae muscle in 52 boys and girls ages 11 to 14 years. In comparison to findings in young adult subjects (mean age 21 years), no differences were observed in muscle force-generating capacity (per cross-sectional area), fatiguability, or speed of contraction and relaxation. These findings imply that muscle fiber composition and function are uniform during the late childhood through young adult years. That is, changes in muscle strength as children grow do not appear to be explained by developmental alterations in the contractile mechanism. In this study, contractile properties were similar by gender as well. This supports the conclusion that differences in strength between boys and girls are related to differences in body composition and hormonal stimulation rather than to gender-related influences on the contractile properties of muscle.

Muscle contractile times do increase with age during early childhood, suggesting maturational changes in the contractile mechanism. Beyond the age of 3 years, however, there appears to be little change (8, 29, 44). A gradual decrease in muscle relaxation time during the course of the childhood years has been reported by Blimkie (8) and McComas et al. (44). But this trend could not be confirmed by Edwards et al., who found no differences in average relaxation rates of quadriceps muscle between children and adults (21). The interpretation of these results is clouded, however, as Blimkie found insignificant correlations between both contraction and relaxation times with strength measures of elbow flexors and knee extensors in males 9 to 18 years old (8).

Muscle Size

The larger the muscle, the greater contractile force it can generate. It is logical to assume, then, that the significant increases in muscle bulk accompanying growth in children should largely, if not completely, explain parallel increases in their muscular strength. Animal studies confirm that force generated by isolated muscle is closely linked to muscle cross-sectional area (16). In children, the gender-related growth curve patterns for body muscle are virtually identical to those for strength (see figs. 13.2 and 13.3). On reviewing research to date, Blimkie concluded, "It is likely that quantitative differences in muscle width account for a large proportion of the observed age and gender differences in strength development during childhood and adolescence" (8,

p. 127). Nonetheless, evidence suggests that simply an increase in muscle bulk is not the entire story.

Dimensionality Theory.
Muscular strength is a direct reflection of muscle cross-sectional area. According to dimensionality theory, muscle cross-sectional area, in turn, should be related to body height squared. By this reasoning, if muscle size is the principal determinant of improvements in strength during childhood, strength measures should scale to body height by an exponent of 2.0.

The few studies that have examined this relationship have found, however, that strength generally improves faster during childhood than can be explained by increases in height squared (4, 5, 12). These investigators have reported, too, that there is a wide variability in the relationship of strength and height for different muscle groups. Asmussen described a mean scaling factor of 2.18 for pulling strength of females 6 to 16 years old relative to body height (4). Carron and Bailey reported that average yearly increase in composite strength in 10-16-year-old boys was 22.7%, as compared to the value of 12.1% that would have been expected from increases in height squared (12).

These discrepancies between experimental and theoretical strength-height relationships in children have lent support to the idea that qualitative as well as quantitative differences in growing muscle may contribute to the development of strength. Blimkie cautioned, however, that these dimensional analyses are predicated on geometric similarity and constancy of body composition across the ages studied, an assumption he labeled as questionable (8).

Disparate Muscle Strength and Size Development.
Rasmussen et al. provided longitudinal data on muscle strength and body muscle mass in 10-year-old boys studied annually until age 16 (62). Muscle mass was estimated via a five-component fractionation of body tissues utilizing standard anthropometric measurements. Muscle strength, evaluated with a cable tensiometer, was measured in flexion and extension for seven joints and summed to create a strength score. Velocity curves indicated that peak muscle mass velocity occurred at an average of 14.3 years, whereas peak strength velocity appeared at age 14.7 years. According to the authors, this observation "supports the view that muscle tissue increases first in mass, then in functional strength. This would seem to suggest a qualitative change in muscle tissue as adolescence progresses and/or perhaps a neuromuscular maturation affecting the volitional demonstration of strength" (p. 32).

Others have observed that peak gain in muscular strength during puberty typically occurs after peak height velocity (24, 71). Blimkie noted, however, that a wide variability existed in both boys and girls for this relationship (8). For instance, these same studies indicate that almost one-fourth of boys and one-half of girls experience peak strength gains before or coincident with peak height velocity.

Relationship Between Muscle Strength and Cross-Sectional Area.
Studies addressing the association of muscle size with measures of strength in children were reviewed in 1975 by Malina (40) and again in 1989 by Blimkie (8). More recent studies utilizing ultrasound and computerized axial tomography presumably provide more accurate estimates of muscle cross-sectional area in examining this relationship. Correlations between isometric evoked and voluntary strength and muscle cross-sectional area in these investigations range from moderate to high (r = 0.60–0.90), the latter more common in studies across wider age ranges.

These data generally support the key role of increasing muscle size in the development of strength in children. Even so, it is apparent that a good deal of variance is still unexplained by the quantitative influence of muscle size itself.

Neural Influences

As reviewed in the preceding pages, increased muscle size does not appear to account entirely for improvements in body strength in children during normal growth; nor does it completely account for such improvement after a period of resistance training (to be discussed later in this chapter). This observation has led to a consideration of alternative factors that might affect the development of strength. That suspicion should fall on changes in neural influences is not surprising, given the importance that nervous innervation plays in muscle contraction. Electromyographic studies in adults undergoing resistance training indicate that increased neurological activation accompanies improvements in strength. Ozmun et al. recently reported similar electromyographic changes after 8 weeks of resistance training in 9-12-year-old children that improved strength but not muscle bulk (55).

Suggested developmental neurological changes that might influence strength in children include the process of myelination (33), increased coordination of muscle synergists and antagonists (64), and improvements in degree of motor unit activation (8). These remain speculative, and only the last hypothesis has been tested experimentally.

Blimkie evaluated the degree of motor unit activation in 10-16-year-old children using the interpolated twitch technique (8). In this method, a supramaximal electric stimulation is applied as the subject produces a peak maximal voluntary isometric contraction. The increment in force output beyond that produced by the voluntary contraction reflects the degree of motor unit activation. In this study, no age-related differences were observed in mean percentage motor activation for the elbow flexors (89.4% and 89.9% for 10- and 16-year-old boys, respectively). For knee extensors, however, activation was substantially higher in the older subjects (77.7% and 95.3%, respectively). These limited data, then, do provide some support for the concept that maturation of neural influences is important in the development of strength in children.

Endocrine Changes

That increased circulating testosterone levels are responsible for the acceleration of muscle mass and strength in males at puberty seems undebatable. The prominent anabolic effects of testosterone are well recognized, and the temporal relationship of muscle mass and strength changes in males at puberty has been a consistent observation. While no study in children has been performed to evaluate the association of strength and testosterone changes in adolescence, some experimental data do support this relationship.

Pratt studied 84 high school boys (mean age 15.7 years) to assess the relationships between lower extremity strength, age, and biological maturity (59). Sexual maturation was determined by Tanner staging, and strength was established by 1 RM maximal lifts for knee extension and flexion. Tanner staging was found to be a better predictor for lower extremity strength (r = 0.53) than chronological age. The authors suggested that the relationship between Tanner staging and strength may be based on the mutual association of these measures with lean body mass.

If testosterone and other androgenic hormones are responsible for accelerating strength in males at puberty, one should expect that early-maturing boys will display precocious strength development compared to late maturers. For the most part, the experimental evidence, reviewed by Malina and Bouchard (42), bears this out. As indicated in figure 13.5, calculated from the data of Beunen et al. (7), the curve for grip strength is higher with age in early maturers in contrast to average and late maturers (by skeletal age).

In summary, the development of strength during the course of childhood and adolescence is multifactorial. Increasing muscle size is the principal determinant driving improvements in strength. At puberty the anabolic influences of testosterone are responsible for acceleration in muscle size and strength. Presumably the maturation of neural influences on muscle contractile force contributes to improvements in strength in children, but there are few experimental studies testing this assump-

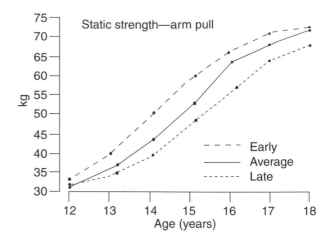

Figure 13.5 Static strength (arm pull) in early-, average-, and late-maturing boys (by skeletal age). Reprinted from Malina and Bouchard 1991.

tion. The force-producing capacity of the muscle fiber (relative to cross-sectional area) appears to be age-independent, at least from beyond the early childhood years. Kraemer et al. have proposed a temporal schema for the various factors contributing to the development of muscle strength in children (33) (see fig. 13.6).

GENETIC INFLUENCES ON STRENGTH

Studies of the heritability of muscle strength in children have produced widely different results, ranging from estimates of small to moderate degrees of heritability. These have been reviewed by Malina (41) and others (10, 31). Blimkie concluded that "it is difficult, based on the existing literature, to provide an unequivocal statement about the importance of genetic influences on the differentiation of strength performance during childhood" (8, p. 150).

Nonetheless, among these studies one can find investigations of twins, siblings, and parents and children that indicate a significant genetic contribution to expressions of muscle strength in children. The degree of heritability in many cases appears to be related to the measure of strength employed. For instance, an investigation of Czechoslovakian male twins 11-25 years old yielded hereditability estimates ranging from .75 for arm static strength to .22 for push-ups (32). Sklad found similar genetic influences on strength in Polish twins ages 8-15 years (70). Heritability estimates were .71, .46, .44, and .68 for elbow flexion and extension and knee flexion and extension, respectively. Malina pointed out that variables such as habitual activity, num-

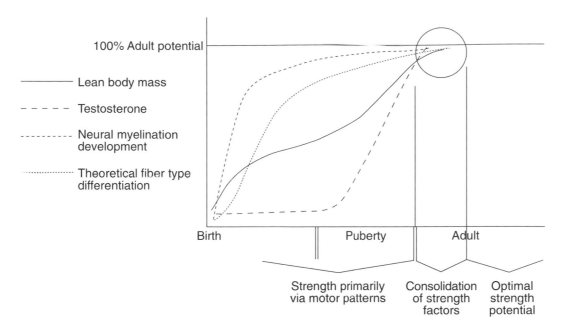

Figure 13.6   Contributions to muscle strength during maturation. Reprinted from Kraemer et al. 1989.

ber of subjects, differential effects of age and sex according to twin types, and differences in means and variances between twin samples can confound the findings in these twin studies (41).

The data from studies of similarities in strength among siblings reveal heritabilities comparable to those of the twin studies. Malina and Mueller examined strength by static testing in 114 pairs of black and 101 pairs of white siblings ages 6-12 years (43). When corrected for weight and test reliability, the estimated heritability based on sibling correlations ranged from .34 to .55 for the four tests. Correlations between brothers were higher than for sisters, but there were no differences in sibling correlation by race. Szopa obtained correlation coefficients of r = .17 to .40 (p < .05) for grip strength in a group of 728 Polish subjects ages 3 to 42 years (73).

Parents tend to be similar to their children in measures of strength (50, 73, 78), and this relationship appears to hold true throughout the life span. Wolanski and Kasprzak reported correlation coefficients of .37 to .62 in grip strength between parent and child in Polish subjects ages 7 to 39 years (78). No significant relationship was observed, however, with shoulder pull and back lift. Szopa found high correlations with arm strength but not grip strength in Polish children 3 to 42 years and their parents, 22 to 78 years of age (73).

CARDIOVASCULAR RESPONSES TO RESISTANCE EXERCISE

The cardiovascular responses to acute bouts of resistance exercise are distinct from those for endurance activities (57). Likewise, the workload placed on the heart is very different in the two forms of exercise. Studies in adults indicate that maximal endurance exercise, such as a progressive treadmill test, produces a volume load on the heart with rise in systolic blood pressure (by about 50% over resting values) and stable or even declining diastolic pressures. The heart responds to the increased systemic venous return in endurance exercise by increasing cardiac output three to five times. Heart rate rises threefold at maximal exercise, and stroke volume increases by a factor of 1.5-2.0.

In contrast, the rise in cardiac output during fatiguing isometric contractions of large muscles in adults is modest, usually increasing to about 8 L/min from resting values of 5 L/min. Heart rate during such exercise rarely exceeds 120 bpm, and increases in stroke volume are minimal.

Sympathetic influences during resistance exercise cause elevation in both systolic and diastolic pressures, the increase being related to the amount of contracting muscle mass and the intensity of contraction. Blood pressure values of 180/130 mmHg are typical in an adult who is performing isometric handgrip exercise at 40% of maximal voluntary contraction to fatigue.

Such blood pressure responses can reach dramatic extremes. Peak pressures as high as 480/350 mmHg, during a double leg press by an experienced body builder, have been reported (38). These responses accompanying static exercise cause an increase in afterload on the heart; consequently these forms of exercise have been proscribed in patients with coronary artery, hypertensive, and valvular heart disease (53).

Studies in children indicate a similar pattern of cardiovascular changes during resistance exercise. Nau et al. measured intraarterial blood pressure responses to bench press weight lifting in children who were undergoing cardiac catheterization for evaluation of dysrhythmias (51). Eight males and three females ages 8 to 16 years old were studied. The day before catheterization, 1 RM values were established for each subject. During catheterization, each subject lifted to fatigue weights equal to 60%, 75%, 90%, and 100% of 1 RM while blood pressure measurements were obtained in the ascending aorta. Mean values for aortic pressure rose from 120/81 mmHg at rest to 162/130 mmHg during the 100% 1 RM lift, with an increase in heart rate from 86 to 139 bpm. When expressed as percentage increase from baseline, these values are comparable to those reported in studies of adult subjects.

It is of interest that the peak blood pressures were not influenced by the lifting condition (i.e., percentage 1 RM) (see fig. 13.7). The 60% 1 RM load was lifted for an average of 16.9 repetitions, the 75% 1 RM load for 8.9 repetitions, and the 90% 1 RM load for 3.7 repetitions. Average peak pressures for these conditions did

not differ significantly from each other nor from that recorded during the 1 RM lift.

Strong et al. measured systolic blood pressure response to isometric exercise in 170 healthy black boys and girls ages 7 to 14 years (72). Each child squeezed a handgrip dynamometer for 30 s at 50% of a previously determined maximal effort. Cuff blood pressure was recorded in the contralateral arm during the last few seconds of exercise. Both resting and exercise blood pressures were directly related to body size. The mean change in systolic blood pressure was 18.3 and 15.7 mmHg for the males and the females, respectively. These values were equivalent to 19.2% and 15.4% increases from resting values. In this study, an inverse relationship was observed between the resting blood pressure and the percentage change with handgrip exercise (r = −.43 for boys and r = −.36 for girls). In other words, the higher the resting systolic pressure, the smaller was the relative increase.

Cassone et al. measured cardiac dimensions during isometric exercise by echocardiography in older adolescent girls who were highly trained volleyball players (13). Subjects performed 75% of maximal handgrip contraction for a period of 1 min. Cardiac output rose by 43%, a change entirely due to increased heart rate. Stroke volume as well as end-diastolic and end-systolic ventricular dimensions did not change with exercise. Systolic and diastolic blood pressures rose 20% and 17%, respectively, with an average peak pressure of 162/91 mmHg.

Gumbiner and Gutgesell performed echocardiography in 18 healthy children ages 9-18 years who were performing isometric exercise (30). Exercise consisted

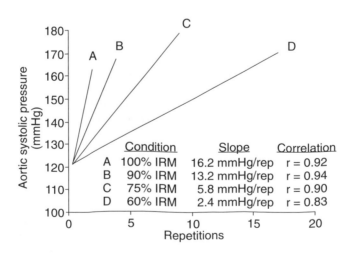

Figure 13.7 Aortic systolic pressure response in children to varying resistance conditions. Reprinted from Nau et al. 1990.

of 3 min of compressing a dynamometer with the dominant hand at 33% of maximal contraction. Mean heart rate rose from 79 bpm at rest to 91 bpm with exercise. Average systolic pressure rose from 115 to 128 mmHg, and diastolic pressure increased from 64 to 76 mmHg. Mean left ventricular end-diastolic and end-systolic dimensions did not change with exercise; consequently there was no average change in left ventricular shortening fraction.

Laird et al. reported similar findings during isometric exercise in a group of healthy 14-16-year-old adolescents (34). Subjects held a grip equal to 25% of maximal for 4 min. Cardiac index rose 22%, due entirely to increased heart rate, while systolic and diastolic ventricular diameters were unchanged. An 18% increase in mean blood pressure was observed.

Most of these studies were performed with relatively low contractile forces using a small muscular volume to allow for accurate measurement of blood pressure and other cardiovascular responses. The extent to which the findings reflect changes that would occur with more intense resistance exercise (e.g., power lifting) is unclear. It does appear that the pattern and magnitude of cardiovascular responses observed in these studies of children mimic those of adults.

STRENGTH TRAINING

In 1978, Vrijens wrote, "The findings of all authors are in general concordant. It seems that strength development is closely related to sexual maturation. Therefore, specific strength training can only be effective in the post-pubescent age" (74, p. 152). This was not an altogether unwarranted expectation. Postpubescent males appeared to demonstrate prominent improvements in muscle bulk with strength training compared to females, and the potent anabolic effects of testosterone seemed to be responsible. Since that time, however, a series of studies in children has consistently proven Vrijens' conclusion to be false (25). Prepubertal subjects, both boys and girls, do demonstrate improvements in strength with resistance training that are quantitatively similar to those of older subjects. Most studies indicate that they accomplish this without concomitant increases in muscle size. Indeed, this is the observation that has implicated the importance of neuromuscular and other adaptations, independent of increases in muscle fiber size, in the development of strength during childhood.

Interest in changes in strength in children with resistance training has partially stemmed from insights that might be gained about the mechanisms of normal development of strength with growth. That is, during the prepubertal years, gains in strength with growth and resistance training both occur in the absence of testosterone and other anabolic hormones. But it cannot be necessarily assumed that the same mechanisms are at play in both situations. Research interest in resistance training in young subjects has also been stimulated from a more pragmatic standpoint, as strength gains from training in children have potential—yet largely unproven—health benefits (9, 33). Improved strength may enhance sport performance and diminish susceptibility to injury (46), and favorable changes in blood lipoproteins have been described after resistance training in children (26, 77). Weight training has been recommended for girls as a means of helping to prevent osteoporosis (37).

Effects of Resistance Training

Most training studies in children have utilized free weights, have involved boys and girls, and have lasted for 8-12 weeks. The reader may consult extensive reviews by Sale (64), Weltman (75), and Duda (20) for details of these studies. Table 13.1 summarizes the findings in recent studies in prepubertal children that have incorporated control subjects in their design. The significant strength gains from resistance training as described in these reports—typically approximating 20-30%—have been similar in boys and girls. Most of the studies that have evaluated alterations in muscle bulk accompanying these strength changes have shown no significant effects on muscle size.

Several studies have been designed to compare the extent of strength gains during resistance training between children and older subjects. As noted by Sale, it is difficult to know what the most legitimate means of expressing strength gains is in this type of study (64). In general, postpubertal subjects demonstrate greater improvements in absolute strength (64, 74). However, when increased strength is expressed as percentage change in pretraining values, gains in strength are usually greater in prepubertal compared to mature subjects (52, 58, 64). Thus, whether children have more or less capacity for augmenting strength with resistance training depends on one's position on which of these ways of expressing changes in strength is most appropriate. Sale concluded that "the issue is not easily resolved" (64, p. 174).

Sale also emphasized the difficulty one encounters in attempting to provide an equivalent training intensity in resistance training programs for children and adults (64). Children obviously need to have a smaller absolute training resistance compared to adults. Sale considered that the training stimulus for adults and children could be equated if resistances were selected relative to maximal effort. This follows the observation noted previously that during maximal voluntary contractions, children and adults develop similar force per unit muscle cross-sectional area.

Table 13.1   Studies of strength changes with resistance training in prepubertal children

Reference	Training	Age	Sex	Weeks	Strength increase	Muscle size increase
Nielsen et al. (52)	Isometric	7–19	F	5	+	
Clarke et al. (15)	Wrestling	7–9	M	12	+	
McGovern (45)	Weights	Grades 4–6	F,M	12	+	—
Servedio et al. (67)	Weights	12	M	8	+	
Pfeiffer and Francis (58)	Weights	8–11	M	8	+	
Sewall and Micheli (68)	Weights	10–11	F,M	9	+	
Weltman et al. (76)	Hydraulic	6–11	M	14	+	—
Siegel et al. (69)	Weights	8	F,M	12	+	
Ozmun et al. (55)	Weights	9–12	F,M	8	+	—
Ramsay et al. (60)	Weights	9–11	M	20	+	—
Fukunga et al. (27)	Isometric	7–11	M,F	12	+	+
Faigenbaum et al. (23)	Weights	8–12	M,F	8	+	

Mechanisms for Strength Gains With Resistance Training

The popular conception—embodied by the male body builder—holds that improvements in strength with resistance training are paralleled by increases in muscle size. Furthermore, testosterone has been considered the hormonal trigger requisite for these changes. Yet adult women improve in their muscular strength with resistance training; children experience progressive improvements in strength as they grow; and, as outlined earlier, there are convincing data that prepubertal subjects exhibit expected increases in strength after training. That all of these subjects demonstrate augmented strength (a) in the absence of much circulating testosterone, and (b) without necessarily showing parallel changes in muscle size has served as evidence that such improvements must be derived through other mechanisms. This section will address the mechanisms for improvements in strength with resistance training prior to the age of puberty.

Muscle Size.   Most studies that have examined changes in muscle size with resistance training in children have shown little or no effect despite significant improvements in muscular strength. In the largest and most comprehensive study on this question, Ramsay et al. had 13 boys ages 9-11 years perform weight training three times a week for 20 weeks (60). Significant improvements in strength measures compared to values for a nontraining control group were observed in 1 RM bench press (35%), leg press (22%), absolute peak torque of the elbow flexors (26%) and knee extensors (21%), and isometric strength. However, no effects of the training were observed on muscle cross-sectional areas of the upper arm and thigh as assessed by computerized axial tomography scans.

Weltman et al. trained 16 prepubertal boys (mean age 8.2 years) using hydraulic resistance equipment for 14 weeks, three sessions per week (76). Significant improvements were seen in isokinetic strength for flexion and extension at the knee and elbow joints compared to the values for controls. Of 15 measured circumferences, only 3 (shoulder, chest, abdomen) increased more in the training subjects. Likewise, Ozmun et al. found no changes in arm circumferences or skinfolds despite a 23% increase in isotonic and a 28% rise in isokinetic strength after 8 weeks of arm weight training in eight 10-year-old subjects (55).

Fukunga et al. used ultrasound to measure cross-sectional muscle area in the upper arm of 52 boys and girls, ages 7-11 years, who underwent a 12-week period of isometric training (27). The training group comprised males and females in the 1st, 3rd, and 5th grades. The males showed significant strength improvements in maximal elbow flexion as compared to the nontraining controls in all 3 grades, but the same pattern was not seen in the females. No differences were observed between training and nontraining groups in changes in elbow extension strength. Lean upper arm cross-sectional area increased significantly with training in both boys and girls in the 3rd and 5th grades, but not the 1st grade. In the control group, increased muscle cross-sectional area was observed in both sexes only in the 5th grade. No clear-cut relationship was found between percentage improvement in muscle strength and percentage increase in muscle area.

Intrinsic Muscle Force Production.   Improvements in strength with training could reflect enhancement of the intrinsic force-producing capacity of muscle. Such changes could reflect alterations in factors like excitation-contraction coupling, myofibril packing density, and muscle compliance associated with fiber damage. Evoked contraction strength, the contraction force created by electrical stimulation of muscle, is a measure of such alterations. Tetanic stimulation would provide the best information on intrinsic muscle contractile strength, but this technique is painful. Therefore, the force produced by a single maximal twitch contraction, a less precise indicator, has been utilized experimentally instead.

Ramsay et al. measured changes in evoked contractile properties of elbow flexors and knee extensors in their study of prepubertal males described previously (60). Training resulted in significant increases in absolute values for both muscle groups (29.6% and 29.7%, respectively); when normalized for cross-sectional area, the increase in evoked twitch torque remained significant for the elbow flexors but not the knee extensors. The absolute increase in elbow flexor torque in the boys was approximately half that for 21-year-old men in a similar study. However, when expressed as percentage change with training, the increase in the boys was over twice that for the men (64).

Neural Adaptations. Some experimental data support the idea that changes in neurological influences on muscle contraction contribute to strength gains from resistance training in children. Ozmun et al. reported that electromyogram activity increased 16.8% in prepubertal boys after an 8-week resistance training program (55). In that study, significant improvements were observed in isotonic (22.6%) and isokinetic (27.8%) strength without changes in arm circumferences. No strength or electromyogram alterations were observed in untrained control children.

Ramsay et al. used the interpolated twitch technique described earlier to estimate the percentage motor unit activation (%MUA) before and after a 20-week resistance training program in 9-11-year-old boys (60). Changes in %MUA with training were not statistically significant, but there was a trend toward increased %MUA for both elbow flexors and knee extensors at mid- and posttesting (13.2% and 17.4%, respectively). Meanwhile, no appreciable changes were observed in control subjects. Strength improvements in this study ranged from 25% to 30% without increase in muscle size. The authors suggested therefore that other neurological adaptations such as changes in motor unit coordination, recruitment, and firing frequency might have also contributed to these strength gains.

SUMMARY

Although far from complete, the available research data are sufficient to provide a reasonably consistent picture of strength gains in children. Muscular strength improves throughout childhood, a reflection of neural adaptations and increases in muscle size. The latter are generated by growth factors (e.g., growth hormone) in the absence of circulating testosterone. At puberty the rapid rise in androgenic steroids in males causes a dramatic acceleration in muscle size and strength in boys.

Resistance training before puberty can enhance muscle strength, with quantitative changes that are gender-independent and are similar to those in adults. Increase in muscle size appears to contribute little to training-induced improvements in strength in children before the age of puberty. Such improvements presumably reflect neural adaptations and improvements in the force generated by the intrinsic contractile mechanism.

What We Know

1. Muscle strength progressively improves during childhood, principally as the result of increasing muscle size.
2. Hormonal influences at puberty are responsible for the dramatic increase in muscle bulk and strength in males.
3. Muscle strength can be improved by resistance training before puberty in both boys and girls. These changes occur without substantive increases in muscle size.
4. Cardiovascular responses to resistance exercise in children are similar to those in adults: both systolic and diastolic blood pressure rises, with limited changes in heart rate and cardiac output.

What We Would Like to Know

1. How influential are factors independent of muscle size (neural, contractile, endocrine) in the development of strength and responses to strength training in children?

2. What test of muscle strength is most predictive of generalized body muscle strength?
3. How important is the development of muscle strength in children as a contributor to health?
4. How important are genetic influences on strength and response to strength training during childhood?

References

1. Aherne, W.; Ayyar, D.R.; Clarke, P.A.; Walton, J.N. Muscle fibre size in normal infants, children, and adolescents: an autopsy study. J. Neurol. Sci. 4:171-182; 1971.
2. Alexander, J.; Molnar, G.E. Muscular strength in children: preliminary report on objective standards. Arch. Phys. Med. Rehab. 54:424-427; 1973.
3. Antonio, J.; Gonyea, W.J. Muscle fiber splitting in stretch-enlarged avian muscle. Med. Sci. Sports Exerc. 26:973-977; 1994.
4. Asmussen, E. Growth in muscular strength and power. In: Rarick, G.L., ed. Physical activity, human growth and development. New York: Academic Press; 1973:p. 60-79.
5. Asmussen, E.; Heeboll-Nielsen, K. A dimensional analysis of physical performance and growth in boys. J. Appl. Physiol. 7:593-603; 1955.
6. Berger, R.A. Applied exercise physiology. Philadelphia: Lea & Febiger; 1982:p. 1-46.
7. Beunen, G.; Ostyn, M.; Simons, J.; Renson, R.; Van Gerven, D. Motorische vaardigheid somatische ontwikkeling en biologische maturiteit [Motor ability, somatic development and biological maturity]. Geneeskunde en Sport 13:36-42; 1980.
8. Blimkie, C.J.R. Age- and sex-associated variation in strength during childhood: anthropometric, morphological, neurologic, biomechanical, endocrinologic, genetic, and physical activity correlates. In: Perspectives in exercise science and sports medicine. Vol. 2, Gisolfi, C.V.; Lamb, D.R., eds. Youth, exercise, and sport. Indianapolis: Benchmark Press; 1989:p. 99-164.
9. Blimkie, C.J.R. Benefits and risks of resistance training in children. In: Cahill, B.R.; Pearl, A.J., eds. Intensive participation in children's sports. Champaign; IL: Human Kinetics; 1993:p. 133-166.
10. Bouchard, C.; Malina, R.M. Genetics of physiological fitness and motor performance. Exerc. Sport Sci. Rev. 11:306-339; 1983.
11. Bowden, D.H.; Goyer, R.A. The size of muscle fibers in infants and children. Arch. Path. 68:188-189; 1960.
12. Carron, A.V.; Bailey, D.A. Strength development in boys from 10 to 16 years. Soc. Res. Child Devel. 39:1-37; 1974.
13. Cassone, R.; Germano, G.; Dalmaso, S.; Corretti, R.; Astarita, C.; Chieco, P.; Corsi, V. Evaluation of cardiac dynamics during isometric exercise in young female athletes: an echocardiographic study. J. Sports Med. 21:359-364; 1981.
14. Chapman, S.J.; Grindrod, S.R.; Jones, D.A. Cross-sectional area and force production of the quadriceps muscle. J. Physiol. 353:53P; 1984.
15. Clarke, D.H.; Vaccaro, P.; Andresen, N.M. Physiological alterations in 7- to 9-year old boys following a season of competitive wrestling. Res. Q. Exerc. Sport 55:318-322; 1984.
16. Close, R.I. Dynamic properties of mammalian skeletal muscle. Phys. Rev. 52:129-197; 1972.
17. Davies, B.N. The relationship of lean limb volume to performance in the handgrip and standing long jump tests in boys and girls, aged 11.6-13.2 years. Eur. J. Appl. Physiol. 60:139-143; 1990.
18. Davies, C.T.M.; White, M.J.; Young, K. Muscle function in children. Eur. J. Appl. Physiol. 52:111-114; 1983.
19. Dempsey, Y. The relationship between the strength of the elbow flexors and muscle size of the upper arm in children [master's thesis]. Madison, WI: University of Wisconsin; 1955.
20. Duda, M. Prepubescent strength training gains support. Phys. Sportsmed. 14:157-161; 1986.
21. Edwards, R.H.T.; Chapman, S.J.; Newham, D.J.; Jones, D.A. Practical analysis of variability of muscle function measurements in Duchenne muscular dystrophy. Muscle Nerve 10:6-14; 1987.
22. Edwards, R.H.T.; Young, A.; Hosking, G.P.; Jones, D.A. Human skeletal muscle function: description of tests and normal values. Clin. Sci. Mol. Med. 52:283-290; 1977.
23. Faigenbaum, A.D.; Zaichkowsky, L.D.; Wescott, W.L.; Micheli, L.J.; Fehlandt, A.F. The effects of a twice-a-week strength training program on children. Pediatr. Exerc. Science 5:339-346; 1993.
24. Faust, M.S. Somatic development of adolescent girls. Soc. Res. Child. Dev. 42:1-90; 1977.
25. Freedson, P.S.; Ward, A.; Rippe, J.M. Resistance training for youth. Adv. Sports Med. Fit. 3:57-65; 1990.
26. Fripp, R.R.; Hodgson, J.L. Effects of resistance straining on plasma lipid and lipoprotein levels in male adolescents. J. Pediatr. 111:926-931; 1987.
27. Fukunga, T.; Funato, K.; Ikegawa, S. The effects of resistance training on muscle area and strength in prepubescent age. An. Physiol. Anthrop. 11:357-364; 1992.
28. Funato, K.; Fukunga, T.; Asami, T.; Ikeda, S. Strength training for prepubescent boys and girls. In: Proceedings of the Department of Sports Sciences, College of Arts and Sciences, University of Tokyo; 21:9-19; 1987.
29. Gatev, V.; Stefanova-Uzunova, M.; Stamatova, L. Influence of vertical posture development on the velocity properties of triceps surae muscle in normal children. J. Neurol. Sci. 52:85-90; 1981.
30. Gumbiner, C.H.; Gutgesell, H.P. Response to isometric exercise in children and young adults with aortic regurgitation. Am. Heart. J. 106:540-547; 1983.

31. Klissouras, V. Heritability of adaptive variation. J. Appl. Physiol. 31:338-344; 1971.

32. Kovar, R. Prispevek ke geneticke pudminenouti lidske motorisky [doctoral dissertation]. Prague: Charles University; 1974.

33. Kraemer, W.J.; Fry, A.C.; Frykman, P.N.; Conroy, B.; Hoffman, J. Resistance training and youth. Pediatr. Exerc. Science 1:336-350; 1989.

34. Laird, W.P.; Fixler, D.D.; Huffines, F.D. Cardiovascular response to isometric exercise in normal adolescents. Circulation 59:651-654; 1979.

35. Lexell, J.; Sjostrom, M.; Nordlund, A.; Taylor, C.C. Growth and development of human muscle: morphological study of whole vastus lateralis from childhood to adult age. Muscle Nerve 15:404-409; 1992.

36. Lodder, M.A.N.; de Haan, A.; Sargeant, A.J. The effect of growth on specific tetanic force in the skeletal muscle of the anaesthetized rat. J. Physiol. 438:15P; 1991.

37. Loucks, A.B. Osteoporosis prevention begins in childhood. In: Brown, E.W.; Branta, C.F., eds. Competitive sports for children and youth. Champaign, IL: Human Kinetics; 1988:p. 213-224.

38. MacDougall, J.D.; Tuxen, D.; Sale, D.G.; Moroz, J.R.; Sutton, J.R. Arterial blood pressure response to heavy resistance exercise. J. Appl. Physiol. 58:785-790; 1985.

39. Malina, R.M. Quantification of fat, muscle and bone in man. Clin. Orthop. 65:9-38; 1969.

40. Malina, R.M. Anthropometric correlates to performance. Exerc. Sport Sci. Rev. 3:249-274; 1975.

41. Malina, R.M. Genetics of motor development and performance. In: Malina, R.M.; Bouchard, C., eds. Sport and human genetics. Champaign, IL: Human Kinetics; 1986:p. 23-58.

42. Malina, R.M.; Bouchard, C. Growth, maturation and physical activity. Champaign, IL: Human Kinetics; 1991:p. 115-131.

43. Malina, R.M.; Mueller, H. Genetic and environmental influences on the strength and performance of Philadelphia schoolchildren. Hum. Biol. 53:163-179; 1981.

44. McComas, A.J.; Sica, R.E.P.; Petito, P. Muscle strength in boys of different ages. J. Neurol. Neurosurg. Psych. 36:171-173; 1973.

45. McGovern, M.B. Effects of circuit weight training on the physical fitness of prepubescent children. Dissert. Abstr. Int. 45:452A-453A; 1984.

46. Micheli, L. Strength training in the young athlete. In: Brown, E.W.; Branta, C.F., eds. Competitive sports for children. Champaign, IL: Human Kinetics; 1988:p. 99-106.

47. Miyashita, M.; Kanehisa, H. Dynamic peak torque related to age, sex, and performance. Res. Q. 50:249-255; 1979.

48. Molnar, G.E.; Alexander, J. Objective, quantitative muscle testing in children: a pilot study. Arch. Phys. Med. Rehab. 54:224-228; 1973.

49. Molnar, G.E.; Alexander, J.; Gutfield, N. Reliability of quantitative strength measurements in children. Arch. Phys. Med. Rehab. 60:218-221; 1979.

50. Montoye, H.J.; Metzner, H.L.; Keller, J.K. Familial aggregation of strength and heart rate responses to exercise. Hum. Biol. 47:17-36; 1975.

51. Nau, K.L.; Katch, V.L.; Beekman, R.H.; Dick, M. Acute intraarterial blood pressure response to bench press weight lifting in children. Pediatr. Exerc. Science 2:37-45; 1990.

52. Nielsen, B.; Nielsen, K.; Behrendt-Hansen, M.; Asmussen, A. Training of functional muscular strength in girls 7-19 years old. In: Berg, K.; Eriksson, B.O., eds. Children and exercise IX. Champaign, IL: Human Kinetics; 1980: p. 69-78.

53. Nutter, D.O.; Schlant, R.C.; Hurst, J.W. Isometric exercise and the cardiovascular system. Mod. Conc. Cardiovasc. Dis. 41:11-15; 1972.

54. Oertel, G. Morphometric analysis of normal skeletal muscles in infancy, childhood and adolescence. J. Neurol. Sci. 88:303-313; 1988.

55. Ozmun, J.C.; Mikesy, A.E.; Surburg, P.R. Neuromuscular adaptations following prepubescent strength training. Med. Sci. Sports Exerc. 26:510-514; 1994.

56. Pate, R.R.; Shephard, R.J. Characteristics of physical fitness in youth. In: Perspectives in exercise science and sports medicine. Vol. 2, Gisolfi, C.V.; Lamb, D.R., eds. Youth, exercise, and sport. Indianapolis: Benchmark Press; 1989:p. 1-46.

57. Petrofsky, J.S.; Phillips, C.A. The physiology of static exercise. Exerc. Sport Sci. Rev. 14:1-44; 1986.

58. Pfeiffer, R.D.; Francis, R.S. Effects of strength training on muscle development in prepubescent, pubescent, and postpubescent males. Phys. Sportsmed. 14:134-143; 1986.

59. Pratt, M. Strength, flexibility, and maturity in adolescent athletes. Am. J. Dis. Child. 143:560-563; 1989.

60. Ramsay, J.A.; Blimkie, C.J.R.; Smith, K.; Garner, S.; MacDougall, J.D.; Sale, D.G. Strength training effects in prepubescent boys. Med. Sci. Sports Exerc. 22:605-614; 1990.

61. Rarick, G.L.; Thompson, J.A.J. Roentgenographic measures of leg muscle size and ankle extensor strength of 7-year old children. Res. Q. 27:321-332; 1956.

62. Rasmussen, R.L.; Faulkner, R.A.; Mirwald, R.L.; Bailey, D.A. A longitudinal analysis of structure/function related variables in 10-16 year old boys. In: Beunen, G.; Ghesquiere, J.; Reybrouck, T.; Claesscus, A.L., eds. Children and exercise. Stuttgart: Ferdinand Enke Verlag; 1990:p. 27-33.

63. Reiff, G.G.; Dixon, W.R.; Jacoby, D.; Ye, G.X.; Spain, C.G.; Hunsicker, P.A. National school population fitness survey. The President's Council on Physical Fitness and Sports; 1985.

64. Sale, D.G. Strength training in children. In: Perspectives in exercise science and sports medicine. Vol. 2, Gisolfi, C.V.; Lamb, D.R., eds. Youth, exercise, and sport. Indianapolis: Benchmark Press; 1989:p. 165-222.

65. Sargeant, A.J. Problems in, and approaches to, the measurement of short term power output in children and adolescents. In: Coudert, J.; Van Praagh, E., eds. Pediatric work physiology. Paris: Masson; 1992:p. 11-18.

66. Schmidt-Nielsen, K. Scaling. Why is animal size so important? Cambridge: Cambridge University Press; 1984:p. 163-164.

67. Servedio, F.J.; Bartels, R.L.; Hamlin, R.L. The effects of weight training using Olympic style lifts on various physiological variables in pre-pubescent boys [abstract]. Med. Sci. Sports Exerc. 17:288; 1985.

68. Sewall, L.; Micheli, L.J. Strength training for children. J. Pediatr. Orthop. 6:143-146; 1986.

69. Siegel, J.A.; Camaione, D.N.; Manfredi, T.G. The effects of upper body resistance training on prepubescent children. Pediatr. Exerc. Science 1:145-154; 1989.

70. Sklad, M. Rozwoj fizyczny I motorcznose blizniat. Materialy I Prace Antropologiczne 85:3-102; 1973.

71. Stolz, H.R.; Stolz, L.M. Somatic development of adolescent boys. New York: Macmillan; 1951.

72. Strong, W.B.; Miller, M.D.; Striplin, M.; Salehbhai, M. Blood pressure response to isometric and dynamic exercise in healthy black children. Am. J. Dis. Child. 132:587-591; 1978.

73. Szopa, J. Familial studies on genetic determination of some manifestations of muscular strength in man. Gen. Polonica 23:65-79; 1982.

74. Vrijens, J. Muscle strength development in the pre- and post-pubescent age. Med. Sport 11:152-158; 1978.

75. Weltman, A. Weight training in prepubertal children: physiological benefit and potential damage. In: Advances in pediatric sport sciences. Vol. 3, Bar-Or, O., ed. Biological issues. Champaign, IL: Human Kinetics; 1989:p. 101-130.

76. Weltman, A.; Janney, C.; Rians, C.B.; Strand, K.; Berg, B.; Tippett, S,; Wise, J.; Cahill, B.R.; Katch, F.I. The effects of hydraulic resistance strength training in pre-pubescent males. Med. Sci. Sports Exerc. 18:629-638; 1986.

77. Weltman, A.; Janney, C.; Rians, C.B.; Strand, K.; Katch, F.I. The effects of hydraulic-resistance training on serum lipid levels in prepubertal boys. Am. J. Dis. Child. 141:777-780; 1987.

78. Wolanski, N.; Kasprzak, E. Similarity in some physiological, biochemical and psychomotor traits between parents and 2-45 years old offspring. Stud. Hum. Ecol. 3:85-131; 1979.

CHAPTER 14

METABOLIC AND ENDOCRINE RESPONSES TO EXERCISE

One of the truly remarkable features of the physiological responses to exercise is the coordinated involvement of virtually all the body's systems. And although the cardiopulmonary and muscular aspects of exercise have drawn the greatest research attention, the critical contributions of other systems cannot be overstated. This chapter addresses the evidence for changes in metabolic fuels as well as the influence of the endocrine system during exercise as children grow. These "supporting actors" in the performance of exercise provide for adequate energy substrate and maintenance of normal fluid and electrolyte balance. Maturity-related differences in these factors have the potential for profoundly influencing exercise performance.

SUBSTRATE UTILIZATION

The energy source for muscle work depends on the intensity and duration of exercise. Short-burst activities rely principally on anaerobic metabolism, with energy derived via glycolytic pathways from the breakdown of glycogen. A different pattern of substrate utilization occurs during low-intensity sustained exercise, which utilizes aerobic metabolism via the Krebs cycle and oxidative phosphorylation. In the early phase of such exercise, muscles rely principally on carbohydrates, derived from glycogenolysis, for their energy source. As exercise continues, however, a progressive shift in substrate utilization occurs, with increasing use of fat. During the latter phase of sustained exercise, in fact, fatty acids become the predominant energy source.

The information presented in chapter 12 indicated that anaerobic capacity improves as children grow, even in relation to body size. Some data incriminate deficiencies in glycogenolysis, particularly decreased activity of the rate-limiting enzyme phosphofructokinase, as responsible for the lower anaerobic fitness observed in younger children. It would not be unreasonable to expect, therefore, that children might rely more than adults on fat metabolism for energy during sustained exercise.

The experimental means that have been used to examine age-related differences in substrate utilization during exercise are reviewed in the sections that follow. Although enhanced utilization of fat for energy substrate during exercise might be expected in children, it is apparent that the data supporting this concept are tenuous. Even if true, this observation would still beg the question: are children less "anaerobic" because of enhanced ability to utilize fats for exercise fuel, or are children forced to rely more on fatty acid oxidation because of an inferior capability to generate such energy through anaerobic metabolic pathways?

Rate of Glycogen Depletion

Little information is available regarding glycogen depletion rates during exercise in children because such studies require serial muscle biopsies during exercise testing. Eriksson et al. reported muscle glycogen depletion during exercise in eight healthy 11-13-year-old boys (see fig. 14.1) (17). Subjects performed a maximal cycle test, and quadriceps femoris muscle biopsies were obtained at each workload and at peak exercise. Muscle glycogen level fell from 54 mmol glucose units per kg

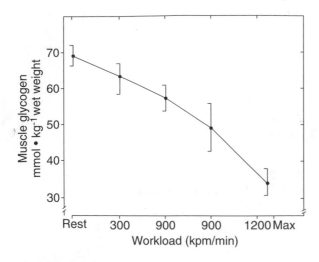

Figure 14.1 Muscle glycogen content in boys during progressive exercise. Reprinted from Eriksson et al. 1973.

to 34 mmol at exhaustion. The authors stated that this decline in muscle glycogen during exercise was "similar to the situation in adults" (p. 494). However, in a later article, Eriksson concluded that glycogen breakdown must be much slower in children than in adults (and younger children compared to older children) because muscle lactate concentrations (a by-product of glycolytic metabolism) during exercise rise with increasing maturity (see chapter 12) (16). Clearly, in the absence of studies directly comparing child and adult subjects, the question of age-related differences in glycogen utilization remains unanswered.

Respiratory Exchange Ratio

The respiratory exchange ratio (RER), or the $\dot{V}CO_2/\dot{V}O_2$ ratio measured at the mouth, has been utilized as an indicator of the respiratory quotient (RQ), the same ratio at the cellular level. The value of the latter reflects substrate utilization, since CO_2 production relative to O_2 consumption is different when fats, carbohydrates, and proteins are used as fuels. The RQ is 1.00 for carbohydrates, 0.70 for fat, and 0.82 for protein. Since protein does not contribute significantly to energy production during exercise, its influence is usually ignored, and RQ is considered an indicator of the relative contributions of carbohydrates and fats as substrate (35).

It is important to recognize that RER is influenced by factors other than RQ. If a subject hyperventilates, breathing in excess of the body's metabolic demands (as with anxiety), CO_2 elimination is increased and RER rises. Lactate production during exercise increases RER as excessive CO_2 is produced by bicarbonate buffering. Respiratory exchange ratio values during moderate-to-high-intensity exercise (i.e., above

the anaerobic threshold) can therefore be expected to exceed those reflecting RQ.

Several authors have assessed RER during prolonged steady state exercise in children and adults as a means of investigating differences in substrate utilization. These studies have produced conflicting results, and no clear picture of maturity-related difference in RER with exercise has emerged.

Martinez and Haymes reported that RER values were lower in 8-10-year-old girls, and declined to a greater extent, during a 30 min treadmill run at 70% $\dot{V}O_2$max compared to values for 20-32-year-old women (see fig. 14.2) (34). The testing was performed after a 12 hr fast; dietary analysis showed no differences between the groups in relative intake of fats, carbohydrates, and protein. No differences were observed in resting RER between the girls and women. Mean RER was 0.93 at 5 min of exercise in the women and changed little during the 30 min run. The girls had an average RER of 0.92 at 5 min with a decline to 0.90 at 30 min. At each 5 min interval between these times, the RER was significantly lower in the girls. At the same time, rise in blood lactate was significantly greater in the women compared to the girls; this may have influenced RER values. Nonetheless, the authors concluded that these data suggest that children rely to a greater extent than young women on fat utilization during treadmill running at 70% $\dot{V}O_2$max.

In a similar study, Rowland and Rimany found no RER differences in girls and women cycling for 40 min at an intensity of 63% $\dot{V}O_2$max (46). The subjects were 11 premenarcheal girls ages 9 to 13 years and 13 women ages 20-31 years. At 10 min of exercise, average RER was 0.95 and 0.97 for the girls and women, respectively ($p > .05$). By 40 min, the mean value had fallen to 0.87 in both groups. Lactate levels were not measured in this study, but 45% of the girls were cycling above their ventilatory threshold compared to 77% of the women.

Asano and Hirakoba reported that adult men (ages 20-34 years) showed a greater fall in RER during 60 min of cycling than 10-12-year-old boys (2). Mean RER declined from 0.92 to 0.88 from the 10th to the 60th min in the men and from 0.88 to 0.87 in the boys. Similarly, Mácek et al. found no significant changes in RER during 60 min of both cycle and treadmill exercise by 10 prepubertal boys at both 36-39% and 60% of $\dot{V}O_2$max (29).

In these studies, subjects were compared at similar exercise intensities. When RER has been measured at the same absolute intensity, conflicting results have also been reported. Robinson had subjects walk on a treadmill at 5.6 km/hr for 15 min (41). The RER at the end of exercise increased with age, with values of 0.87, 0.90, and 0.93 in males 6, 17, and 45 years of age, respectively. Martinez and Haymes found no significant differences in RER between nine women and nine prepu-

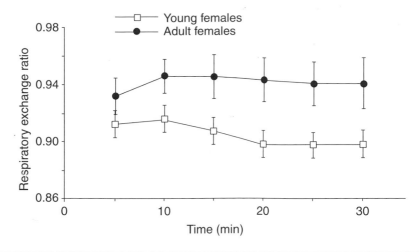

Figure 14.2 Respiratory exchange ratios in girls and women exercising at 70% $\dot{V}O_2$max for 30 min. Reprinted from Martinez and Haymes 1992.

bertal girls running horizontally at 7.2 km/hr for 30 min (except for a higher value in the girls at the initial 5 min measurement) (34). The rate of decline was greater in the girls, however.

Plasma Free Fatty Acids and Glycerol

The concentrations of free fatty acids (FFA) and glycerol in the blood reflect the degree of fat mobilization from peripheral stores. These values have consequently been used as markers of the rate of fat metabolism during exercise. Studies comparing the exercise-induced responses in FFA and glycerol levels in children and adults have generally shown no significant differences. In the study by Martinez and Haymes described in the last section, FFA and glycerol levels rose similarly with sustained treadmill running in both girls and young adult women (34). Free fatty acid values increased by 54% and 82%, and glycerol concentrations rose 621% and 796%, respectively (p > .05).

Wirth et al. reported no difference in the rise of FFA concentration during 15 min of constant-load cycling (70% $\dot{V}O_2$max) in pre-, circum-, and postpubertal swim-trained boys and girls (52). Eriksson et al. found similar concentrations of FFA or glycerol in four 12-13-year-old boys and four 23-year-old men while they cycled at 55-73% $\dot{V}O_2$max for 1 hr (18). Mácek et al. considered the increases in blood glycerol observed during prolonged treadmill and cycle exercise in prepubertal boys to be comparable to those of adults in parallel studies (30).

However, Berg and Keul reported that children have a lower FFA:glycerol ratio during exercise, an observation interpreted as suggesting that children have improved FFA utilization compared to adults (see fig. 14.3) (6). In contrast, the girls and women studied by

Martinez and Haymes had similar FFA:glycerol ratios (34). Delamarche et al. measured FFA and glycerol levels in 10 prepubertal boys during 60 min of cycling at 60% $\dot{V}O_2$max (15). They estimated FFA turnover by relative changes in glycerol and FFA (13). When turnover was expressed per liter $\dot{V}O_2$, the value was 10% greater than that obtained in previous investigations of adults.

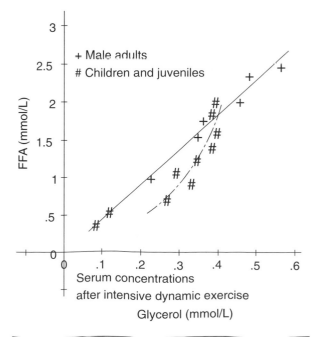

Figure 14.3 Relationship of serum concentrations of free fatty acids and glycerol after intensive dynamic exercise in boys and men. Reprinted from Berg and Keul 1988.

Blood Glucose

Exercising muscle depends on circulating glucose for a substantial portion of its energy requirements. Glucose is the immediate substrate for glycolysis, the chain of chemical reactions responsible for anaerobic adenosine triphosphate production as well as aerobic metabolism through subsequent involvement of the Krebs cycle and oxidative phosphorylation. Since the latter sequence serves as an alternative metabolic process to fatty acid oxidation, it is of interest to examine maturity-related differences in blood glucose with exercise.

Blood glucose levels during exercise represent the balance between muscle glucose uptake and release of glucose from the liver by the process of glycogenolysis. Responses of blood glucose to exercise do not appear to be substantially different in children and adults, indicating that the mechanisms contributing to these two processes function in a maturity-independent manner. This observation also suggests that if children do have inferior capacity during exercise to generate energy by glycolytic metabolism (see chapter 12), lack of availability of circulating glucose is not the explanation.

Blood glucose levels were essentially stable throughout 15 min cycling at 70% $\dot{V}O_2max$ in pre-, circum-, and postpubertal subjects reported by Wirth et al. (52). Eriksson et al. found a similar pattern when comparing 13-year-old boys and adult men during 1 hr of cycling (18). The 10 prepubertal boys described by Delamarche et al. showed a slight dip in blood glucose at 15 min of steady-load cycling (60% $\dot{V}O_2max$) but stable values during the remainder of 60 min exercise (15). When glucose concentrations were corrected for alterations in plasma volume, Martinez and Haymes could find no differences in girls and women performing treadmill running at 70% $\dot{V}O_2max$ for 30 min (34). Submaximal and maximal blood glucose levels were not significantly different in the boys and men during a progressive treadmill run to exhaustion reported by Lehmann et al. (28).

PLASMA VOLUME

During bouts of acute exercise, plasma volume decreases as a result of increased capillary hydrostatic pressure, rising intramuscular osmotic pressure, and dehydration (51). Since changes in plasma volume will affect concentrations of blood constituents, it is important to know whether or not such alterations are similar in children and adults. Studies of plasma volume during acute bouts of exercise in children have generally been conducted through measurement of changes in blood hematocrit. These reports suggest that quantitative differences in the decline in plasma volume with exercise may exist between children and adults. Such differences may be important in comparisons of concentrations of blood-borne substances between groups.

When the prepubertal girls and young adult women studied by Martinez and Haymes ran for 30 min, their plasma volume (estimated by hematocrit changes) declined by an average of 9.6% and 14.3%, respectively ($p < .05$) (34). The importance of this difference was underscored by comparison of blood glucose levels, which rose to significantly higher levels in the women than in the girls. But when the differences in decline in plasma volume were considered, the glucose changes with exercise in the two groups became similar.

Mácek et al. found little change in hematocrit in a group of prepubertal boys who exercised for 60 min on both the cycle and treadmill at 36-39% and 60% $\dot{V}O_2max$ (30). This contrasts with findings for adults showing an initial hemoconcentration at onset of heavy exercise. Mácek et al. suggested that the lower muscle lactate concentrations in children during exercise might result in lower muscle cell osmolarity, lessening shifts of fluid out of the vascular bed.

The 10 prepubertal boys described by Delamarche et al. experienced an average 6.6% increase in packed red cell volume during the first 15 min of cycle exercise, but no changes over the remaining 45 min (15). No comparisons were made with adult subjects in this study, but the pattern (early hemoconcentration) mimics that described in older individuals.

ENDOCRINE RESPONSES TO EXERCISE

The endocrine system, a set of glands that secrete hormones directly into the bloodstream, provides for numerous homeostatic functions during exercise, including the following:

1. Maintenance of energy substrate, including mobilization of fats from body stores, stabilization of circulating glucose, and uptake of blood glucose by muscle cells
2. Control of fluid-electrolyte balance to stabilize blood osmolality
3. Stimulation of heart rate and force of myocardial contraction
4. Regulation of peripheral vascular tone to control distribution of blood flow

Endocrine function during exercise has been reviewed by Wilmore and Costill (51). This section will cover the characteristics of these responses in children.

Insulin

Insulin is secreted by the islet cells of the pancreas and is responsible for facilitating the entry of glucose from the blood into muscle. In adults, plasma insulin levels decline during sustained exercise, while cell receptors become more sensitive to insulin actions. Consequently, blood glucose concentrations remain relatively constant. Studies of insulin response to sustained exercise in children, both with and without direct adult comparisons, have so far failed to indicate a consistent pattern of maturity-related differences.

Wirth et al. reported blood insulin activity during 15 min of steady-load cycle exercise at 70% $\dot{V}O_2$max in pre-, circum-, and postpubertal boys and girls (52). Insulin levels rose during exercise in the prepubertal subjects, was stable in the circumpubertal group, and declined in the postpubertal subjects. Meanwhile, blood glucose concentrations remained essentially unchanged in all groups. The authors suggested that "if the alterations in insulin concentration during exercise are due to changes in insulin secretion influenced by catecholamines, higher catecholamine concentrations or a higher sensitivity to catecholamines could be assumed" (p. 238).

Eriksson et al. examined plasma insulin levels in two groups of four boys and men, 12-13 and 23-24 years old, during 60 min of cycling at 63% $\dot{V}O_2$max (18). Values remained at low levels in both groups and showed no consistent changes.

Oseid and Hermansen described plasma insulin levels in 23 prepubertal boys who ran on a treadmill at approximately 70% $\dot{V}O_2$max for 1 hr (38). While mean plasma glucose slowly rose, insulin levels declined, with the greatest fall occurring during the first 20 min of exercise. The authors considered the magnitude of this decrease in insulin levels comparable to that previously reported in other studies using adult subjects.

Growth Hormone and Endorphins

Growth hormone levels rise during acute exercise, and this response has been utilized in the clinical setting as a provocative test for patients with suspected abnormalities of growth hormone production. Type and duration of exercise affect this response of growth hormone secretion, as does level of physical fitness. In adults the increase in growth hormone level is greater in unfit individuals compared to athletes, and the fall is more precipitous during recovery. The physiological implications of the rise of growth hormone during exercise are not clear, but this hormone appears to play a role in mobilizing fats from body deposits.

Seip et al. examined the clinical usefulness of cycle exercise as a stimulus for growth hormone release in 10 healthy children ages 9 to 15 years (47). Growth hormone levels were determined immediately before, and twice at 5 min intervals after, 15 min of high-intensity cycling on two occasions. After exercise, growth hormone concentrations exceeded the suggested diagnostic threshold levels (7 µg/L) on both tests in 9 of the 10 children.

However, Marin et al. found that growth hormone responses to exercise were strongly related to pubertal status, and normal prepubertal subjects did not often satisfy the 7 µg/L criterion (32). Subjects ran on a treadmill at an intensity producing a heart rate of 170-190 bpm for 15 min. The mean peak growth hormone level for prepubertal children was 5.7 µg/L; for subjects with Tanner stages 2, 3, 4, and 5 the average values were 7.6, 15.9, 11.3, and 17.2 µg/L.

Amirav et al. reported changes in growth hormone concentration in eight healthy adolescents (mean age 15 years) during 6 min of cycling at 60 rpm (intensity approximately two-thirds of predicted maximal O_2 uptake) (1). Values rose with a mean peak of approximately 7-8 ng/ml. That greater levels can be expected with more intense, sustained exercise is suggested by the findings in prepubertal boys studied by Oseid and Hermansen (38). These subjects increased average growth hormone levels to 20.6 ng/ml (eight times resting values) after 1 hr of treadmill running at 70% $\dot{V}O_2$max.

As indicated in the study by Marin et al. (32), resting (mean 24 hr concentrations) and exercise growth hormone concentrations are lower in prepubertal compared to postpubertal subjects (33, 52). In the study of Wirth et al. just described, growth hormone levels were almost three times higher in postpubertal (mean age 16 years) compared to prepubertal swimmers after 15 min of cycle exercise (52). This impaired capacity of exercise to stimulate growth hormone production in children is similar to age differences seen with other provocative tests of growth hormone production (arginine infusion, hypoglycemia) (see fig. 14.4). It is interesting to note, however, that the ratio of exercise to resting growth hormone levels in the study by Wirth et al. was greater in the younger subjects. That is, exercise stimulated a more pronounced change in growth hormone level in the prepubertal children. The authors suggested that the maturity-related differences in growth hormone secretion could be explained by differences in sex hormone concentrations.

Plasma levels of the opiate beta-endorphin are considered to reflect concentrations in the central nervous system that may affect mood states during and after exercise. Adult athletes who have been given naloxone, an opiate antagonist, show an inhibition of growth hormone release during exercise. It has been suggested, then, that plasma beta-endorphin might play a key role in the response of growth hormone to physical activity.

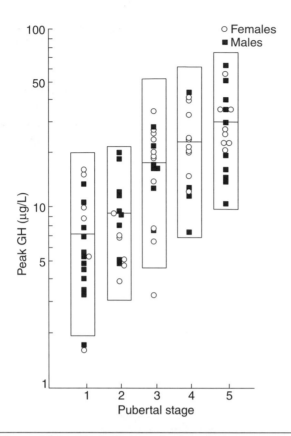

Figure 14.4 The influence of pubertal stage on responses of growth hormone to exercise, arginine, or insulin stimulation. The boxes extend to the lower and upper 95% confidence limits. Reprinted from Marin 1994.

To test this hypothesis and also to examine maturity-related differences in endorphin response, Bouix et al. studied the changes in both growth hormone and beta-endorphin after cycle exercise in 30 prepubertal and 30 circumpubertal children (7). A standardized progressive exercise protocol was used to bring the subjects to 90% of maximal heart rate after 15 min of cycling. As expected, growth hormone responses were significantly greater in the older children. Exercise caused a rise in beta-endorphin (mean 4.26 to 5.74 fmol/ml), but there was no significant difference in the magnitude of the rise in the two groups. In addition, a relationship was observed between increases in growth hormone and beta-endorphin. These findings fail to support the hypothesis that beta-endorphin is important in triggering growth hormone release during exercise in children. Moreover, the results suggest that the beta-endorphin response to exercise, in contradistinction to that of growth hormone, is independent of subject maturity.

Epinephrine

Epinephrine is secreted from the adrenal medulla during exercise and plays a key role in sustaining blood glu-

cose levels and mobilizing fatty acids from peripheral lipid stores. In addition, it acts as both an inotropic and chronotropic cardiac stimulant, a function shared with norepinephrine released from sympathetic nerve endings. The cardiovascular effects of these catecholamines have been reviewed in chapter 8; this section will be devoted only to the metabolic aspects of epinephrine activity during exercise in children.

Much research has focused on epinephrine as a glycogenolytic agent. Since this hormone acts to initiate glycogenolysis, data indicating that children have a lower capacity for anaerobic metabolism than adults have been explained as possibly attributable to age-related differences in epinephrine release. Indeed, a close relationship between plasma catecholamines and blood lactate during progressive exercise has been demonstrated for both children and adults (6) (see fig. 12.7, page 197).

However, in the only study that has directly compared child and adult epinephrine responses to exercise, no significant differences were observed. Lehmann et al. compared epinephrine responses in eight boys (mean age 12.8 years) with those of seven adult males (mean age 27.8 years) during progressive treadmill exercise (28). Mean epinephrine level in the boys increased from a pre-exercise value of .115 ng/ml to .970 ng/ml at exhaustion. Respective concentrations for the men were .092 and 1.028 (p > .05).

Delamarche et al. measured epinephrine, glucose, and FFA levels in 10 boys ages 8.5 to 11 years during 60 min of constant-load cycling at about 60% $\dot{V}O_2$max (15). Epinephrine rose progressively and linearly during the exercise, with a maximal concentration at the 60th min of exercise that was 1.6 times the resting pre-exercise sitting value. As expected, there was a close correlation between epinephrine level and both blood glycerol and FFA concentrations.

Adult subjects were not included in this study, but the findings can be compared to those of Hoelzer et al., who investigated epinephrine responses in eight untrained young adult men and women using the identical experimental design (26). In that study, mean epinephrine values rose from 59 pg/ml pre-exercise to 165 pg/ml at the end of 60 min (2.8-fold rise). Blood glucose levels remained essentially stable in both of these studies. The significance of the child-adult differences in magnitude of epinephrine response during sustained exercise in the two investigations is difficult to interpret.

Renin, Angiotensin, and Aldosterone

As noted previously, contraction of plasma volume occurs early in exercise from increased vascular pressure, a rise in extravascular osmotic pressure, and the effects of dehydration. Since maintenance of adequate blood volume is critical for exercise performance, the endocrine system provides for adaptations that counter this shrinkage of intravascular volume. The kidneys respond to such changes by secreting renin, a substance that converts angiotensinogen in the blood to angiotensin. Angiotensin acts as a peripheral arteriolar vasoconstrictor to maintain blood pressure and triggers the release of aldosterone from the adrenal cortex. Aldosterone increases sodium reabsorption in the kidneys and expands body fluid volume. The end result of this cascade of events is support of blood pressure and intravascular volume.

Basal recumbent levels of plasma renin activity (PRA) and plasma aldosterone concentration (PAC) normally decrease throughout childhood (9, 25). Fukushige et al., for instance, reported that basal PRA values in 13-15-year-old subjects were 60% of those for 4-6-year-olds (24). Little is known about changes of these factors in children during exercise. When the 4- to 15-year-old subjects studied by Fukushige et al. assumed the standing position for 60 min, PRA and PAC increased in all age groups (24). The increment of PRA (two to four times basal) was greater in the older than in the younger children, but the rise in PAC was age-independent.

Falk et al. measured PAC in 30 children while they cycled at 50% $\dot{V}O_2$max (19); 11 of the subjects were prepubertal, 12 midpubertal, and 7 late pubertal by Tanner staging. Subjects cycled for three 20 min bouts with a 10 min rest between bouts. Exercise was performed in a warm environment (42° C with 20% relative humidity), as the study was designed to determine whether maturity-related differences in temperature control during exercise might influence hormonal responses. Percentage plasma volume decrease was not significantly different in the three groups (about 5%). No changes were observed in serum osmolality in any of the groups. Before exercise there were no significant differences in mean PAC between the three groups, and the exercise provoked similar rises in levels (7-8-fold rise). A direct relationship was seen between the increase in aldosterone and the fall in plasma volume (r = 0.46, p < .05). This limited information suggests that responses of the renin-angiotensin system to exercise are independent of subject maturation.

Reproductive Hormones

The "awakening" of the reproductive organs at puberty is a reflection of increased production of male and female sex hormones. In the male, luteinizing hormone (LH) and follicle-stimulating hormone (FSH) are secreted by the pituitary gland, triggering testosterone release by the testes, sperm production, and secondary sexual characteristics (voice change, anabolic effects on bone and muscle, facial and axillary hair). Follicle-stimulating hormone, luteinizing hormone, and prolactin from the pituitary gland are necessary for development of the ovarian follicles and ovulation in the female. These hormones also trigger the production of estrogen and progesterone by the ovary, the former being responsible for secondary sexual characteristics of the female (breast development, increased body fat) and the latter for preparing the uterus for implantation of a fertilized ovum.

Two observations have prompted an interest in the effect of exercise and sport training on these sex hormones and reproductive function, particularly in females. First, menarche (the initiation of menses) occurs at a later age in young athletes, a phenomenon observed in a wide variety of sports (8). The average age of menarche in the United States is approximately 12.3 to 12.8 years, while that for trained athletes is typically 13 to 14 years. There is some evidence that the age of menarche is related to the number of years of training before initiation of menses. Frisch et al. reported that on average, a 0.4-year delay in menarche can be expected for each year of training prior to puberty (22).

This phenomenon has been explained by at least two theories: (a) intense exercise in the prepubertal years delays reproductive function by creating energy loss or preventing the attainment of a critical body weight or fat content (23), or (b) the physical characteristics associated with later pubertal onset (slender body habitus, less body fat, long legs) are those more likely to be related to athletic success (31). Whether later onset of menarche in athletes can be adequately explained by the "energy drain" or the "preselection" hypothesis remains unclear.

The second observation drawing attention to hormonal status in athletes is disruption or elimination of normal menstrual cycles in intensely training females, particularly those involved in endurance sports (42). Irregular menstrual periods or amenorrhea generally occur only with highly intense training; in one study of adult distance runners, this effect was not observed in women who were training less than 15-20 miles/week (20). Cessation of training causes normal menstrual periods to resume, and ultimate fertility does not appear to be affected (48). As with delayed menarche, it has been proposed that leanness, low body weight, energy drain, or emotional stress are contributing factors to menstrual changes with training, but the precise mechanisms remain uncertain (5).

Females. A number of investigators have examined hormonal characteristics of adult female athletes, but no clear-cut picture of the profile related to the cause or effect of menstrual changes with exercise training has emerged (5). The same can be said for studies of young adolescents. As noted by Plowman (40), experimental evidence on this question is scant, and the studies that have been performed usually involved resting values and were limited to information from single blood specimens.

Warren studied pubertal progression and reproductive function in 15 ballet dancers (initially 13-15 years old) over a period of 4 years (48). Menarche occurred at an average age of 15.4 years compared to 12.6 years in nonathletic control girls. Of the 12 subjects who experienced menarche during the study, 11 later developed secondary amenorrhea for at least a 6-month period. While they were premenarcheal, sex hormone levels were low, and those who subsequently developed amenorrhea showed the same pattern.

Creatsas et al. assessed the endocrinologic status of 20 oligomenorrheic 17-year-old ballet dancers (14). Among these subjects, 10 had started training at age 10 years, before menarche (group A), while the other 10 began training 1 year following menarche (group B). Hormonal values were compared to those of a group undergoing short-term low-intensity training and having normal menstrual cycles (group C). No significant differences in FSH levels were observed between the groups; LH was lower in group A than in group C, but no significant difference was seen between groups A and B. Prolactin and estradiol levels were similar in groups A and B, but both were lower than in group C. The authors concluded that no appreciable endocrinological differences exist in oligomenorrheic athletes relative to menarche.

Baer and Taper compared estrogen levels in six amenorrheic and six eumenorrheic distance runners (mean ages 16.1 and 15.5 years, respectively) (4). The amenorrheic girls trained for more miles a week than those who were eumenorrheic (average 40.7 vs. 20.1, respectively), but caloric intake was not significantly differ-

ent. Mean plasma estradiol concentration (mmol/L) was 113 in the amenorrheic runners and 243 in the eumenorrheic girls. In a similar study of 10 amenorrheic and eumenorrheic runners (16.0 and 16.5 years old, respectively), Baer described not only depressed estradiol levels but also low concentrations of FSH and LH in the amenorrheic subjects (3).

Peltenburg et al. compared hormonal status in prepubertal and early pubertal (based on breast development) gymnasts and swimmers (39). Levels of FSH, LH, and estradiol were not significantly different between subjects in the two sports but were, as expected, greater in the early pubertal girls. There was no relationship between any hormonal value and body composition. Carli et al. found that 6 months of swim training produced similar increases in prolactin and decreases in testosterone in premenarcheal and eumenorrheic girls (10).

Plowman concluded that "no obvious pattern emerges from these collective sketchy data" (40, p. 308). These studies appear to indicate, as observed in adult athletic women, that oligomenorrhea in teenage athletes is associated with depression of hypothalamic-pituitary-ovarian function. It remains to be clarified just how vigorous repetitive physical activity is linked to these endocrine changes.

Males. Little information is available on the influence of athletic training on sex hormones in boys. Rowland et al. reported serum levels of total and free testosterone in 15 adolescent postpubertal male cross-country runners during the course of a competitive season (see fig. 14.5) (45). Mean age was 16.1 years. Training mileage was approximately 200 km/month. No significant changes in testosterone concentrations were observed over the 8-week period, suggesting that distance

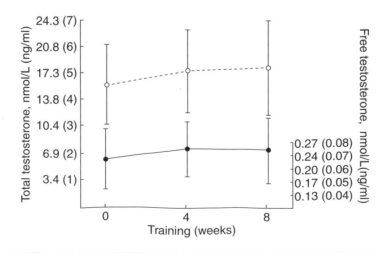

Figure 14.5 Serum testosterone changes during 8 weeks of cross-country training in postpubertal adolescents. Reprinted from Rowland et al. 1987.

running training of this intensity does not influence the hypothalamic-pituitary-gonadal axis at this age. However, Wheeler et al. have reported that middle-aged men who run at least 64 km/week can show depressed levels of serum testosterone and prolactin (50).

Mero et al. examined serum testosterone levels at the beginning, middle, and end of 1 year of running (n = 4), sprint running (n = 4), weight-lifting (n = 4), and tennis (n = 7) training in male athletes 10-12 years old (36). The initial testosterone levels were approximately three times greater than those of a control group of nontraining boys. Mean testosterone almost doubled during the training year (2.92 to 5.81 nmol/L), exceeding the rise in the control group.

CHANGES IN SERUM ELECTROLYTES AND MINERALS

During intense bouts of physical activity, alterations in serum electrolyte concentrations can reflect spillage of intracellular cations from exercising muscle into the extracellular fluids, hemoconcentration from decrease in plasma volume, or both. Some evidence suggests that these responses may be different in children and adults.

Potassium

Berg and Keul found that serum potassium levels in children and adolescents were almost twice those of adults after equal periods of participation in endurance sports (see fig. 14.6) (6). Since such electrolyte shifts from intra- to extracellular fluid spaces increase potassium excretion, the authors suggested that "an investigation of serum electrolyte concentrations in the days after intensive excretion and a substitution of these electrolytes as in adults [is warranted in children]" (p. 72).

Mácek et al. reported increases in serum potassium concentration from 0.2 to 0.5 mEq/L in 10 prepubertal boys performing 60 min of both cycling and treadmill exercise at two levels of work (approximately 40% and 60% $\dot{V}O_2$max) (30). Such changes were interpreted as reflecting increased membrane permeability of muscle cells with contraction. However, no statistically significant differences could be ascertained in serum potassium changes between the high- and low-intensity workloads.

Magnesium

In adults, serum magnesium levels during acute exercise have been reported to follow the same pattern of increase as potassium. However, Berg and Keul reported lower magnesium levels after cross-country skiing in children and adolescents 8 to 17 years of age (6). For example, values in the 10-11-year-old group declined from a pre-exercise mean of 2.10 mg/dl to 1.90 mg/dl after 60 min of skiing. There were no apparent age trends in either pre-exercise serum magnesium concentration or amount of decline with exercise.

Conn et al. compared findings in 22 competitive prepubertal swimmers with those in nonathletic children to determine whether or not serum magnesium levels were related to level of aerobic fitness (12). Subjects were 9.5 to 12.9 years old. Both male and female swimmers had greater $\dot{V}O_2$max than their respective controls. No significant differences were observed in any of the magnesium concentrations between swimmers and controls. $\dot{V}O_2$max and plasma magnesium concentrations were positively correlated in the male controls but not the male swimmers. On the other hand, plasma magnesium

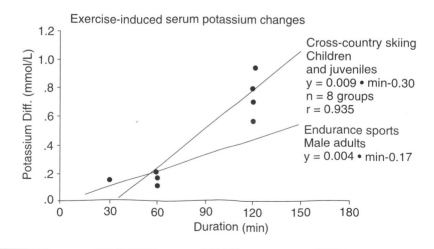

Figure 14.6 Differences in serum potassium concentrations in men and boys after intensive endurance exercise. Reprinted from Berg and Keul 1988.

levels and $\dot{V}O_2$max were inversely related in the female swimmers but not in the controls. The authors concluded that the relationship between plasma magnesium concentrations and maximal aerobic power in children remains uncertain.

Iron

Iron plays a critical role in optimizing exercise performance. This mineral is important in the synthesis of hemoglobin, and iron deficiency anemia reduces O_2-carrying capacity and diminishes exercise tolerance. Iron is also important in the intracellular utilization of energy, serving as a cofactor for enzymatic reactions within the Krebs cycle as well as a component of myoglobin (necessary for cellular O_2 storage) and the cytochromes (in phosphorylative oxidation pathways).

Studies in animals suggest that the state of nonanemic iron deficiency (low iron stores with adequate hemoglobin levels) can seriously compromise endurance exercise performance (21). It has been postulated that this effect reflects depletion of intracellular iron. Unfortunately, while iron deficiency anemia is easy to detect by blood analysis, the role of iron in aerobic metabolism within the cell is difficult to assess by any method short of muscle biopsies. Iron stores, however, are accurately estimated by determination of serum ferritin levels.

These data bear potential importance for adolescent athletes, particularly females, who have a high frequency of nonanemic iron deficiency (ferritin < 12 ng/ml, hemoglobin > 12 g percent). In any group of high school female athletes, approximately one-third can be expected to show low ferritin levels, considered secondary to a combination of low dietary iron and menses at a time of accelerated iron need due to growth (43). The frequency of nonanemic iron deficiency in males is much less.

Studies in adolescent distance runners demonstrate that training accelerates iron losses. The cause of declining ferritin levels in training athletes is not certain but may reflect a combination of gastrointestinal and sweat losses coupled with hemolysis from repetitive foot strikes (43).

Studies evaluating the impact of nonanemic iron deficiency in adolescents and adults on athletic performance and $\dot{V}O_2$max have generally shown, in contrast to investigations in animals, no effect (11, 27, 37). However, Yoshida et al. demonstrated a significant improvement in 300 m run performance in female college-aged runners with nonanemic iron deficiency who were treated with iron (53). And Rowland et al. reported an improvement in treadmill endurance time to exhaustion when a group of high school female cross-country runners with low ferritin levels were provided iron treatment (44).

SERUM ENZYMES

High-intensity exercise has been observed to elicit a rise in the serum levels of certain muscle cell enzymes, particularly creatinine phosphokinase (CK) and lactic dehydrogenase. This response is presumed to reflect skeletal muscle cell damage or increased membrane permeability during exercise. The degree of enzyme rise is greater in untrained individuals and is more pronounced in adult men than women. Limited experimental data suggest that the increase observed in children is less than that in adult subjects.

Webber et al. measured serum CK levels in 16 children (mean age 10.4 years) and 15 adults (mean age 27.1 years) immediately before and 24 hr after a single 30 min bout of downhill treadmill running (–10% grade) (49). Mean pre-exercise CK activities were not significantly different between the children and adults (91.7 vs. 77.1 μmol $\cdot$ L^{-1} $\cdot$ min^{-1}, respectively). However, CK activities 24 hr postexercise were lower in the children (160.3 vs. 265.8 μmol $\cdot$ L^{-1} $\cdot$ min^{-1}, respectively) (see fig. 14.7). Mean enzyme activity was significantly higher for males regardless of age category. The authors suggested several possible mechanisms for child-adult differences in CK response to downhill running in this study: (a) because of their greater body weight, adults generate more force per unit muscle fiber area, resulting in greater muscle cell damage and consequently more enzyme release; (b) the muscle cells of adults may contain more CK than those of children; (c) the time course of CK release after exercise may be different in children and adults; and (d) mechanisms of CK clearance from the blood may be age-related.

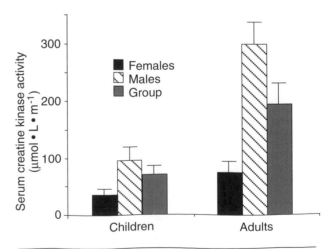

Figure 14.7 Amount of increase in serum creatine kinase activity (SCKA) from pre-exercise to 24 hr postexercise in children and adults. Reprinted from Webber et al. 1989.

Berg and Keul also noted that serum CK responses to exercise were depressed in children compared to adults (6). Serum CK activity after sustained cross-country skiing in child and adolescent subjects was significantly lower than in adult athletes performing the same exercise. The authors felt that "this observation may reflect lower mechanical stress of the foot muscles according to the weight and height of the children" and cautioned that "the reduced CK activity changes should not be interpreted as an indication of a reduced peripheral stress and lower efflux of muscle enzymes" as has been described in highly trained adult athletes (p. 71).

SUMMARY

The available research information offers only limited insights into the influence of biological maturity on metabolic and endocrine responses to exercise. There are theoretical reasons to expect that children should rely more than adults on fatty acids for energy substrate during sustained exercise. However, the research data supporting this concept are not strong and in many cases are conflicting.

Children may demonstrate a smaller decline in plasma volume during acute exercise compared to adults. This question deserves further research attention, since such differences might significantly influence studies comparing concentrations of blood-borne substances during exercise in children and adults.

There is some evidence that electrolyte leakage from muscle cells during exercise is greater in children than in adults, but the mechanism for this observation and its implications are obscure. Blood levels of creatine phosphokinase, a marker of skeletal muscle cell damage, show a greater rise after exercise in adults than in children. This may result from a greater force per muscle fiber area or a greater muscle CK content in mature individuals.

What We Know

1. Responses of blood glucose to exercise are not different in children and adults.
2. Growth hormone response to exercise is directly related to pubertal status.
3. Function of the renin-angiotensin system appears to be independent of level of biological maturation.
4. The onset of menarche is later in trained athletes than in nonathletes.
5. Nonanemic iron deficiency is common in both female high school athletes and nonathletes.

What We Would Like to Know

1. Do children rely more on fatty acids for energy substrate during exercise than adults? If so, does this mean that they have an enhanced capacity to do so or that they are "forced" to rely more on fats for energy because of relatively impaired glycolytic capacity?
2. Is rate of glycogen depletion during endurance exercise different in children than in adults?
3. Are there maturity differences in RER during exercise?
4. How are changes in plasma volume during exercise influenced by growth and biological maturation?
5. Is the later onset of menses in athletes a result of self-selection or exercise training?
6. What is the effect of nonanemic iron deficiency on athletic performance?

References

1. Amirav, I.; Dowdeswell, R.J.; Plit, M.; Panz, V.R.; Joffe, B.I.; Seftel, H.C. Growth hormone response to exercise in asthmatic and normal children. Eur. J. Pediatr. 149:443-446; 1990.
2. Asano, K.; Hirakoba, K. Respiratory and circulatory adaptation during prolonged exercise in 10-12 year-old children and adults. In: Ilmarinen, J.; Valimaki, I., eds. Children and sport. Berlin: Springer-Verlag; 1984:p. 119-128.
3. Baer, J.T. Endocrine parameters in amenorrheic and eumenorrheic adolescent female runners. Int. J. Sports Med. 14:191-195; 1993.

4. Baer, J.T.; Taper, J. Amenorrheic and eumenorrheic adolescent runners: dietary intake and exercise training status. J. Am. Diet. Ass. 92:89-91; 1992.

5. Baker, E.R. Menstrual dysfunction and hormonal status in athletic women: a review. Fert. Steril. 36:691-696; 1981.

6. Berg, A.; Keul, J. Biochemical changes during exercise in children. In: Malina, R.M., ed. Young athletes. Biological, psychological, and educational perspectives. Champaign, IL: Human Kinetics; 1988:p. 61-77.

7. Bouix, O.; Brun, J.F.; Fedou, C.; Raynaud, E.; Kerdelhue, B.; Lenoir, V.; Orsetti, A. Plasma beta-endorphin, corticotrophin and growth hormone responses to exercise in pubertal and prepubertal children. Horm. Metab. Res. 26:195-199; 1994.

8. Brisson, G.R.; Dulac, S.; Peronnet, F.; Ledoux, M. The onset of menarche: a late event in pubertal progression to be affected by physical training. Can. J. Appl. Sports Science 7:61-67; 1982.

9. Brons, M.; Thayssen, P. Plasma renin concentration, activity and substrate in normal children. Int. J. Pediatr. Nephrol. 4:43-46; 1983.

10. Carli, G.; Martinelli, G.; Viti, A.; Baldi, L.; Bonafazi, M.; Lupo di Prisco, C. The effect of swimming training on hormonal levels in girls. J. Sports Med. Phys. Fit. 23:45-51; 1983.

11. Celsing, F.; Blomstrand, E.; Werner, B.; Pihlstedt, P.; Ekblom, B. Effects of iron deficiency on endurance and muscle enzyme activity in man. Med. Sci. Sports Exerc. 18:156-161; 1986.

12. Conn, C.A.; Schemmel, R.A.; Smith, B.W.; Ryder, E.; Heusner, W.W.; Ku, P. K. Plasma and erythrocyte magnesium concentrations and correlations with maximum oxygen consumption in nine-to-twelve year old competitive swimmers. Magnesium 7:27-36; 1988.

13. Costill, D.L.; Fink, W.J.; Getchell, L.H.; Ivy, J.L.; Witzman, A. Lipid metabolism in skeletal muscle of endurance-trained males and females. J. Appl. Physiol. 61:1796-1801; 1979.

14. Creatsas, G.; Salakos, N.; Averkiou, M.; Miras, K.; Aravantinos, D. Endocrinological profile of oligomenorrheic strenuously exercising adolescents. Int. J. Gynecol. Obstet. 38:215-221; 1992.

15. Delamarche, P.; Monnier, M.; Gratas-Delamarche, A.; Koubi, H.E.; Mayet, M.H.; Favier, R. Glucose and free fatty acid utilization during prolonged exercise in prepubertal boys in relation to catecholamine responses. Eur. J. Appl. Physiol. 65:66-72; 1992.

16. Eriksson, B.O. Muscle metabolism in children—a review. Acta Paediatr. Scand. Suppl. 283:20-27; 1980.

17. Eriksson, B.O.; Gollnick, P.D.; Saltin, B. Muscle metabolism and enzyme activities after training in boys 11-13 years old. Acta Physiol. Scand. 87:485-497; 1973.

18. Eriksson, B.O.; Persson, B.; Thorell, J.I. The effects of repeated prolonged exercise on plasma growth hormone, insulin, glucose, free fatty acids, glycerol, lactate, and beta-hydroxybutyric acid in 13 year old boys and in adults. Acta Paediat. Scand. Suppl. 217:142-146; 1971.

19. Falk, B.; Bar-Or, O.; MacDougall, J.D. Aldosterone and prolactin response to exercise in the heat in circumpubertal boys. J. Appl. Physiol. 71:1741-1745; 1991.

20. Feicht, C.B.; Johnson, T.S.; Martin, B.J.; Sparkes, K.E.; Wagner, W.W. Secondary amenorrhea in athletes. Lancet 2:1145-1146; 1978.

21. Finch, C.A.; Miller, L.R.; Inamidar, A.R.; Person, R.; Seiler, K.; Mackler, B. Iron deficiency in the rat. Physiological and biochemical studies of muscle dysfunction. J. Clin. Invest. 58:447-453; 1976.

22. Frisch, R.E.; Gotz-Welbergen, A.V.; McArthur, J.W.; Albright, T.; Witschi, J.; Bullen, B.; Birnholz, J.; Reed, R.B.; Hermann, H. Delayed menarche and amenorrhea of college athletes in relation to age of onset of training. JAMA 246:1559-1563; 1981.

23. Frisch, R.E.; Revelle, R. Height and weight at menarche and a hypothesis of menarche. Arch. Dis. Child. 46:695-701; 1971.

24. Fukushige, J.; Shimomura, K.; Uda, K. Influence of upright activity on plasma renin activity and aldosterone concentration in children. Eur. J. Pediatr. 153:284-286; 1994.

25. Harshfield, G.A.; Alpert, B.A.; Pulliam, D.A. Renin-angiotensin-aldosterone system in healthy subjects aged ten to eighteen years. J. Pediatr. 122:563-567; 1993.

26. Hoelzer, D.R.; Dalsky, G.P.; Clutter, W.E.; Shah, S.D.; Holloszy, J.H.; Cryer, P.E. Glucoregulation during exercise: hypoglycemia is prevented by redundant glucoregulatory systems, sympathochromaffin activation, and changes in islet hormone secretion. J. Clin. Invest. 77:212-221; 1986.

27. Klingshirn, L.A.; Pate, R.R.; Bourque, S.P.; Davis, J.M.; Sargent, R.G. Effect of iron supplementation on endurance capacity in iron-depleted female runners. Med. Sci. Sports Exerc. 24:819-824; 1992.

28. Lehmann, M.; Keul, J.; Korsten-Reck, U. The influence of graduated treadmill exercise on plasma catecholamines, aerobic and anaerobic capacity in boys and adults. Eur. J. Appl. Physiol. 47:301-311; 1981.

29. Mácek, M.; Vavra, J.; Novosadova, J. Prolonged exercise in prepubertal boys. I. Cardiovascular and metabolic adjustment. Europ. J. Appl. Physiol. 35:291-298; 1976.

30. Mácek, M.; Vavra, J.; Novosadova, J. Prolonged exercise in prepubertal boys. II. Changes in plasma volume and in some blood constituents. Europ. J. Appl. Physiol. 35:299-303; 1976.

31. Malina, R.M. Menarche in athletes: a synthesis and hypothesis. Ann. Human Biol. 10:1-24; 1983.

32. Marin, G.; Domene, H.M.; Barnes, K.M.; Blackwell, B.J.; Cassorla, F.G.; Cutler, G.B. The effects of estrogen priming and puberty on the growth hormone response to standardized treadmill exercise and arginine-insulin in normal girls and boys. J. Clin. Endocrinol. Metab. 79:537-541; 1994.

33. Martha, P.M.; Rogol, A.D.; Veldius, J.D.; Kerrigan, J.R.; Goodman, D.W.; Blizzard, R.M. Alterations in the pulsatile properties of circulating growth hormone concentrations during puberty in boys. J. Clin. Endocrin. Metab. 69:563-570; 1989.

34. Martinez, L.R.; Haymes, E.M. Substrate utilization during treadmill running in prepubertal girls and women. Med. Sci. Sports Exerc. 24:975-983; 1992.
35. McArdle, W.D.; Katch, F.I.; Katch, V.L. Exercise Physiology. Energy, nutrition, and human performance. Philadelphia: Lea & Febiger; 1981:p. 98-102.
36. Mero, A.; Jaakkola, L.; Komi, P.V. Serum hormones and physical performance capacity in young boy athletes during a 1-year training period. Eur. J. Appl. Physiol. 60:32-37; 1990.
37. Newhouse, I.J.; Clement, D.B.; Taunton, J.E.; McKenzie, D.C. The effects of prelatent/latent iron deficiency on physical work capacity. Med. Sci. Sports Exerc. 21:263-268; 1989.
38. Oseid, S.; Hermansen, L. Hormonal and metabolic changes during and after prolonged muscular work in pre-pubertal boys. Acta Pediatr. Scand. Suppl. 217:147-153; 1971.
39. Peltenburg, A.L.; Erich, W.B.M.; Thijssen, J.J.H.; Veeman, W.; Jansen, M.; Bernink, M.J.E.; Zonderland, M.L.; VanderBrande, J.L.; Huisveld, I.A. Sex hormone profiles of premenarcheal athletes. Eur. J. Appl. Physiol. 52:385-392; 1984.
40. Plowman, S. Maturation and exercise training in children. Pediatr. Exerc. Science 1:303-312; 1989.
41. Robinson, S. Experimental studies of physical fitness in relation to age. Arbeitsphysiologie 10:250-321; 1938.
42. Rogol, A. Pubertal development in endurance-trained female athletes. In: Brown, E.W.; Branta, C.F., eds. Competitive sports for children and youth. Champaign, IL: Human Kinetics; 1988:p. 173-193.
43. Rowland, T.W. Iron deficiency and supplementation in the young endurance athlete. In: Advances in pediatric sport sciences. Vol. 2, Bar-Or, O., ed. Biological issues. Champaign, IL: Human Kinetics; 1989:p. 169-190.
44. Rowland, T.W.; Deisroth, M.B.; Green, G.M.; Kelleher, J.F. The effect of iron therapy on the exercise capacity of non-anemic iron-deficient adolescent runners. Am. J. Dis. Child. 142:165-169; 1988.
45. Rowland, T.W.; Morris, A.H.; Kelleher, J.F.; Haag, B.L.; Reiter, E.O. Serum testosterone response to training in adolescent runners. Am. J. Dis. Child. 141:881-883; 1987.
46. Rowland, T.W.; Rimany, T.A. Physiological responses to prolonged exercise in premenarcheal and adult females. Pediatr. Exerc. Science 7:183-191; 1995.
47. Seip, R.L.; Weltman, A.; Goodman, D.; Rogol, A. Clinical utility of cycle exercise for the physiological assessment of growth hormone release in children. AJDC 144:998-1000; 1990.
48. Warren, M.P. The effects of exercise on pubertal progression and reproductive function in girls. J. Clin. Endocrinol. Metab. 51:1150-1157; 1980.
49. Webber, L.; Byrnes, W.; Rowland, T.; Foster, V. Serum CK activity and delayed onset of muscle soreness in prepubescent children. Pediatr. Exerc. Science 1:351-359; 1989.
50. Wheeler, G.D.; Wall, S.R.; Belcastro, A.N.; Cumming, D.C. Reduced serum testosterone and prolactin levels in male distance runners. JAMA 252:514-516; 1984.
51. Wilmore, J.H.; Costill, D.L. Physiology of sport and exercise. Champaign, IL: Human Kinetics; 1994:p. 184-185.
52. Wirth, A.; Trager, E.; Scheele, K.; Mayer, D.; Diehm, K.; Reischle, K.; Weicker, H. Cardiopulmonary adjustment and metabolic response to maximal and submaximal physical exercise of boys and girls at different stages of maturity. Eur. J. Appl. Physiol. 39:229-240; 1978.
53. Yoshida, T.; Udo, M.; Chida, M.; Ichioka, M.; Makiguchi, K. Dietary iron supplement during severe physical training in competitive female distance runners. Sports Train. Med. Rehabil. 1:279-285; 1990.

CHAPTER 15

ADAPTATIONS TO THERMAL STRESS

The "fires" of cellular metabolism create heat. This warmth is critically important in maintaining a constant body temperature, but excessive rise of metabolic heat is clearly detrimental to thermal homeostasis. The human body works within a relatively narrow temperature range (about 35 to 41 °C); an excess creates signs and symptoms of heat stress—weakness, dizziness, muscle cramps, disorientation—and, in extremes, leads to cardiovascular collapse and death. To prevent this, a set of adaptations is brought into play that facilitates heat loss from the body. In humans this occurs at the body surface by evaporative cooling from sweat as well as by convective and radiation heat loss from the skin.

Exercise stokes the metabolic furnace, and the resultant increase in heat production must be counterbalanced by these mechanisms for heat loss. There is evidence to indicate that adaptations to the rise of body heat during exercise are different in children and adults. It's an issue that has drawn considerable research attention, given (1) the potential for such differences to place the child at greater risk for heat stress and (2) the possibility that deciphering maturity-related responses might help improve our basic understanding of temperature homeostasis. This chapter will review the experimental evidence indicating that differences in thermal adaptations to exercise exist between children and adults. Whether such differences might have clinical implications is not clear, since an increased incidence of heat stress injury during sport participation in children has not yet been identified. Reviews have addressed thermal stresses during exercise (3, 32, 38) as well as the unique responses in children (2, 4, 5). The reader is referred to these sources for additional information.

THE ADULT MODEL

Human skeletal muscle operates at an efficiency of about 20%. This means that a fifth of the chemical energy entering into the metabolic machinery of the muscle cell is converted into mechanical work while the rest is released as heat. The problem of dealing with this heat becomes compounded during physical activity, given the dramatic rise in the metabolic rate of muscle exercising at high intensity. It is not difficult, then, to understand the stresses that are placed on the body's cooling systems, which act to prevent the buildup of excessive body heat during exercise.

Human beings lose heat through their body surface area (BSA) by two principal mechanisms: (1) skin cooling by the evaporation of sweat and (2) increased cutaneous blood flow that carries core heat to the skin for convective heat loss to the air. Both of these responses are largely mediated through changes in the autonomic nervous system.

The amount of evaporation from the skin is dependent upon the gradient between the skin and ambient vapor pressure. That is, evaporation of sweat will serve as a less effective means of heat dispersion on highly humid days. The amount of sweat produced is dependent on both the number of sweat glands and the rate of sweat produced per gland. Glands are stimulated to create sweat principally by cholinergic postganglionic sympathetic fibers (i.e., acetylcholine rather than norepinephrine acts as the neurotransmitter), but circulating epinephrine also plays a role.

Heat is dissipated from the body's core to the periphery for convective heat loss by increasing cutaneous blood flow. This occurs through vasodilation of vessels at the skin surface, a result largely of sympathetic withdrawal. This rise in skin blood flow for thermoregulation can be substantial, causing a diminished central blood volume and reduced cardiac filling. Stroke volume may be compromised, triggering an increase in heart rate. In extreme conditions, decreased central blood volume from this "steal" to the cutaneous circulation, combined with large fluid volumes lost through brisk sweating, can lead to dehydration and compromise of cardiac output.

During an acute bout of dynamic exercise, the core temperature rises as a result of increased intensity of muscle contraction. This initial increase is independent of the environmental temperature. As the mechanisms for heat loss (evaporation, convection) come into play, the core temperature reaches a plateau. However, if these responses are unable to compensate for heat production from intense exercise because of environmental conditions of high heat or humidity, the core temperature will continue to rise and signs of heat stress will occur.

In adults, changes in core temperature are related to the relative rather than the absolute intensity of exercise. That is, the rise in core temperature in response to a given workload is associated with percentage $\dot{V}O_2$max at that level of exercise. It would seem to follow that more highly aerobically fit individuals with a greater $\dot{V}O_2$max should show a lower rise in body temperature while doing the same work as subjects with lower fitness levels. Although most studies have supported this concept, the literature has not always been consistent (3).

When an adult exercises in the heat, $\dot{V}O_2$max is reduced in comparison to that measured when the same subject is tested in a cooler environment. This probably occurs because of the diversion of blood flow to the cutaneous circulation for heat loss, reducing central blood flow and maximal stroke volume and cardiac output. During a given level of submaximal exercise, the total energy expenditure is probably increased in the heat. There is evidence, too, that in a warm environment there is a shift from aerobic to a greater reliance on anaerobic metabolic pathways.

Adults who exercise regularly in the heat become more able to tolerate physical activity without fatigue and signs of heat stress. This acclimatization is an expression of a set of adaptations that include an earlier and higher sweating rate as well as a slower rise in core temperature and diminished tachycardia at a given exercise intensity. This appears to reflect a lowering of the thermoregulatory "set point" that triggers cooling mechanisms (38). Such changes of acclimatization can be triggered by 7-10 days of daily exercise in the heat. Although all the research is not consistent, most data

support the concept that physical fitness or training improves the rate of heat acclimatization (3).

CHILDREN ARE DIFFERENT

Children are equally obliged to obey the laws of thermodynamics, and the mechanisms for maintaining thermal homeostasis during exercise are no different for children than for adults. However, there is a considerable body of experimental evidence indicating that quantitative differences in thermal responses to exercise exist between prepubertal and mature individuals (2, 5), including the following:

1. At a given level of work, children produce a greater amount of heat relative to their body mass than adults. Younger subjects are able to maintain thermal balance by heat loss from their relatively larger BSA.
2. Children do not sweat as much during exercise as adults. The sweat glands of prepubertal subjects produce less sweat and are activated at a higher exercise intensity threshold than those of adults.
3. To compensate for diminished sweating rate, children rely on a greater cutaneous blood flow for convective heat loss during exercise. It has been suggested, too, that cardiac output relative to O_2 uptake (i.e., a given metabolic rate) is lower in children.
4. The content of sweat is different in children, who have lower chloride and higher lactate concentrations.
5. Children tolerate exercise in very hot conditions more poorly than adults. This appears to be related to cardiovascular factors rather than heat stress per se.
6. While their adaptive responses to repeated exercise in warm conditions are similar to those in adults, children require a longer period of time for heat acclimatization.

These maturity-related differences suggest that children are at a disadvantage compared to adults in thermal regulation during exercise in hot environments. However, there are no epidemiological data to indicate that prepubertal competitors are, in fact, more susceptible to heat injury during sport participation. But as pointed out by Bar-Or, the thermal regulation characteristics of children may have particular relevance to pediatric patients with diseases that place them at higher risk for heat stress. These include cystic fibrosis (excessive sodium-rich sweat), obesity (higher core temperatures) (16), and anorexia nervosa (dehydration) (5). For young people with these diseases, attention to adequate hydration and avoidance of activity in hot environments are particularly important.

The discussions that follow will address the experimental evidence for each of the maturity-related differences in thermal response to exercise that have been outlined.

ANIMAL STUDIES

The dynamics of heat exchange are closely linked to differences in body size. Considering the dramatic change of body dimensions in growing children, an appreciation of this relationship is important for developmental physiologists. It is therefore useful to examine evidence in adult animals that has been accumulating for over 100 years regarding the influence of body size on heat production and loss.

The core temperature of mammals is similar, regardless of body size (33). It doesn't matter whether you are a 10 g shrew living in the Arctic tundra or an elephant in central Africa—core temperature is consistently about 36-38 °C. This observation signifies that over the enormous range of mammal size (a factor of 10^7), physiological mechanisms must be in place to create a balance between heat production and heat loss, and this balance, which must be struck at the same requisite temperature for optimal tissue function, is size-independent.

This fact becomes all the more remarkable when one considers that small animals produce significantly greater amounts of metabolic heat for their size than larger animals. This has been recognized since the late 1800s, when Rubner demonstrated that a dog weighing 3 kg has a metabolic rate per kg body mass more than twice that of a dog weighing 31 kg (33). How does the smaller animal get rid of this extra heat load? Rubner's findings seemed to provide the answer, as metabolic rate when expressed relative to BSA did not differ appreciably between dogs of different sizes. This conformed nicely to earlier ideas that the rate of cooling of animals is proportional to their surface area. Smaller animals possess a greater ratio of surface area to mass. This, the argument goes, allows them to dissipate their relatively greater amounts of metabolic heat through their relatively greater surface area.

As reviewed in chapter 6, this "surface law" has been utilized to explain this phenomenon in reverse. That is, at rest, smaller animals have a greater relative metabolic rate *because* they possess a higher surface area:mass ratio. Viewed from this perspective, the smaller mammal is required to generate more metabolic heat per kg to maintain constant core temperature since the relative greater surface area creates a more rapid heat loss to the environment. During exercise, of course, the reverse is true: a means must be established for eliminating the extra metabolic heat created by muscular contractions, and the avenue for this loss is through the body surface.

These concepts are all intuitively attractive. However, they run into a snag when we observe that across many mammalian species the rate of heat production at rest is empirically related to $mass^{.75}$, while body surface is expected to vary by $mass^{.67}$. There is, it appears, a discrepancy between heat in and heat out. Does this mean that the surface law is invalid? Or are there ways to account for this difference?

Much energy has been expended on debating this issue in the literature. Perhaps the concept of heat loss through surface area is overly simplistic, as different portions of the surface dissipate varying amounts of heat. As Schmidt-Nielsen asked, "Does the true surface of an animal include the skin area between the legs that is not exposed to the outside? Does it include the ears, and if so, both sides? . . . These questions mean an uncertainty of perhaps 20%" (33, p. 82). Others have suggested the importance of differences between large and small animals in geometric or elastic properties as well as differential effects of gravity. Schmidt-Nielsen concluded, "Most of the explanations that have been proposed [for the discrepancy between scaling factors for heat production and BSA] have been unsatisfactory and have had a somewhat metaphysical quality" (33, p. 84).

However one might explain the disparity of heat production and surface area mass exponents, both large and small animals appear capable of balancing heat production and loss and maintaining a stable core temperature. At the same time, if heat production increases with $mass^{.75}$ and "effective" surface area truly relates to $mass^{.67}$, the larger animal will have greater difficulty dispersing body heat (since heat production increases more rapidly with body size than does surface area). By this argument, the larger mammal would be at a disadvantage for maintaining heat balance during conditions, such as physical exercise, that increase heat production.

THERMAL RESPONSES IN CHILDREN

The issues of size outlined are important for an understanding of thermal responses of children to exercise. At the same time, other size-independent developmental changes are also evident that separate such responses in children from those in adults.

Heat Production

The work efficiency of skeletal muscle in children is equivalent to that in adults (31). Values during cycle exercise of 20-25% have been reported in both groups, depending on whether absolute, net, or rate of change of efficiency is being described. Therefore, the heat load relative to metabolic rate during exercise can be expected to be age-independent. From this fact one can surmise that $\dot{V}O_2$ is a valid marker for comparing heat production during exercise in children and adults. This assumption, however, neglects (a) possible maturity-related differences in substrate utilization that would alter the relationship of $\dot{V}O_2$ to caloric expenditure, and (b) the influence of variations between children and adults in anaerobically derived energy (see chapter 12).

Rest.   Metabolic heat production in the resting state decreases relative to body size during childhood, at least after the 1st year of life. For example, basal metabolic rate declines on the average from 53 to 44 calories/hour per square meter BSA in boys between ages 6 and 18 years (23). Holliday et al. demonstrated that the relationship between resting metabolic heat and size is not constant as a child grows (17). Below a mass of 10 kg, metabolic rate relates to mass by an exponent of 1.02 (i.e., the increases in heat production with growth are closely linked to body mass). But beyond this weight the slope changes to 0.58, indicating that heat production declines with age relative to either body mass or surface area. The relatively greater resting heat production at younger ages is effectively countered by enhanced heat loss, as body core temperature is essentially constant throughout the course of childhood.

Heat produced at rest reflects the metabolic activities of the large internal organs. The combined metabolic rates of brain, heart, kidney, liver, and lung account for 79% of the total body metabolic rate (17), and this percentage is constant regardless of body size. Holliday et al. argued that consequently the higher relative resting heat production at younger ages is attributable to the fact that these same organs account for a larger proportion of body mass in younger compared to older subjects (17). The authors calculated that these five organs contributed 14.6% of body weight in a 10 kg child but 6.2% in a 70 kg adult.

Exercise.   Heat production during exercise, a reflection of increased skeletal muscle metabolism, is either greater, the same, or less in children compared to adults depending on the mode of exercise, its intensity, and the means of expression relative to body size.

On a cycle ergometer, in which an external resistance creates the workload, the metabolic heat produced at a given absolute workload is similar in children and adults (31). This means that the heat burden will depend on body size: that is, relative to his body mass, a 30 kg boy will have approximately three times as much heat to disperse during a given submaximal cycle workload as

a 90 kg man. Since $\dot{V}O_2$max per kg is relatively stable throughout childhood and adolescence, heat production at exhaustion is directly associated with body mass. The relative heat burden at maximal exercise does not therefore change appreciably as a child grows. Compared to young adults (who typically have a lower $\dot{V}O_2$max per kg), however, children have greater mass-relative heat production at maximal exercise.

During submaximal weight-bearing exercise, such as horizontal treadmill running at a given speed, heat production is greater in older children because they have a greater mass to move. When expressed relative to body mass, however, heat production progressively decreases as a child ages (25). Initial allometric analyses have suggested that submaximal $\dot{V}O_2$ during weight-bearing exercise relates to mass by an exponent of approximately 0.75 (interestingly, this is the same exponent as for resting heat production in animals, but—as noted above—not in humans) (34). The possible mechanisms for this improvement in economy with growth have been reviewed in chapter 11.

The end result of this trend is an increased heat burden during submaximal exercise in smaller children. For instance, Bar-Or calculated that the relative heat production in a 6-year-old girl running at a speed of 10 km/hr is 20% greater than that of a 16-year-old (5). At maximal exercise, the same relationships of heat production to body mass and maturity should hold true for weight-bearing as for cycle exercise (outlined earlier).

In summary, the younger child produces more heat relative to body mass, and this is true at rest as well as during exercise. Mechanisms must be in place, therefore, to counterbalance this high heat burden with augmented heat loss to maintain thermal homeostasis. The next section outlines the means by which this is accomplished.

Body Surface Area

Heat loss—by radiation, convection, or evaporative cooling—is a surface phenomenon, and humans disperse heat relative to their external BSA. It is clear, then, that the major means by which small children are able to match heat loss to their greater heat burden during exercise is through a relatively greater BSA.

The laws of dimensionality dictate that as geometrically similar (i.e., proportionally identical) structures become larger, their mass or volume increases by a factor of length cubed, while surface area increases by height squared. That is, BSA relates to mass by the equation $BSA = kM^{.67}$. And so it is with growing children. As demonstrated in figure 1.6 (page 10), the ratio of BSA to mass falls dramatically during childhood. The decrease amounts to a 33% decline between the ages of 2 and 16 years.

However, as Kleiber noted, it is precarious to utilize mathematical models of surface area in quantitating heat balance, since BSA is "ill-defined" (22, p. 183). The portion of a subject's skin that is truly effective in heat transfer is unclear, and accurate measurement is problematic. The influence of insulation (body fat) and, in animals, fur and feathers, in altering heat loss by surface area must be considered. In addition, small children are not truly geometrically similar to adults (they have proportionally bigger heads and shorter legs).

The importance of the BSA:mass ratio as well as the amount of subcutaneous fat in governing heat loss in children was demonstrated by Sloan and Keatinge (35). They reported body temperature (sublingual) in 28 boys and girls before and after 33-40 min of swimming in water at a mean temperature of 20.3 °C. Average body temperature declined from 37.5 °C before the swim to 36.2 °C afterward. The rate of decline in temperature was closely associated with the reciprocal of skinfold thickness measurements (r = 0.85), and the relationship was improved when variations in BSA were considered (r = 0.91).

The relatively greater BSA of small children represents an advantage for heat loss only as long as the temperature of the skin exceeds that of the surrounding air. As Drinkwater et al. (10) summarized this principle:

Since children have a higher BSA/wt ratio than adults, they should have an advantage in heat transfer when working in an environment where mean skin temperature (T_{sk}) is higher than the ambient temperature (T_a), be at a disadvantage when T_a exceeds T_{sk}, and be on par with adults when $T_{sk} = T_a$. (p. 1064)

The findings of these authors in comparing responses of girls and women to exercise in the heat suggested that ambient temperature begins to exceed skin temperature at approximately 35 °C (95 °F). Above this threshold, heat is absorbed by the body from the surrounding air, and the relatively greater area for surface heat transfer in children becomes disadvantageous. When the air temperature is greater than that of the skin, convective heat loss becomes ineffective. In such conditions, evaporative cooling must serve as the principal means of expelling body heat load. However, as will be seen in the following sections, evidence indicates that evaporative mechanisms are inferior in children compared to adults. Moreover, evaporative loss is depressed in highly humid conditions. In short, the advantages of a greater relative BSA in small children, their major means of compensating for a greater heat burden, may be lost in extreme environmental conditions of high heat and humidity.

Evaporative Heat Loss

Investigators who exercise children have long recognized that prepubertal subjects—although flushed and breathless—sweat little during testing, even at exhaustive levels. Scientific inquiry into this observation has indicated several deficiencies of sweat production in children compared to responses in adults. While children do not have a lower number of sweat glands, they produce less sweat per gland during exercise. This results in a lower sweating rate per surface area. In addition, the exercise intensity that triggers sweating is higher in children. There are maturational differences in content of sweat as well. The sweat of children has a lower concentration of sodium chloride and greater lactate than that of adults.

Considerable research attention has focused on maturity-related differences in sweating patterns. Evaporation of sweat is an important source of heat loss and, as just noted, is particularly critical in very hot ambient conditions. Patterns of sweating during exercise in children have been reviewed comprehensively by Bar-Or (5) and will be summarized here.

Sweating Rate.
Studies comparing sweating rates between boys and men (measured as milliliters per square meter per hour) indicate that, in general, rates in male adults are approximately twice those of prepubertal boys (5). Interestingly, no obvious differences are described between girls and adult females. Data from the study of Araki et al., comparing sweating rates in boys and young adult men, are shown in figure 15.1 (1).

Falk et al. investigated the influence of biological maturation on sweating during exercise (11). Sweating

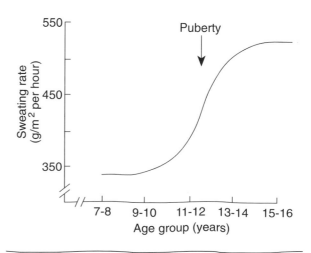

Figure 15.1 Sweating rate in boys during moderate-intensity exercise relative to age. Reprinted from Smith 1983.

response to cycle exercise in the heat was examined in 16 healthy prepubertal (Tanner stage 1), 15 midpubertal (Tanner stages 2-4), and 5 late pubertal (Tanner stage 5) boys. Mean ages for the groups were 10.8, 13.6, and 16.2 years, respectively. Subjects cycled at 50% $\dot{V}O_2$max at 42 °C ambient temperature and 20% relative humidity in a climatic chamber. There were no differences in the increases of heart rate, skin temperature, or rectal temperature during exercise between the three groups. Whole-body sweating rate was calculated from change in body mass after correction for fluid intake and change in weight of clothes as well as for urine and respiratory water loss. Sweating rate expressed relative to BSA was found to be directly related to level of biological maturity.

Sweat Gland Density and Secretion Rate. If total body sweating rate rises with maturation, either an increased number of sweat glands or an augmented secretion rate per gland (or both) must be responsible. In the study by Falk et al. cited earlier, sweat gland population density and mean area of sweat drops (a marker of gland activity) were determined by skin photographic techniques (11). Population density was greater in the prepubertal subjects than in mid- or late-pubertal boys, while the mean area of sweat drops rose with increasing maturation level. The calculated sweat rate per gland was significantly lower in the prepubertal boys than in the older groups (see fig. 15.2).

These findings support conclusions of other investigators who compared children and adults. Bar-Or et al. found that the population density of sweat glands was inversely proportional to BSA when they compared 60 children 10-12 years old with 19 adults 18-27 years old

(6). Kawahata reported the same relationship in subjects ranging from 1 month to 35 years of age (20). Children therefore have a *greater* concentration of sweat glands than adults. This makes sense, since the total number of sweat glands remains constant in humans beyond the age of 2 years and since children have a smaller BSA than adults (24).

The rate of sweat production per gland, on the other hand, is decidedly less in prepubertal subjects than in adults, at least for males. Each individual sweat gland of a typical prepubertal boy produces only about 45% of the sweating rate produced by the sweat gland of a young adult (19, 21). This is true both at rest and during exercise in warm environments, as well as when sweating is induced in a thermoneutral environment by pilocarpine iontophoresis (18).

There may be significant gender differences in maturity-related sweating responses. Kawahata investigated sweating responses in 9-year-old girls and 21–27-year-old women while they were resting in ambient conditions of 34 °C and 40% relative humidity (20). No significant differences were observed in either total body sweating rate or sweating rate per gland.

At least for males, then, children have lower body sweating rates at rest and exercise compared to adult men. This finding is a reflection of diminished rate of sweat production per gland. The explanation for augmented sweat production with advancing biological maturation is unknown. Falk et al. noted that both expansion of BSA and sweat gland size may contribute to the increased sweating rate per gland (11). In their study, sweat rate per gland was closely associated with BSA ($r = 0.76$). Regression analysis indicated that BSA accounted for 42% of the variance in sweat rate per gland.

But there is evidence that factors other than simply an increase in size are responsible for variations in sweat gland production. The data from the study of Falk et al. strongly suggest that biological maturation is linked to sweat production and hormonal influences at puberty. Indeed, their regression analysis indicated that a combination of BSA and physical maturity accounted for 66% of the variance in sweat production per gland. Falk et al. concluded, "Although it may be difficult to separate the effect of growth and maturation, the greater proportion of explained variance (66% to 42%) [when maturity is entered into the equation] supports the notion that qualitative changes, which occur during puberty and accompany physical growth, contribute to changes in sweat gland function" (11, p. 317).

The limited data suggesting that such changes occur in males but not in females imply that testosterone may be the trigger for augmented sweat gland function during puberty. However, this inference awaits experimental confirmation (5).

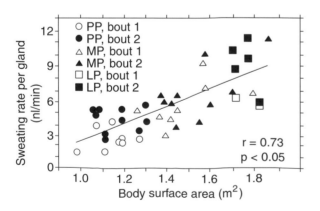

Figure 15.2 Relationship of body surface area and sweating rate (per gland) during two exercise bouts in the heat in prepubertal (PP), midpubertal (MP), and late-pubertal (LP) subjects. Reprinted from Falk et al. 1992.

Electrolyte and Lactate Concentration. Other results suggest qualitative changes in sweat gland function during maturation. Araki et al. found that chloride concentrations in prepubertal boys were about 60% those of pubertal subjects during intense physical exercise (1). This result suggests maturational differences in electrolyte reabsorption within the sweat duct. Falk et al. reported significantly greater sweat chloride concentrations during exercise in the heat in postpubertal compared to midpubertal and prepubertal boys (13). They suggested that this result might be explained by the greater sweating rate in the older boys, since sweating rate and sweat chloride concentrations are closely related. Meyer et al. confirmed this finding in their study of prepubertal, pubertal, and young adult males and females cycling at 50% $\dot{V}O_2$max in 40-42 °C temperature (27). Sweat sodium and chloride concentrations were directly related to maturational status, while sweat potassium concentrations were lower in both male and female adults than in prepubertal children.

Lactate concentration in sweat can be used as a marker of anaerobic sweat gland metabolism. Fellman et al. found similar sweat lactate concentrations in children and adults exposed to a 45 °C environment (14, 15). Falk et al. compared sweat lactate concentration and lactate excretion rate per gland in groups of pre-, mid-, and postpubertal boys cycling for three 20 min bouts at 50% $\dot{V}O_2$max (12). Sweat lactate concentration was inversely related to pubertal status, but the differences reached statistical significance only during the first exercise bout (see fig. 15.3). Lactate excretion rate per gland, considered a more appropriate index of gland anaerobic metabolism, showed a trend for increasing values with greater maturity. However, the differences were significant only between pre- and midpubertal groups during the first exercise bout. The authors concluded that increasing biological maturation is charac-terized by a lower sweat lactate concentration but a trend towards elevated lactate excretion per gland. The implications of these findings regarding sweat gland metabolism at puberty remain uncertain.

Sweating Threshold. It takes less of a rise in core temperature to trigger onset of sweating in adults than in children. Araki et al. exercised seven young men and an equal number of 9-year-old boys at 29 °C (1). A rise of 0.2 °C in rectal temperature stimulated sweating in the men, compared to a threshold rise of 0.7 °C in the boys. Similarly, Inbar demonstrated that the mean sweating rate per degree rise in rectal temperature above 37 °C in young men was more than twice that observed in 8-10-year-old boys (19).

Cutaneous Blood Flow and Convective Heat Loss

Given the dampened sweating response of children to exercise as compared to that of adults, it might be anticipated that children would rely more on convective heat loss through their relatively greater BSA. This idea is supported by the observation, noted by several authors, that children maintain a stable core temperature during exercise that is similar to that of adults despite lower evaporative heat loss (7, 8, 13). From such findings, Davies estimated that 44% of heat loss in children running for 1 hr at 68% $\dot{V}O_2$max at 21 °C was due to radiation and convection, compared to 33% in adults (7).

Greater convective losses require a larger skin blood flow. There are some experimental data to indicate that in fact cutaneous blood flow is relatively more pronounced in children than in adults during exercise. Measurement of forearm blood flow by venous plethysmography has been used as an estimate of blood flow to the skin during treadmill or cycle exercise (since muscles of

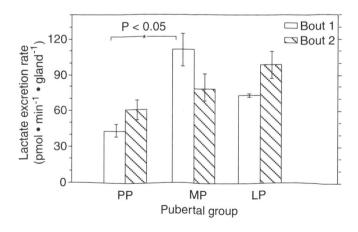

Figure 15.3 Lactate excretion rate per gland during two exercise bouts in prepubertal (PP), midpubertal (MP), and late-pubertal (LP) boys. Reprinted from Falk et al. 1991.

the upper arm will be relatively inactive). Falk et al. found that forearm flow was significantly greater in prepubertal than in postpubertal boys both at rest and during cycling at 50% $\dot{V}O_2$max in a 42 °C environment (13) (see fig. 15.4). Drinkwater et al. found greater postexercise forearm blood flow in girls compared to women (10).

Cardiovascular Responses

During exercise, the central and cutaneous circulations "compete" for blood flow to accomplish their respective tasks of muscle perfusion and thermoregulation. There is some evidence that the greater reliance on convective heat loss by augmented cutaneous flow in children might prove detrimental by diverting blood from the central circulation.

Drinkwater et al. described physiological responses of five prepubertal girls and five college women who performed treadmill walking at approximately 30% $\dot{V}O_2$max for two 50 min periods in three climatic conditions: (1) 28 °C and 45% relative humidity, (2) 35 °C and 65% humidity, and (3) 48 °C and 10% humidity (10). While exercising in each of the three environments the girls showed a higher mean heart rate and lower stroke index (measured by acetylene rebreathing). Rise in heart rate to values exceeding 90%max associated with severe fatigue, facial flushing, and dizziness caused four of the five girls to be removed from the treadmill between 12 and 46 min of exercise. Since only modest elevations in core temperatures were observed at the time, the authors considered this exercise limitation to be related to cardiovascular rather than thermal factors. Resting blood volume per kg body mass was not significantly different between the girls and the women. However, when blood volume was expressed

relative to BSA, mean values were 2.269 L/m² for the girls and 3.095 L/m² in the women. These data, plus the limited endurance capacity of the girls compared to the women, were interpreted as suggesting that the maintenance of appropriate cutaneous blood flow for thermoregulation required a greater proportion of the total blood volume in the girls to be diverted to the skin. The study indicated that this might limit exercise tolerance of children in the heat by more significantly reducing central blood volume.

This problem would be compounded if, as suggested by some, the cardiac output at a given metabolic rate is less in children than in adults (4). This question has been reviewed in chapter 8. Most research data suggest that maximal cardiac index (cardiac output relative to BSA) does not change appreciably during childhood and adolescence. Direct comparisons of submaximal cardiac output relative to $\dot{V}O_2$ in children and adults have not been made. Further investigation into maturity-related differences in cardiac responses to exercise will be necessary before the issue is resolved.

Thermal Homeostasis

Given the differential influences of surface area, sweating rates, and cutaneous blood flow, how does the ability of the child to maintain thermal balance during exercise compare to that of adults? In general, no significant differences have been observed in stability of core temperature during exercise between children and adults, regardless of ambient temperature. As noted in an earlier section, however, there is some evidence that prepubertal subjects have a greater impairment of endurance capacity when exercising in very hot environments.

When the pre-, mid- and late-pubertal subjects studied by Falk et al. cycled at 50% $\dot{V}O_2$max at 42 °C, no

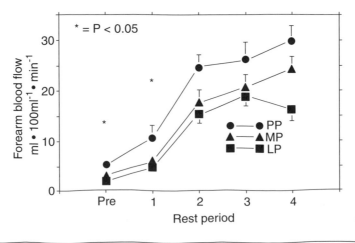

Figure 15.4 Forearm blood flow in prepubertal (PP), midpubertal (MP), and late-pubertal (LP) boys at rest and immediately following progressive exercise bouts in the heat. Reprinted from Falk et al. 1992.

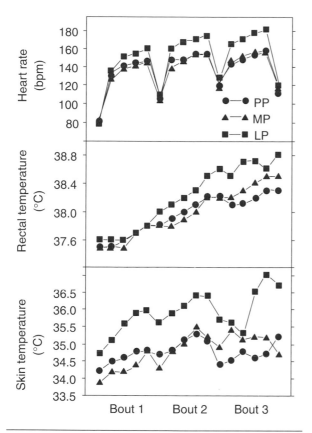

Figure 15.5 Heart rate and rectal temperatures during three exercise bouts in the heat in prepubertal (PP), midpubertal (MP), and late-pubertal (LP) boys. Reprinted from Falk et al. 1992.

difference in rate of rise of rectal temperature was observed between the three groups (see fig. 15.5) (13). Other studies directly comparing thermal responses to exercise between prepubertal and mature subjects have demonstrated the same finding at ambient temperatures of 20-22 °C (30), 28 °C (10), 35 °C (10), 42 °C (27), and 49 °C (36).

Piekarski et al. performed a longitudinal study of thermal responses to exercise in four children over a period of 5 years, beginning at age 10 (28). Subjects walked on a horizontal treadmill at 4 km/hr in temperatures ranging from 25 to 55 °C. No significant trend was observed in mean annual change in rectal temperature for all environmental conditions in three of the four subjects (the exception had a mean annual decrease of 0.08 °C) (p < 0.02).

Wagner et al. compared thermal responses to exercise in groups of 11-14-year-old boys, 15-16-year-old adolescents, and 25-30-year-old men (37). While exercising at the same absolute workload (level treadmill walking at 5.6 km/hr) in 49 °C heat, mean endurance time was 50, 67, and 79 min for the three groups, respectively.

If core temperature responses to exercise are independent of age, what is the explanation for the relative intolerance of children to exercise in very hot surroundings? Bar-Or concluded that "the three main culprits are probably the child's higher area-to-mass ratio, lower sweating capacity, and less effective cardiovascular adjustment to exercise in the heat (perhaps inability to maintain arterial blood pressure due to low central blood volume and cardiac output)" (5, p. 353). He also noted that the studies outlined above were typically conducted in dry heat. The added influence of high humidity, particularly as it depresses sweating rate, on age-related differences in heat intolerance remains to be examined.

Aerobic Fitness and Heat Tolerance

Studies in adults indicate that physiological adaptations to exercise in the heat are better in trained compared to untrained individuals (3). People who have undergone physical training or who have a higher $\dot{V}O_2max$ often demonstrate enhanced sweat responsiveness, greater cutaneous blood flow, and delayed rises in heart rate and rectal temperature. These responses are in fact similar to those of heat acclimatization, suggesting possible common triggering mechanisms.

There are few data regarding this issue in children. The available information suggests, however, that prepubertal subjects in contrast to adults do not exhibit an association between fitness and thermal responses to exercise.

Delamarche et al. studied 11 boys ages 10-12 years who varied in $\dot{V}O_2max$ from 43 to 65 ml · kg^{-1} · min^{-1} (8). Subjects exercised on a cycle ergometer for 60 min at 60% $\dot{V}O_2max$ in 20 °C and 20% relative humidity. No relationship was observed between $\dot{V}O_2max$ and either evaporative rate or changes in rectal temperatures. Docherty et al. exercised 10-13-year-old boys on a flat treadmill at 6 km/hr for 60 min in 30 °C and 80% relative humidity (9). $\dot{V}O_2max$ of the subjects accounted for only 16% of the variance in the rise of rectal temperatures during exercise. Matsushita and Araki reported no changes in exercise rectal temperature or sweating rate after a 40-day running program in a group of prepubertal boys (26).

Heat Acclimatization

Prepubertal children are capable of adaptive changes that improve tolerance to heat after a period of exercise in high temperatures. There is evidence to suggest, however, that children may achieve acclimatization at a slower rate than adults.

Wagner et al. compared physiological adaptations to repeated exercise in the heat in nonathletic males who were prepubertal (11-14 years old), postpubertal (15-16 years old), and adult (ages 25-30 years) (37). Subjects performed eight consecutive daily treadmill walks of 45-90 min in 47.7 to 49 °C conditions. Test walks were conducted in a 22 °C room before and after the eight walks in the heat.

The repeated walks produced significant acclimatization effects in all groups. Reduction in rectal and skin temperature, decline in heart rate, and improved evaporative loss during exercise were qualitatively and quantitatively similar regardless of maturity status. However, compared to the postpubertal boys and men, the young boys showed these changes to a lesser extent by the 2nd day. Similarly, Inbar showed that 8-10-year-old boys and young men exhibited no differences in adaptation to repeated exercise at 43 °C but that the response was slower in the boys (19). The explanation for this apparent retarded acclimatization in children is obscure.

EXERCISE IN COLD TEMPERATURES

During exercise in cold environments, the added heat produced from the rise in metabolic rate is advantageous in helping prevent hypothermia (fall in body core temperature). At least three factors are important in determining thermal balance and risk of hypothermia during exercise in the cold:

1. Location of exercise. Thermal conductivity of water is many times greater than that of air. Therefore, heat loss is more exaggerated during swimming than during exercising in cold air (e.g., ice hockey), and the chance of hypothermia is greater.
2. Amount of body fat. Fat acts as a thermal insulator and protects against heat loss in cold ambient conditions.
3. Body surface area. Heat is lost through the body's surface. Therefore, people with a greater BSA: mass ratio will be at greater risk for hypothermia in the cold.

The last of these factors is the one that should place small children at particular risk for hypothermia in cold environments, especially during swimming. The study of young swimmers by Sloan and Keatinge, described previously, supports this concept (35). Rate of body cooling with swimming in that study was inversely related to age and skinfold thicknesses and directly correlated with BSA:mass ratio.

The only other study addressing age-related thermal responses to exercise in the cold in children failed to reveal such differences in air. Smolander et al. described core temperatures in 11-12-year-old boys and 19-34-year-old men who first were exposed to 5 °C air for 20

min and then cycled in the same condition at 30% $\dot{V}O_2$max for 40 min (36). During this 60 min exposure, rectal temperatures were stable in the men and actually increased slightly in the boys. These findings suggest that, at least within the conditions of this study, children are able to compensate for their increased heat loss through their relatively larger BSA. Additional research will be important for understanding the limits of this adaptive capacity.

SUMMARY

There are differences in the thermal responses to exercise that set children apart from adults. In most climatic conditions these maturity-related differences appear to bear little clinical significance for healthy children. However, in extremely hot environments, or during performance of exercise in the heat without adequate acclimatization, the differences should be expected to place the child at greater risk for heat stress injury. Still, there are currently no epidemiological data to confirm that heat stress injury during sport participation in the heat is more common in children.

At rest and during exercise at equal absolute workloads, children generate more heat relative to their body mass than do adults. This greater heat production in respect to body mass during exercise in children is compensated for by losses to the environment via their relatively larger BSA.

Children and adults possess an equal number of sweat glands, and since children have a smaller BSA they possess a greater density of sweat glands. This fact notwithstanding, the sweat rate per surface area is less in children, indicating that adults are capable of producing more sweat per gland. The differences between the child and the adult sweating pattern appear to emerge at puberty, suggesting that hormonal influences may be influential. Limited information suggests that pubertal influences on sweating rates with exercise are not as great in girls as in boys.

Since children sweat less than adults, they can dissipate heat to a lesser degree by evaporative cooling. Consequently, children rely more on convective heat loss from the skin to maintain thermal homeostasis. In very hot environments, however, ambient temperature may exceed skin temperature and prevent convective heat loss. This places the child at a disadvantage for maintaining thermal balance.

Despite the potential maturity-related differences in ability to tolerate heat during exercise, children show stable core temperatures in all reported environmental testing conditions. However, prepubertal subjects are not as capable of sustaining exercise in very hot conditions as adults. This appears to relate to cardiovascular rather than thermal instability.

In contrast to the situation for adults, children who possess greater aerobic fitness do not appear to tolerate exercise in the heat better than those who have low levels of fitness. Children acclimatize to repeated exercise in the heat equally well as adults, but the rate of thermal adaptations may be slower in prepubertal subjects.

What We Know

1. Heat production relative to body mass at rest and during exercise is inversely related to age during childhood.
2. The excessive mass-relative heat production during exercise in younger subjects is dissipated through a relatively larger BSA.
3. The greater BSA:mass ratio in small children is advantageous for heat loss when ambient temperature is less than body core temperature (except in cold environments), but disadvantageous in the reverse condition.
4. Children sweat less than adults during exercise, and this is a result of less sweat production per gland.
5. Children become fatigued sooner than adults during exercise in the heat. This appears to be related to cardiovascular rather than thermal factors, as core temperature in such exercise studies are independent of age.

What We Would Like to Know

1. Is the incidence of heat injury with exercise truly greater in children than in adults?
2. Why do children demonstrate lower exercise endurance in the heat than adults?
3. What are the mechanisms that delay heat acclimatization in children?
4. How do the hormonal influences of puberty affect thermal regulation?

References

1. Araki, T.; Toda, Y.; Matsushita, K.; Tsujino, A. Age differences in sweating during muscular exercise. Jap. J. Phys. Fit. Sports Med. 28:239-248; 1979.
2. Armstrong, L.E.; Maresh, C.M. Exercise-heat tolerance of children and adolescents. Pediatr. Exerc. Science 7:239-252; 1995.
3. Armstrong, L.E.; Pandolf, K.B. Physical training, cardiorespiratory physical fitness and exercise-heat tolerance. In: Pandolf, K.B.; Sawka, M.N.; Gonzalez, R.R., eds. Human performance physiology and environmental medicine at terrestrial extremes. Indianapolis: Benchmark Press; 1988:p.199-226.
4. Bar-Or, O. Pediatric sports medicine for the practitioner. New York: Springer-Verlag; 1983.
5. Bar-Or, O. Temperature regulation during exercise in children and adolescents. In: Perspectives in exercise science and sports medicine. Vol. 2, Gisolfi, C.V.; Lamb, D.R., eds. Youth, exercise, and sport. Indianapolis: Benchmark Press; 1989:p. 335-368.
6. Bar-Or, O.; Lundegren, H.M.; Buskirk, E.R. Heat tolerance of exercising obese and lean women. J. Appl. Physiol. 26:403-409; 1969.
7. Davies, C.T.M. Thermoregulation during exercise in relation to sex and age. Eur. J. Appl. Physiol. 42:71-79; 1979.
8. Delamarche, P.; Bittel, J.; La Cour, J.R.; Flandrois, R. Thermoregulation at rest and during exercise in prepubertal boys. Eur. J. Appl. Physiol. 60:436-440; 1990.
9. Docherty, D.; Eckerson, J.D.; Hayward, J.S. Physique and thermoregulation in pre-pubertal males during exercise in a warm, humid environment. Am. J. Phys. Anthropol. 70:19-23; 1986.
10. Drinkwater, B.L.; Kupprat, I.C.; Denton, J.E.; Crist, J.L.; Horvath, S.M. Response of prepubertal girls and college women to work in the heat. J. Appl. Physiol. 43:1046-1053; 1977.
11. Falk, B.; Bar-Or, O.; Calvert. R.; MacDougall, J.D. Sweat gland response to exercise in the heat among pre-, mid-, and late-pubertal boys. Med. Sci. Sports Exerc. 24:313-319; 1992.
12. Falk, B.; Bar-Or, O.; MacDougall, J.D. Thermoregulatory responses of pre-, mid-, and late-pubertal boys to exercise in dry heat. Med. Sci. Sports Exerc. 24:688-694; 1992.

13. Falk, B.; Bar-Or, O.; MacDougall, J.D.; McGillis, L.; Calvert, R.; Meyer, F. Sweat lactate in exercising children and adolescents of varying physical maturity. J. Appl. Physiol. 71:1735-1740; 1991.

14. Fellman, N.; Grizard, G.; Coudert, J. Human frontal sweat rate and lactate concentration during heat exposure and exercise. J. Appl. Physiol. 54:355-360; 1983.

15. Fellman, N.; Labbe, A.; Gachon, A.M.; Coudert, J. Thermal sweat lactate in cystic fibrosis and in normal children. Eur. J. Appl. Physiol. 54:511-516; 1985.

16. Haymes, E.M.; Buskirk, E.R.; Hodgson, J.L.; Lundegren, H.M.; Nicholas, W.C. Heat tolerance of exercising lean and heavy prepubertal girls. J. Appl. Physiol. 36:566-571; 1974.

17. Holliday, M.A.; Potter, D.; Jarrah, A.; Bearg, S. The relation of metabolic rate to body weight and organ size. Pediat. Res. 1:185-195; 1967.

18. Huebner, D.E.; Lobeck, C.C.; McSherry, N.R. Density and secretory activity of eccrine sweat glands. Pediatrics 38:613-618; 1966.

19. Inbar, O. Acclimitization to dry and hot environment in young adults and children 8- to 10-years old [EdD dissertation]. New York: Columbia University Press; 1981.

20. Kawahata, A. Variation in the number of active human sweat glands with age. J. Physiol. Soc. Jap. 4:438-444; 1939.

21. Kawahata, A. Sex differences in sweating. In: Yoshimura, H.; Ogata, K.; Itch, S., eds. Essential problems in climatic physiology. Kyoto: Nankodo; 1960:p. 169-184.

22. Kleiber, M. The fire of life. New York: Wiley; 1961.

23. Knoebel, L.K. Energy metabolism. In: Selkurt, E.E., ed. Physiology. Boston: Little, Brown; 1963:p. 564-579.

24. Kuno, Y. Human perspiration. Springfield, IL: Charles C Thomas; 1956:p. 68.

25. MacDougall, J.D.; Roche, P.D.; Bar-Or, O.; Moroz, J.R. Maximal aerobic capacity of Canadian school children: prediction based on age related oxygen cost of running. Int. J. Sports Med. 4:194-198; 1983.

26. Matsushita, K.; Araki, T. The effect of physical training on thermoregulatory responses of pre-adolescent boys to heat and cold. Jap. J. Phys. Fit. Sports Med. 29:69-74.

27. Meyer, F.; Bar-Or, O.; MacDougall, D.; Heigenhauser, G.J.F. Sweat electrolyte loss during exercise in the heat: effects of gender and maturation. Med. Sci. Sports Exerc. 24:776-781; 1992.

28. Piekarski, C.; Morfield, P.; Kampmann, B.; Ilmarinen, R.; Wenzel, H.G. Heat-stress reactions of the growing child. In: Rutenfranz, J.; Mocellin, R.; Klimt, F., eds. Children and exercise XII. Champaign, IL: Human Kinetics; 1986:p. 403-412.

29. Rees, J.; Shuster, S. Pubertal induction of sweat gland activity. Clin. Sci. 60:689-692; 1981.

30. Rowland, T.W.; Rimany, T.A. Physiological responses to prolonged exercise in premenarcheal and adult females. Pediatr. Exerc. Science 7:183-191; 1995.

31. Rowland, T.W.; Staab, J.S.; Unnithan, V.B.; Rambusch, J.M.; Siconolfi, S.F. Mechanical efficiency during cycling in prepubertal and adult males. Int. J. Sports Med. 11:452-455; 1990.

32. Sawka, M.N.; Wenger, C.B. Physiological responses to acute exercise-heat stress. In: Pandolf, K.B.; Sawka, M.N.; Gonzalez, R.R., eds. Human performance physiology and environmental medicine at terrestrial extremes. Indianapolis: Benchmark Press; 1988:p. 97-152.

33. Schmidt-Nielsen, K. Scaling. Why is animal size so important? Cambridge: Cambridge University Press; 1984.

34. Sjodin, B.; Svedenhag, J. Oxygen uptake during running is related to body mass in circumpubertal boys: a longitudinal study. Eur. J. Appl. Physiol. 65:150-157; 1993.

35. Sloan, R.E.G.; Keatinge, W.R. Cooling rates of young people swimming in cold water. J. Appl. Physiol. 35:371-375; 1973.

36. Smolander, J.; Bar-Or, O.; Korhonen, O.; Ilmarinen, J. Thermoregulation during rest and exercise in the cold in pre- and early-pubescent boys and young men. J. Appl. Physiol. 72:1589-1594; 1992.

37. Wagner, J.A.; Robinson, S.; Tzankoff, S.P.; Marino, R.P. Heat tolerance and acclimitization to work in the heat in relation to age. J. Appl. Physiol. 33:616-622; 1972.

38. Wenger, C.B. Human heat acclimatization. In: Pandolf, K.B; Sawka, M.N.; Gonzalez, R.R., eds. Human performance physiology and environmental medicine at terrestrial extremes. Indianapolis: Benchmark Press; 1988:p. 153-198.

CREDITS

Figures

Figure 1.1: Adapted, by permission, from R.E. Scammon, 1930, The measurement of the body in childhood. In *The measurement of man*, edited by J.A. Harris et al. (Minneapolis: University of Minnesota Press), 193.

Figure 1.3: Reprinted, by permission, from J.M. Tanner, R.H. Whitehouse, and M. Takaishi, 1966, "Standards from birth to maturity for height, weight, height velocity, and weight velocity: British children," *Archives of Disease in Childhood* 41:454–471.

Figure 1.4: Adapted from: Hamill PVV, Drizd TA, Johnson CL, Reed RB, Roche AF, Moore WM: Physical growth: National Center for Health Statistics percentiles. AM J CLIN NUTR 32:607-629, 1979. Data from the National Center for Health Statistics (NCHS), Hyattsville, Maryland. Used with permission of Ross Products Division, Abbott Laboratories, Columbus OH 43216 from NCHS Growth Charts. ©1982 Ross Products Division, Abbott Laboratories.

Figure 1.5: Adapted from: Hamill PVV, Drizd TA, Johnson CL, Reed RB, Roche AF, Moore WM: Physical growth: National Center for Health Statistics percentiles. AM J CLIN NUTR 32:607-629, 1979. Data from the National Center for Health Statistics (NCHS), Hyattsville, Maryland. Used with permission of Ross Products Division, Abbott Laboratories, Columbus OH 43216 from NCHS Growth Charts. ©1982 Ross Products Division, Abbott Laboratories.

Figure 2.2: Adapted, by permission, from V.L. Katch, 1973, "Use of the oxygen/body weight ratio in correlational analyses," *Medicine and Science in Sports* 5: 255.

Figure 2.3: Reprinted, by permission, from W.A. Calder, 1984, *Size, function, and life history* (Cambridge, Mass: Harvard University Press), 11.

Figure 3.1: Reprinted, by permission, from O. Bar-Or, 1987, "The Wingate Anaerobic Test: An update on methodology, reliability and validity," *Sports Medicine* 4: 382.

Figure 4.1a: Reprinted, by permission, from R.A. Boileau, 1988, Problems associated with determining body composition in maturing youngsters. In *Competitive sports for children and youth*, edited by E.W. Brown and C.F. Branta (Champaign, Ill.: Human Kinetics), 8.

Figure 4.1b: Reprinted, by permission, from R.A. Boileau, 1988, Problems associated with determining body composition in maturing youngsters. In *Competitive sports for children and youth*, edited by E.W. Brown and C.F. Branta (Champaign, Ill.: Human Kinetics), 9.

Figure 4.1c: Reprinted, by permission, from R.A. Boileau, 1988, Problems associated with determining body composition in maturing youngsters. In *Competitive sports for children and youth*, edited by E.W. Brown and C.F. Branta (Champaign, Ill.: Human Kinetics), 6.

Figure 4.2: Reprinted, by permission, from R.A. Boileau, 1988, Problems associated with determining body composition in maturing youngsters. In *Competitive sports for children and youth*, edited by E.W. Brown and C.F. Branta (Champaign, Ill.: Human Kinetics), 11.

Figure 4.3: Reprinted, by permission, from R.M. Malina and C. Bouchard, 1991, *Growth, maturation and physical activity* (Champaign, Ill.: Human Kinetics), 97.

Figure 6.1: Reprinted, by permission, from O. Bar-Or, 1986, "Pathophysiological factors which limit the exercise capacity of the sick child," *Medicine and Science in Sports and Exercise* 18: 277.

Figure 6.2: Reprinted, by permission, from T.A. McMahon, 1984, *Muscles, reflexes, and locomotion* (Princeton, N.J.: Princeton University Press), 281.

Figure 6.3: Reprinted, by permission, from T.W. Rowland, 1990, *Exercise and children's health* (Champaign, Ill.: Human Kinetics), 67.

Figure 6.4: Reprinted, by permission, from M.A. Holliday et al., 1967, "The relation of metabolic rate to body weight and organ size," *Pediatric Research* 1: 188.

Figure 6.5: Reprinted, by permission, from G.S. Krahenbuhl et al., 1985, "Developmental aspects of maximal aerobic power in children," *Exercise and Sports Science Reviews* 13: 513.

Figure 6.6: Reprinted, by permission, from G.S. Krahenbuhl et al., 1985, "Developmental aspects of maximal aerobic power in children," *Exercise and Sports Science Reviews* 13: 514.

Figure 6.8: Reprinted by permission of the publisher from R.L. Mirwald and D.A. Bailey, 1986, *Maximal aerobic power* (Eastbourne, England: Sports Dynamics), 27.

Figure 6.12: Reprinted, by permission, from T.W. Rowland, 1990, *Exercise and children's health* (Champaign, Ill.: Human Kinetics), 51.

Figure 6.13: Reprinted by permission of the publisher from Cumming: "Bruce treadmill tests in children: Normal values in a clinic population," *American Journal of Cardiology*, 4:70. Copyright 1978 by Excerpta Medica Inc.

Figure 7.1: Reprinted, by permission, from T.W. Rowland, 1990, *Exercise and children's health* (Champaign, Ill.: Human Kinetics), 35.

Figure 7.3: Reprinted, by permission, from T.B. Gilliam et al., 1981, "Physical activity patterns determined by heart rate monitoring in 6-7 year old children," *Medicine and Science in Sports and Exercise* 13: 66.

Figure 7.4: Reprinted, by permission, from L.B. Rowell, 1986, *Human circulation: Regulation during physical stress* (New York: Oxford University Press), 261.

Figure 8.1: Reprinted, by permission, from T.W. Rowland, 1991, " 'Normalizing' maximal oxygen uptake, or the search for the holy grail (per kg)," *Pediatric Exercise Science* 3(2): 98.

Figure 8.2: Reprinted, by permission, from A. Sproul and E. Simpson, 1964, "Stroke volume and related homodynamic data in normal children," *Pediatrics* 33: 916.

Figure 8.3: Reprinted, by permission, from R.M. Malina and C. Bouchard, 1991, *Growth, maturation and physical activity* (Champaign, Ill.: Human Kinetics), 157.

Figure 8.4: Reprinted, by permission, from B. Marcus et al., 1990, "Intrinsic heart rate in children and young adults," *American Heart Journal* 112: 914.

Figure 8.5: Reprinted with permission from the American College of Cardiology, *Journal of the American College of Cardiology*, 1992, vol. 19, p. 624.

Figure 8.6: Reprinted, by permission, from R.A. Hurwitz et al., 1984, "Right ventricular and left ventricular ejection fraction in pediatric patients," *American Heart Journal* 107: 730.

Figure 8.7: Reproduced from *The Journal of Experimental Medicine*, 1979, vol. 128, p. 380 by copyright permission of The Rockefeller University Press.

Figure 8.8: Reprinted, by permission, from R.M. Malina and C. Bouchard, 1991, *Growth, maturation and physical activity* (Champaign, Ill.: Human Kinetics), 158.

Figure 8.10: This figure is reprinted with permission from the *Research Quarterly for Exercise and Sport,* 1983, volume 54, page 57. *RQES* is a publication of the American Alliance for Health, Physical Education, Recreation and Dance, 1900 Association Drive, Reston, VA 22091.

Figure 8.11: Reprinted from *International Journal of Cardiology,* vol. 1, E.M. Oyen, p. 149, 1987, with kind permission from Elsevier Science Ireland Ltd., Bay 15K, Shannon Industrial Estate, Co. Clare, Ireland.

Figure 8.12: Reprinted, by permission, from M. Miyamura and Y. Honda, 1973, "Maximum cardiac output related to sex and age," *Japanese Journal of Physiology* 23: 648.

Figure 8.13: Reprinted, by permission, from O. Bar-Or, 1983, *Pediatric sports medicine for the practitioner* (New York: Springer-Verlag), 20.

Figure 8.15: Reprinted, by permission, from B.S. Alpert et al., 1982, "Responses to ergometry exercise in a healthy biracial population of children," *Journal of Pediatrics* 101: 538.

Figure 9.1: Reprinted, by permission, from E. Asmussen et al., 1981, "Heart rate and ventilatory frequency as dimension-dependent variables," *European Journal of Applied Physiology* 46: 383.

Figure 9.3: Reprinted, by permission, from K.L. Andersen et al., 1974, "Physical performance capacity of children in Norway," *European Journal of Applied Physiology* 33: 270.

Figure 9.4: Reprinted, by permission, from Y. Armon et al., 1991, "Maturation of ventilatory responses to 1-minute exercise," *Pediatric Research* 29: 366.

Figure 9.5: Reprinted, by permission, from S. Godfrey, 1974, *Exercise testing in children* (London: W.B. Saunders), 78.

Figure 9.6: Reprinted, by permission, from I. Mercier et al., 1991, "Influence of anthropometric characteristics on changes in maximal exercise ventilation," *European Journal of Applied Physiology* 63: 239.

Figure 9.7: Reprinted, by permission, from S. Godfrey, 1974, *Exercise testing in children* (London: W.B. Saunders), 69.

Figure 9.8: Reprinted, by permission, from S. Godfrey, 1974, *Exercise testing in children* (London: W.B. Saunders), 80.

Figure 9.9: Reprinted, by permission, from M. Boule et al., 1989, "Breathing pattern during exercise in untrained children," *Respiration Physiology* 75: 227.

Figure 9.10: Reprinted, by permission, from T.W. Rowland and T.A. Rimany, 1995, "Physiological responses to prolonged exercise in premenarcheal and adult females," *Pediatric Exercise Science* 7: 183-191.

Figure 10.2: Reprinted, by permission, from P.R. Dallman et al., 1979, "Percentile curves for hemoglobin and red cell volume in infancy and childhood," *Journal of Pediatrics* 94: 28.

Figure 10.4: Reprinted, by permission, from P.O. Åstrand, 1952, *Experimental studies of physical working capacity in relationship to sex and age* (Copenhagen: Munksgaard), 48.

Figure 10.5: From Cassels, *Cardiopulmonary data for children and young adults*, 1962. Courtesy of Charles C Thomas, Publisher, Springfield, Illinois.

Figure 10.7: Reprinted, by permission, from Schmidt-Nielsen, K. 1984, *Scaling: Why is animal size so important?* (New York: Cambridge University Press), 120.

Figure 10.8: Reprinted, by permission, from A. Berg, S.S. Kim, and J. Keul, 1986, "Skeletal muscle enzyme activities in healthy young subjects," *International Journal of Sports Medicine* 7: 236-239.

Figure 10.9: Reprinted, by permission, from R.D. Bell et al., 1980, "Muscle fiber types and morphometric analysis of skeletal muscle in six-year-old children," *Medicine and Science in Sports and Exercise* 12: 28-31.

Figure 10.10: Reprinted, by permission, from R.D. Bell et al., 1980, "Muscle fiber types and morphometric analysis of skeletal muscle in six-year-old children," *Medicine and Science in Sports and Exercise* 12: 28-31.

Figure 11.1: Reprinted, by permission, from Schmidt-Nielsen, K. 1984, *Scaling: Why is animal size so important?* (New York: Cambridge University Press), 168.

Figure 11.2: Reprinted, by permission, from Schmidt-Nielsen, K. 1984, *Scaling: Why is animal size so important?* (New York: Cambridge University Press), 169.

Figure 11.4: Reprinted, by permission, from R.L. Waters et al., 1983, "Energy cost of walking in normal children and teenagers," *Developmental Medicine and Child Neurology* 25: 185.

Figure 11.6: Reprinted, by permission, from T.W. Rowland et al., 1990, "Mechanical efficiency during cycling in prepubertal and adult males," *International Journal of Sports Medicine* 11: 454.

Figure 11.8: Reprinted, by permission, from T.J. Dawson and C.R. Taylor, 1973, "Energetic cost of locomotion in kangaroos," *Nature* 246: 314.

Figure 11.9: Reprinted, by permission, from D.M. Cooper et al., 1985, "Kinetics of oxygen uptake at the onset of exercise as a function of growth in children," *Journal of Applied Physiology* 59: 214.

Figure 11.10 Reprinted, by permission, from T.W. Rowland and T.A. Rimany, 1995, "Physiological responses to prolonged exercise in premenarcheal and adult females," *Pediatric Exercise Science* 7: 183-191.

Figure 12.1: From *AAHPERD youth fitness test manual* (1976), page 26. Reproduced with permission from the American Alliance for Health, Physical Education, Recreation and Dance.

Figure 12.2: Reprinted, by permission, from O. Bar-Or, 1983, *Pediatric sports medicine for the practitioner* (New York: Springer-Verlag), 311-314.

Figure 12.3: Reprinted, by permission, from O. Bar-Or, 1983, *Pediatric sports medicine for the practitioner* (New York: Springer-Verlag), 311-314.

Figure 12.4: Reprinted, by permission, from O. Bar-Or, 1983, *Pediatric sports medicine for the practitioner* (New York: Springer-Verlag), 311-314.

Figure 12.5: Reprinted, by permission, from O. Bar-Or, 1983, *Pediatric sports medicine for the practitioner* (New York: Springer-Verlag), 311-314.

Figure 12.6: Reprinted, by permission, from C.J.R. Blimkie, P. Roche, and O. Bar-Or, 1986, The anaerobic-to-aerobic power ratio in adolescent boys and girls. In *Children and exercise XII*, vol. 17, edited by J. Rutenfranz, R. Mocellin, and F. Klimt (Champaign, Ill.: Human Kinetics), 35.

Figure 12.7: Reprinted, by permission, from P. Duche et al., 1992, Longitudinal approach of bioenergetic profile in boys before and during puberty. In *Pediatric work physiology*, edited by J. Coudert and E. Van Praagh (New York: Masson), 45.

Figure 12.8: Reprinted, by permission, from D.H. Paterson et al., 1986, "Recovery O_2 and blood acid: Longitudinal analysis in boys aged 11 to 15 years," *European Journal of Applied Physiology* 55: 95.

Figure 12.9: Reprinted, by permission, from B.O. Eriksson et al., 1971, "Muscle metabolites during exercise in pubertal boys," *Acta Paediatrica, Scandinavian Supplement* 217: 154-157.

Figure 12.12: Reprinted, by permission, from O. Bar-Or, 1983, *Pediatric sports medicine for the practitioner* (New York: Springer-Verlag), 14.

Figure 12.13: Reprinted, by permission, from D.H. Paterson et al., 1986, "Recovery O_2 and blood acid: Longitudinal analysis in boys aged 11 to 15 years," *European Journal of Applied Physiology* 55: 95.

Figure 12.14: Reprinted, by permission, from T. Reybrouck et al., 1985, "Ventilatory anaerobic threshold in healthy children," *European Journal of Applied Physiology* 54: 280.

Figure 12.15: Reprinted, by permission, from B.Vanden Eynde et al., 1989, Endurance fitness and peak height velocity in Belgian boys. In *Children and exercise XIII*, vol. 19, edited by S. Oseid and K.-H. Carlson (Champaign, Ill.: Human Kinetics), 23.

Figure 12.16: Reprinted, by permission, from B. Emmett and P.W. Hochachka, 1986, "Scaling of oxidative and glycolytic enzymes in mammals," *Respiration Physiology* 45: 267.

Figure 12.17: Reprinted, by permission, from A. Berg and J. Keul, 1988, Biochemical changes during exercise in children. In *Young athletes: Biological, psychological and educational perspectives*, edited by R.M. Malina (Champaign, Ill.: Human Kinetics), 65.

Figure 13.1: Reprinted, by permission, from J. Lexell et al., 1992, "Growth and development of human muscle," *Muscle Nerve* 15: 406.

Figure 13.2: Reprinted, by permission, from R.M. Malina and C. Bouchard, 1991, *Growth, maturation and physical activity* (Champaign, Ill.: Human Kinetics), 127.

Figure 13.3: Reprinted, by permission, from R.M. Malina and C. Bouchard, 1991, *Growth, maturation and physical activity* (Champaign, Ill.: Human Kinetics), 191.

Figure 13.4: Reprinted, by permission, from B.N. Davies, 1990, "The relationship of lean limb volume to performance in the handgrip and standing long jump tests," *European Journal of Applied Physiology* 60: 141.

Figure 13.5: Reprinted, by permission, from R.M. Malina and C. Bouchard, 1991, *Growth, maturation and physical activity* (Champaign, Ill.: Human Kinetics), 296.

Figure 13.6: Reprinted, by permission, from W.J. Kraemer et al., 1989, "Resistance training and youth," *Pediatric Exercise Science* 1(4): 342.

Figure 13.7: Reprinted, by permission, from K.L. Nau et al., 1990, "Acute intraarterial blood pressure response to bench press weight lifting in children," *Pediatric Exercise Science* 2(1):42.

Figure 14.1: Reprinted, by permission, from N.O. Eriksson et al., 1973, "Muscle metabolism and enzyme activities after training in boys 11-13 years old," *Acta Physiologica Scandinavica* 87: 486.

Figure 14.2: Reprinted, by permission, from L.R. Martinez and E.M. Haymes, 1992, "Substrate utilization during treadmill running in prepubertal girls and women," *Medicine and Science in Sports and Exercise* 24: 978.

Figure 14.3: Reprinted, by permission, from A. Berg and J. Keul, 1988, Biochemical changes during exercise in children. In *Young athletes: Biological, psychological and educational perspectives*, edited by R.M. Malina (Champaign, Ill.: Human Kinetics), 68.

Figure 14.4: Reprinted, by permission, from G. Marin, 1994, "The effects of estrogen priming and puberty on the growth hormone response to standard treadmill exercise," *Journal of Clinical Endocrinology and Metabolism* 79:539.

Figure 14.5: Reprinted, by permission, from T.W. Rowland et al., 1987, "Serum testosterone response to training in adolescent runners," *American Journal of Disabled Children* 141: 882. Copyright 1987, American Medical Association.

Figure 14.6: Reprinted, by permission, from A. Berg and J. Keul, 1988, Biochemical changes during exercise in children. In *Young athletes: Biological, psychological and educational perspectives*, edited by R. Malina (Champaign, Ill.: Human Kinetics), 73.

Figure 14.7: Reprinted, by permission, from L.M. Webber et al., 1989, "Serum creatine kinase activity and delayed onset muscle soreness in prepubescent children: A preliminary study," *Pediatric Exercise Science* 1(4): 356.

Figure 15.1: American Academy of Pediatrics. Sports Medicine: Health Care for Young Athletes. Evanston, Ill.: AAP; 1983.

Figure 15.2: Reprinted, by permission, from B. Falk et al., 1992, "Sweat gland response to exercise in the heat among pre-, mid-, and late-pubertal boys," *Medicine and Science in Sports and Exercise* 24: 316.

Figure 15.3: Reprinted, by permission, from B. Falk et al., 1991, "Sweat lactate in exercising children and adolescents of varying physical maturity," *Journal of Applied Physiology* 71: 1737.

Figure 15.4: Reprinted, by permission, from B. Falk et al., 1992, "Thermoregulatory responses of pre-, mid-, and late-pubertal boys to exercise in dry heat," *Medicine and Science in Sports and Exercise* 24: 691.

Figure 15.5: Reprinted, by permission, from B. Falk et al., 1992, "Thermoregulatory responses of pre-, mid-, and late-pubertal boys to exercise in dry heat," *Medicine and Science in Sports and Exercise* 24: 691.

Tables

Table 1.1: Adapted, by permission, from W.A. Marshall and J.M. Tanner, 1969, "Variations in pattern of pubertal changes in girls," *Archives of Disease in Childhood* 44: 291-303, and from W.A. Marshall and J.M. Tanner, 1970, "Variations in pattern of pubertal changes in boys," *Archives of Disease in Childhood* 45: 13-23.

Table 3.1: Reprinted, by permission, from T.W. Rowland, 1993, *Laboratory exercise testing: Clinical guidelines* (Champaign, Ill.: Human Kinetics), 23.

Table 3.2: Reprinted, by permission, from T.W. Rowland, 1993, *Laboratory exercise testing: Clinical guidelines* (Champaign, Ill.: Human Kinetics), 36.

Table 3.3: Reprinted, by permission, from T.W. Rowland, 1993, *Laboratory exercise testing: Clinical guidelines* (Champaign, Ill.: Human Kinetics), 20.

Table 3.5: Reprinted, by permission, from T.W. Rowland, 1993, *Laboratory exercise testing: Clinical guidelines* (Champaign, Ill.: Human Kinetics), 169.

Table 3.6: Reprinted, by permission, from T.W. Rowland, 1993, *Laboratory exercise testing: Clinical guidelines* (Champaign, Ill.: Human Kinetics), 169.

Table 4.1: Reprinted, by permission, from T.G. Lohman, 1989, "Assessment of body composition in children," *Pediatric Exercise Science* 1:22.

Table 4.2: Reprinted, by permission, from R. M. Malina and C. Bouchard, 1991, *Growth, maturation and physical activity* (Champaign, Ill.: Human Kinetics), 94.

Table 4.3: Reprinted, by permission, from T.G. Lohman, 1992, *Advances in body composition assessment* (Champaign, Ill.: Human Kinetics), 74.

Table 4.4: Reprinted, by permission, from T.G. Lohman, 1989, "Assessment of body composition in children" *Pediatric Exercise Science* 1:20.

Table 4.5: Reprinted, by permission, from T.G. Lohman, 1992, *Advances in body composition assessment* (Champaign, Ill.: Human Kinetics), 56.

Table 7.3: Reprinted, by permission, from O. Bar-Or, 1989, "Trainability of the prepubescent child," *The Physician and Sportsmedicine* 17(5): 75.

Table 7.4: Reprinted, by permission, from T.W. Rowland, 1985, "Aerobic response to endurance training in prepubescent children: a critical analysis," *Medicine and Science in Sports and Exercise* 17: 495.

INDEX

ABOUT THE AUTHOR

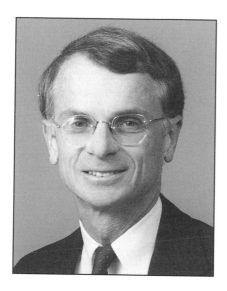

Thomas W. Rowland, MD, is director of pediatric cardiology at the Baystate Medical Center in Springfield, Massachusetts, where he established an exercise testing laboratory. The author of *Exercise and Children's Health* and editor of *Pediatric Exercise Science*, he is also associate editor of *Medicine and Science in Sports and Exercise*.

Dr. Rowland is president of the North American Society for Pediatric Exercise Medicine (NASPEM) and a member of the American College of Sports Medicine (ACSM). He received the Honor Award from the New England Chapter of the ACSM in 1992.

Since receiving BS and MD degrees from the University of Michigan in 1965 and 1969, Dr. Rowland has been an assistant and associate professor of pediatrics at the University of Massachusetts Medical School in Worchester (1977 to 1990) and an assistant and associate clinical professor of pediatrics at Tufts University School of Medicine in Boston (1975 to the present). In 1995 he became adjunct professor of exercise science at the University of Massachusetts in Amherst.

In addition to conducting extensive research, Dr. Rowland has written and spoken widely on developmental exercise physiology, the effects of lifestyle on cardiovascular function in children, iron deficiency in adolescent athletes, and the determinants of exercise performance in children.

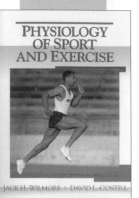
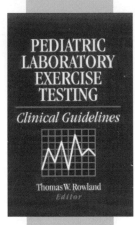
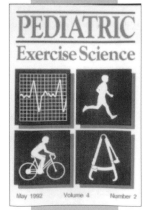